Living Cuisine

Living Cuisine

THE ART AND SPIRIT OF RAW FOODS

Renée Loux Underkoffler

AVERY

a member of Penguin Group (USA) Inc.

New York

Neither the publisher nor the author is engaged in rendering professional advice or services to the individual reader. The ideas, procedures, and suggestions contained in this book are not intended as a substitute for consulting with your physician. All matters regarding health require medical supervision. Neither the author nor the publisher shall be liable or responsible for any loss, injury, or damage allegedly arising from any information or suggestion in this book. The opinions expressed in this book represent the personal views of the author and not of the publisher.

The recipes contained in this book are to be followed exactly as written. Neither the publisher nor the author is responsible for your specific health or allergy needs that may require medical supervision, or for any adverse reactions to the recipes contained in this book.

While the author has made every effort to provide accurate telephone numbers and Internet addresses at the time of publication, neither the publisher nor the author assumes any responsibility for errors or for changes that occur after publication.

Most Avery books are available at special quantity discounts for bulk purchase for sales promotions, premiums, fund-raising, and educational needs. Special books or book excerpts also can be created to fit specific needs. For details, write Penguin Group (USA) Inc. Special Markets, 375 Hudson Street, New York, NY 10014.

a member of
Penguin Group (USA) Inc.
375 Hudson Street
New York, NY 10014
www.penguin.com

Library of Congress Cataloging-in-Publication Data

Underkoffler, Renée Loux.
Living cuisine : the art and spirit of raw foods / Renée Loux Underkoffler.
p. cm.
Includes bibliographical references and index.
ISBN 1-58333-171-9
1. Cookery (Natural foods). 2. Raw foods. I. Title.
TX741.U53   2003   2003051927
641.5'63—dc21

This book is printed on acid-free, recycled paper. ♾ ♻

Printed in the United States of America
13 15 17 19 20 18 16 14

Book design by Stephanie Huntwork

CONTENTS

Part Three: Raw Foods Preparation Techniques

Part Four: The Recipes

This is what should be done
by those who are skilled in goodness,
and those who know the path of peace:
Let them be able and upright,
straightforward and gentle in speech.
Humble and not conceited,
contented and easily satisfied,
unburdened with duties and frugal in their ways.
Peaceful and calm, and wise and skillful,
not proud and demanding in nature.
Let them do not the slightest thing
that the wise would later reprove.
Wishing: in gladness and in safety,
may all beings be at ease.
Whatever living beings there may be;
whether they are weak or strong, omitting none,
the great or the mighty, medium, short or small,
the seen and unseen,
those living near and far away,
those born and to-be-born,
may all beings be at ease!
Let none deceive another,
or despise any being in any state.

Let none through anger or ill-will
wish harm upon another.
Even as a mother protects with her life,
her child, her only child,
so with a boundless heart
should one cherish all beings;
radiating kindness over the entire world:
spreading upward to the skies,
and downward to the depths,
outward and unbounded,
freed from hatred and ill-will.
Whether standing or walking, seated or lying
*   down.*
Free from drowsiness,
one should sustain this recollection.
This is said to be sublime abiding.
By not holding to fixed veins,
the pure-hearted one, having clarity of vision,
being freed from all sense desires,
is not born again into this world.

—THE BUDDHA'S WORDS ON LOVING-
KINDNESS (METTA SUTRA)

ACKNOWLEDGMENTS

Thank you:

To Mom and Dad, who have shown me the meaning of unconditional love
   and an integral work ethic
To my lamb-brother, Lyle
To counselor Thomas John Ballanco, for love deeper than the days between
To my yoga gurus and dearest friends, Eddie Modestini and Nicki Doane
To the light, love, and SOL partners, Woody and Laura
To my sweet, spunky Alicia
To Lynn Shauwecker, my bunny-love and balance for lifetimes before and to come
To my soul-sister, Alecks Evanguelidi
To Valerie Reiss, whose brilliance and talent I hope is contagious
To Roger Lewis, who always saw me
To the light of New York, Joy and Bart and the Candle Cafe
To my sweet lady Lavinia and my good man Joel
To my cosmic partner in cahoots, Fernando
To my sister of light and integrity, Julia Butterfly Hill
To true angels Cherie and Terri, Chad Sarno, and The Living Light Institute
To the wild memory of Jonathan Bailey
To the great yogis, seen and unseen

To the loving support of Elam

To the gorgeous brothers Eli and Ethan

To the torch of Dr. Gabriel Cousens

To the spark awakened in me by Viktoras Kulvinskas and Dr. Ann Wigmore

To the loving support and productive example of Jacob Freydont-Attie

To Jerry, always grateful

To my fuzzy man Dan

To Dave Frankel, who reminds me of the beauty of humanity and change

To the timeless light and wisdom of Krishnamacharya

To the whole Raw Experience, especially Christopher, Suzie, and Jeremy

To my Sundance brothers and sisters for strength and return

To my kung-fu master, Kevin Terpsma

To the sweet spirit of Tyler and the buckets of love from Drew and Oceana

To the memory of a kind and generous mentor, Csilla Jacobson

To the extraordinary vision of Roxanne and Michael Klein

To the clairvoyant insight of Yeshe

To the heart wisdom of Margaret

To Jim Fitzgerald. I knew if you could get this out there, the world would be just
the place I want to live.

Last, and perhaps most important, thank you, Dara Stewart, my editing hero at Avery.
You are a gem. Your insight, savvy mechanics, trust, and ease have made these pages possible and my perspective of the future bright.

FOREWORD

Though it was years ago, I still remember that meal. I had heard about a master raw chef named Renée. Long before I met her, I had heard rave reviews from various friends about her "rawesome" culinary skills, and in particular, her raw pies. Though I wasn't raw at the time, I knew enough to know that raw food and its emphasis on enzymes being the life force of the food is the way to go for optimum health and energy. Still, you can talk theory all you want; if the taste isn't there, color me a cooked-food junkie. A life of lettuce, cucumbers, and garbanzo sprouts just *wasn't* happening for this meat-and-potato-raised Texan. I mean, I admire Gandhi, but I didn't want to eat like him. So I was still taking in a hefty percentage of cooked and processed foods at the time, but eyeballing the benefits of a raw diet from a respectable and flavor-filled distance.

In my pursuit of knowledge (while yearning for taste), I had the opportunity to meet someone whom I greatly admire, Gabriel Cousens, well-respected author of some of the quintessential books on vibrant health and possibly the world's leading expert on nutrition and the raw foods diet. We had dinner in Paia, Maui, at a sweet little restaurant called the Raw Experience.

That night, I discovered what raw food could taste like if you could sit and dream a little dream with your tongue. Up came a striking green-eyed wonder, full of energy and confidence. Little did I know at the time that while I was sitting at the feet of the raw knowledge master, the raw taste master had appeared. Renée began dropping one amazing, sumptuous dish after another onto our table. Gabriel and I were ecstatic about the food to the point where we stopped talking and were solely focused on the edible delights before us. We were struck dumb by our taste buds. All energy in the mouth was devoted to mastication. The coup de grâce was one of Renée's coconut cream pies, which, I confess, almost brought Gabriel and me to blows over the last piece.

I joke with Renée that her raw pies could "take over the world," but, in a sense, they could stimulate a change in the way people think about desserts. Most folks, around dessert time, start to feel an almost twisted pleasure—the sinful act of desecrating the body temporarily overshadowed by the enjoyment of the taste buds. Renée has a "chocolate" pie made with carob and avocado that is better than any pie I have ever tasted, and it's actually good for you! She drops that chocolate pie on the table, and people get primal, attacking it with bare hands. Anyone who has tasted Renée's pies knows that desserts can taste great and don't have to be bad for you. That is the beginning of revolutionary thinking about food. Understanding the impact that eating right has on the planet, I would love to see her pies take over the world.

After dinner, I said goodbye to Gabriel and spent hours talking with Renée. I was amazed at her depth of knowledge and passion for preparing beautiful, wholesome, living meals. That night began a friendship, which I am sure will last a lifetime, to the benefit of my heart, mind, and taste buds.

Renée has been working on this book for years, always off in a corner with her laptop while the rest of us played. At long last, she is finished, and I am proud to say that you are holding the most exciting, comprehensive, and up-to-date collection of information on the thrills and importance of vibrant health, along with hundreds of delicious recipes that will leave you and your family and friends smiling, speechless, and ready to fight for the last piece of pie.

—WOODY HARRELSON

Living Cuisine

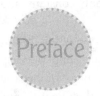

The Integration of Science and Spirit

We are the miraculous integration of the world around us. The air we breathe, the food we eat, the people we join with, and the actions we take and make are the very source of our existence.

It is by the grace and knowledge of the great minds before us and among us that we begin to understand the vast assimilation of life. There may be more information available these days than there ever has been to reveal the mysteries of life, health, and harmony, yet the simple task of feeding ourselves properly is as confusing as ever.

Ancient and modern sciences have deciphered planes of understanding that hint at the greater meaning of things, with the humble respect that we are only scratching the surface of understanding. For all of the days that people have roamed the earth, our deepest scientific inquiry cannot exactly explain the magic of how a cell works. Yet each of us is made of more than a trillion cells, working in symphony to grant a walking, talking, loving, complex reality of multiplicity day after day.

Empirical knowledge is not absolute. The greatest theorems and laws are subject to change and evolution. Einstein's general theory of relativity revolutionized our understanding of energy in the last century to such a great degree that the "laws" of physics have been fundamentally changed. Prior to Einstein's theory ($E = mc^2$), it was scientifically agreed that energy is immutable, meaning that it can never change. Einstein, who admitted he was only scratching the surface, revealed that energy is a variable in the formula of life. My theory is that change is the only constant; take what you know and go with your gut (especially with food where your guts are at stake). Mix in time as the only constant, and the revelation is a growing, changing universe, within and without.

The eye of science beholds an intricate system of laws and formulas that governs our natural and physical world. The intelligence of imperical explanation is only a part of the union of life. Only you know what is right. The magic of love is unable to be specified by a microscope. It is sense and intuition that integrate the scientific and spiritual worlds to balance personal, physical, intellectual, emotional, and spiritual evolution.

The conditions of our individual lives determine the translation of information and concepts on a very personal level. There is no magic word or miracle pill that will bring good health to every individual of the growing population of the planet, faced with an increasingly complex world. It is with regular, honest inquiry for information, cross-referenced with our own experience and intuition, that our own master formula will come into focus.

Yoga is a very appropriate analogy. Yoga is the integration of an ancient science and spirit. The word *yoga* has many meanings. It is from a Sanskrit root that translates to mean "union" or "to join." The yoga of food is simply our union with food. We literally become our food, and our food becomes us. This union happens every day without regard to the conscious acknowledgment of this simple and profound veracity. The enormous importance of food in relationship to health is evident in every bite.

Homeostasis

We exist in homeostasis: the dance of maintaining a dynamic balance inside the body in the ever-changing environment outside the body. The literal translation is "unchanging" (*homeo:* the same; *stasis:* still) and more accurately describes the miraculous equilibrium inside the body. It requires the cooperation of every cell of every tissue, gland, organ, and bone for life to function. The spectrum and quality of life in our internal universe are vast and resilient.

The more aware we become of our bodies, the more aware our bodies become. There are more than a trillion cells in our bodies communicating with integral intelligence. A clear line of communication with each of those cells may be beyond our cognitive capacity; however, a conscious effort of what is collectively going on in our bodies is a course for freedom. Knowledge is power.

Change is the only constant. Cells are dividing and growing every moment. It is generally understood that our bodies are able to rebuild more than 90 percent of their cells every two years. We are constantly changing organisms in a state of renewal and decay shaped by our internal and external environments.

There are several factors that fundamentally influence our health and vitality. These are discussed below.

External Factors

Global-Systemic Issues

Externally, there are many environmental elements and factors that are not in our immediate control. The external environment we live in is in various states of disarray and cooperation that influence our personal health and well-being. These are global issues that affect the system of the whole world.

The greater state of the planet has a significant impact on each of us. The quality of air and water is consequential. There are global changes at hand: environmental policies, the price of gas and bottled water, waste disposal, global politics, water treatment, mandatory vaccinations, clean-air acts, commercial farming, and the pervasive manipulation of the media.

The ecology of inequality is the rampant unjust distribution of wealth and denial of access to good food, clean water, and unpolluted air that affect the poor in this country and around the world. The ecology of inequality begins with poor educational systems that feed a cycle of oppression. The poor and impoverished feel the brunt of pollution and the poor availability of food and clean water due to geographical circumstance and lack of assistance. The "out of sight, out of mind" policy for waste, chemical, and nuclear disposal ends up in the backyard of poor, rural areas. In urban areas, access to good food is out of the monetary reach of many. It is difficult to consider buying expensive organic food and health tools when paying the rent is a struggle. It is difficult to consider exercising or practicing yoga when working two jobs. There are inexpensive ways to eat healthily, like sprouting and eating whole grains and beans, but without education, these possibilities remain out of reach. It is an uphill battle for many to make choices for health and break the cycle of oppression. The ecology of inequality is an issue deeply rooted in sociological and economic injustice. Mahatma Gandhi said, "Prejudices cannot be removed by legislation—they yield to patient toil and education."

Individual-Systemic Issues

Individual-systemic issues are influenced by global systemic conditions. These are external causes that we have a little more influence over (than, say, global-domestic policy) and principally affect our health and well-being.

Externally, where we live has a huge influence on our health and lives. Cities and urban sprawl are a rough dominion to endure. Air pollution, car pollution, treated water, radiation, and stress are only a few variables to contend with. To some degree, geographical and bioregional circumstance are within the margin of our control, but family, career, and opportunities are only a few decisive factors with very real influence. Not everyone can live in the pristine countryside, pumping their own water and growing their own food. There is valuable recognition that living in cities has a much lighter impact on the environment. There are ways to strike an educated compromise for clean living in every circumstance.

Where we live determines the availability of right-minded choices that begin with education. Access to housing and building materials that are not detrimental to our health and the environment, efficient appliances, responsible fuel for appliances and cars, and recycling and waste-disposal programs are greatly decided by where we live.

Internal Factors

Internal conditions begin with fundamental genetic predisposition, rearing and education, and the belief systems instilled from birth into adulthood.

Internally, our genetic disposition is a fundamental determinant of our constitutional propensity. The genes we came in with greatly determine our health, vitality, and fortitude. These are systemic elements that we do not have much influence over. Regardless of the resolve of our genetic complexion and circumstantial living conditions, the ultimate equation of health is orchestrated by our lifestyles and habits, diet and exercise, stress, and enjoyment of life.

Education has profound influence on the way we carry out our lives. The structure of how we are raised and educated begins the program and relationship to mental and spiritual health, concepts about community and resources, and ultimately the foundation of consumerism.

Personal consumerism is an essential responsibility (especially in America) that impacts personal and planetary health. Household and building materials are more toxic today than ever before. Off-gassing carpets and couches, chemically treated wood, synthetic clothing, chemical products for cleaning the house and car, exposure to radiation from cell phones, and pharmaceutical medications all have significant impact on personal health. These are elements that we each have more say and influence over than internal factors like genetic disposition and how we were raised before we had a say in the process. Personal consumerism and choices influence outside and external elements that in turn influence us.

Personal health practice will enforce or change tendencies of genetic disposition and bioregional circumstance. If diabetes, high blood pressure, heart disease, or obesity runs rampant in your family gene pool, and you take the initiative to eat well, exercise, and rest, it is likely that these disorders will not plague you as easily.

Diet is the only variable we have complete control of, internally and externally, and one that touches the near and far reaches of personal and global health. Diet is the primary factor that influences health. The five leading causes of death in America are all diet-related. Diet is a real tool for physical, mental, and spiritual health. You are what you eat.

What Is Diet? Mind, Body, and Spirit Union

Every cell in our bodies is made up of food, air, and water. The miraculous process of biological life hinges on our diet. Diet is far more than what goes into our mouths. Our lifestyle, exercise and rest, emotional well-being, thoughts, and love are meaningful variables in the formula of health. We can think ourselves sick or love ourselves well. Thoughts alone can be as acid-causing as a bad meal.

There are more than 6.5 billion of us and just as many possible formulas for health. Health is ultimately a personal journey. There is an overwhelming amount of nutritional information available, much of which is directly contradictory. Everyone has a stance on what is the right diet. The general public has been sold on a swinging pendulum of expertise. From low-fat, high-fiber diets to high-protein diets to eating according to blood type, many people are buying it. The truth is that we need to know ourselves. Trusting our bodies and loving how they serve us is the beginning. The body will reside long after the fad diet has been dispelled. Lifestyles work. Diets are a phase.

We want to feel good. We want to look good. We want balance. We want comfort in our bodies and to source a sustainable level of natural energy. Real health is not a lofty ideal. Health is available underneath the misalignment and mismanagement of neglect. Given a chance, the body will heal. Tissues and organs come to balance. Blood clears. Strength comes. Systems function properly. Homeostasis can be realized, and the symphony will celebrate.

Get Educated!

These days, when we have such an incredible amount of information and options, we can "hybridize" our own formula. Just as it is wise to eat a wide variety from the generous cornucopia of natural food, it is wise to learn about different approaches to nutrition and health for the changing needs of a long life.

There is a freedom in education. Learning to know the body helps us diagnose our needs and when we need to improve our health. Learning about our bodies and what we are putting in them and on them makes it easier to know what to do. Do you know where your gallbladder is? Do you know what your liver does? Do you know what essential fatty acids are? Do you know how to make delicious and nutritious meals that will feed all of your senses? There is an incredible liberation in independence. There is a confidence in helping ourselves. It is possible to live in pleasure and be free of the whims of imbalance and trepidation. We all start somewhere, and, yes, we *can* have it all.

Part One

*

The Basics

1

Food for Life

Truth is rarely black and white. We are colorful people, and there are infinite shades of gray in the discussion of just what is the optimal diet and which food choices are best. There are 6.5 billion people on our planet, and this number is growing. There are so many variables and factors that affect health. Drawing blanket conclusions about the proper diet for all might be better reserved for a cloned monoculture, not for the complex, changing world we live in. We are a brilliant, dynamic tapestry woven from fabric from the near and far reaches of the genetic and geographical pool. The formula for good health is a personal one.

Respect for micro- and macro-integration is my house prescription. This means to take a thoughtful look at your personal lifestyle to find ways to realistically and responsibly make changes for the better in day-to-day life and for the world as a whole. Small changes add up to healthy transformation.

There is no highfalutin pedestal for the preacher in these pages. There is just information and knowledge that are meant to be translated into truth for each of us. And there are some fabulously delicious recipes in these pages. Eating food that makes sense and tastes good is the name of the game. Choose, chew, and leave room for the dessert of wisdom and experience.

What Are Living Foods?

Raw foods—or live foods—are whole and unprocessed and make a brilliant prescription for vital health. Cooking and processing deplete food of some of its nutrients. Raw foods contain their full complement of nutrients and are complete with the enzymes needed to turn the food into energy that the body can use. They make optimal assimilation of nutrition easy, provide pure, clean energy for the body, and do not require a lot of energy for digestion. Fresh fruits and vegetables, fresh juices, nuts and seeds, sprouted beans and grains, fermented and cultured foods, and low-temperature dehydrated crackers, breads, and treats are delicious examples of the cornucopia of raw living food.

Living foods have the energy of life force. Life force is the essence of energy. Energy can be measured only by its effects on life. Life force is what activates *chemical energy* in our bodies. Life force can be called the *electrical energy* in our bodies that enables the *mechanical energy* of every action in our cells, tissues, bones, and blood.

The raw and living foods discussed in this book are plant-based. A plant-based diet is an intelligent choice for micro- and macro-energy. Plants have the "magical" ability to *photosynthesize* energy from the sun to be stored in every cell. This energy remains intact for some time after the plant is harvested. The fresher the food, the more energy it has. The more energy within the food, the easier it is for our bodies to assimilate the energy. Alternatively, electrical energy is not present in dead tissue. Dead flesh does not have life force or the available energy for a vibrant transformation of energy for a beautiful body.

Living foods provide the most out of matter. They are a sound investment for the body: the temple of health. The net worth of anything else is in their shadow: Cooked, processed, and flesh foods require more energy *from* the body to yield less energy *for* the body. Live food is at an optimal peak, requiring minimal energy from the body to give maximum energy to the body. Less work, more yield. Everybody wins.

Assimilation

The most important aspect of eating is *assimilation*, the body's taking in of the food's nutrients. Our bodies must be able to identify, digest, and assimilate nutrients from food in order to use it for building and regenerating cells, tissue, blood, and bones. A certain food may contain all the nutrients in the world, but if the body cannot assimilate those nutrients, they are useless. Good health from a balanced diet is founded in assimilating the good stuff.

Healthy digestion is an essential part of promoting health and optimal assimilation. Chewing well, proper food combinations, maintaining a healthy balance of intestinal flora, and choosing foods suited to individual needs all play an important part of good assimilation and happy digestion.

Eating a fresh, sensibly balanced diet yields good health for the long run. Crash diets and quick results are fleeting answers compared with the real deal of enjoying a lifetime of eating well. A good diet is a maintenance system for a long life. And when it tastes as good as the dishes I will present to you, there'll be no denying it.

Enzymes

Enzymes are responsible for every metabolic action in the body, including digestion. All fresh raw and living foods, including fresh, cold-pressed oils, have the enzymes necessary to aid their digestion. It is widely accepted that heating food above 110°F destroys its enzymes. When foods that are lacking enzymes are eaten, the pancreas must compensate by producing additional digestive enzymes to help with digestion. A diet composed exclusively of cooked food puts stress on the pancreas and requires a lot of energy to be expended for digestion. Alternatively, fresh raw foods are teeming with enzymes for easy digestion and assimilation and provide ample clean energy without diminishing returns.

Does Food Lose Nutrients When It Is Cooked?

The direct answer to whether food loses its nutrients when cooked is yes. All nutrients, vitamins, minerals, and enzymes are sensitive and destroyed by heat.

Many studies suggest that a predominantly raw foods diet is the optimal diet and promotes health. Raw foods have more nutrition available in a simpler state than the diminished nutritional value of cooked and processed food.

Cooking affects a given food's nutrients on a sliding scale. Steaming vegetables does not damage the precious goods too much. Baking and grilling are more damaging. Microwaving and deep-frying are very destructive.

The fresher the better. The sooner after harvest a food is eaten, the more nutrients and life force it has available. Eating fruits and vegetables that are in season or grown in your region is a smart bet for the freshest food available. A wide variety of fruits and vegetables provides a cornucopia of nutrition to nourish every body.

Nutrients are miraculous and delicate compounds. Many vitamins are heat- and light-sensitive, meaning they begin to diminish soon after they are harvested. Nutrients break down exponentially the longer they are exposed to oxygen and the food sits around. Besides, fresher food just tastes better.

Viriditas

Hildegard von Bingen was a twelfth-century German philosopher, writer, and mystic who saw the principle of *viriditas,* or "greenness," in every aspect of life. This is simply the principle that a life force moves us, makes things grow, and inspires passion, emotion, and creativity. She saw this divine energy "penetrating into all places, in the heights, on earth and in every abyss," giving the earth and all living things an effervescence of life and spirit.

Hildegard recognized *viriditas* to be an essential part of the natural relationship of symbiotic life. Unfamiliar with this sage, hundreds of years later, in the twentieth century, Dr. Weston Price confirmed the principle of greenness through anthropological and botanical study.

Dr. Price studied indigenous people and native diets in many remote places around the world. He discovered that much of the wild food in native diets contained at least four times the minerals and ten times the fat-soluble nutrients of a twentieth-century American diet.

Dr. Price recognized an element he called the "X-factor," a potent catalyst for mineral absorption. This factor was found in wild-growing food. It was also found in animal products such as fish, eggs, butter, organs, and meat of animals *only* if these foods came from animals that consumed green, growing food—algae and plankton for fish and green grass for land animals. Farmed fish and animals fed dry and processed feed provided no X-factor. Subsequently, generations of factory-farmed diets resulted in disease and fertility problems never seen in indigenous people prior to this introduction.

Even our food that once had *viriditas* growing in the fields withers during industrial processing. This is seen in industrial farming and processing of foods like soy, wheat, and corn. Ground and smashed, pressed and extracted, exposed to solvents and heat, irradiated and homogenized, emulsified and rearranged, foods once containing *viriditas* are stripped of it to reach the market shelves.

The preparation of our food begins on the farm, in managing and sowing the soil, and continues through careful preparation in the kitchen with love. It is only with mindful care through every step that *viriditas* is conserved.

As Hildegard recognized centuries ago, "greenness" is necessary for healthy life on earth. Ultimately, the presence or absence of *viriditas* in our diet and farming is the barometer for the future of humanity and our land.

Whole Food versus Processed Food

Whole food is better than processed food for many reasons. Food in its natural state is designed in a complementary balance. The proteins, minerals, vitamins, phytonutrients, carbohydrates, and oils are in a natural relationship for optimum nutrition and assimilation. For example, vitamins require cofactors and the presence of other vitamins to be available for absorption; to build protein from food, all of the essential amino acids must be present. Whole food provides a delicate formula for sound nutrition, found in plants in their whole, natural state.

A common example can be seen with whole grains versus processed flours, cereal, pasta, and breads. A whole grain has *bran, germ,* and *gluten* or *endosperm.* The *bran* has essential fiber and B vitamins. The *germ* has precious vitamins, minerals, protein, and valuable oils. And the *gluten* or *endosperm* has complex carbohydrates and protein. Shortly after a grain is milled into flour, the germ loses the precious vitamin E and valuable oils. The minerals and vitamins are in a broken home and begin to deteriorate, leaving a pasty filler with little to offer.

Flour that has been freshly milled by stone, without heat, and refrigerated in airtight containers, potentially maintains valuable nutrition. This kind of fresh flour is rarely available in stores. More commonly, flour that is bought in the store is shipped and stored for months without much care because flour is not considered to be perishable food. Flour that is exposed to air will turn rancid. Unfortunately, rancid flour is hard to detect as it does not look or smell any different. This undetectable rancidity is a common culprit in wheat allergies. By the time store-bought flour reaches the loyal consumer, it is devoid of almost any nutrition.

Alternatively, fresh, whole grain is a much heartier package. Whole grains have fiber and are rich in vitamins, minerals, and nutrients. Dry grain is designed by nature to stay vital and weather months of a freezing winter and drought. Surviving the bulk bins at the health food store is small potatoes for whole grain.

Sprouting and Steaming for Optimal Assimilation

Even a hearty digestive system has a hard time breaking down some food. Foods like beans and grains have a complex nutritional portfolio to manage. Sprouting beans and grains breaks down the protein and carbohydrates into a simpler, more available state for the body to use.

Some vegetables have a large proportion of cellulose (an indigestible fiber) and are also difficult to properly digest. The *Brassica* genus, including cabbage, broccoli, cauliflower, Brussels sprouts, and kale, tends to be tough to suitably digest. Blending, fermenting, and lightly steaming "tough" vegetables are good solutions for easier digestion.

- Blending tougher vegetables into a soup or chopping them finely and marinating them in lemon juice helps for easier digestion.
- Fermenting "tough" vegetables into kimchi or sauerkraut breaks down the cellulose and predigests the nutrition. Fermented food is escorted by a teeming flurry of healthy bacteria that supports digestion, assimilation, and elimination.
- Lightly steaming "tough" vegetables and sprouted beans and grains is very helpful for delicate or transitioning digestive systems. Light steaming is not a crime in raw foods preparation. Although some nutrients and enzymes are lost, the steaming also breaks down the cellulose, the main constituent of cell walls, allowing the nutrients inside those cells to be accessed and assimilated. Good deal.

Cultured and Fermented Food

Cultured vegetables like sauerkraut and kimchi, miso, and raw shoyu (soy sauce) are great digestive aids and are easy to digest, even for weakened systems. In the fermenting and culturing process, food is partially digested by live cultures. The cultured food's enzyme count is tremendous, making the nutrition readily available. Cultured food is naturally rich in probiotics, such as *L. acidophilus* and *L. bifidus*—healthy bacteria that support good intestinal ecology for optimal digestion, assimilation, and elimination. (See Chapter 17 for culturing and fermenting techniques.)

Dehydrating Food

Dehydrating food is a responsible way to enjoy crispy crackers, savory flat breads, sweet cookies and biscotti, and other treats. Sprouting grains for these tasty morsels amps up the nutritional values, which are preserved by low-temperature (below 120°F) dehydrating. (See Chapter 18 for more information and dehydrating techniques.)

2

Modern Farm
to Modern Table

Choosing organically grown food is fast becoming the most important investment in the future. Up until the mid-twentieth century, there was always a symbiotic relationship, feeding the earth to grow food to feed us. In the last century, human food has so radically changed that it is relatively unrecognizable as food at all. From growing to processing, most of us have become foreigners to the most essential and natural cycle for life: sustainable food.

There are so many reasons to support organic farming and sustainable agriculture, not the least of which is dependable nutrition free from chemicals. Buying and eating organically grown food is a direct vote for our personal health and for domestic and world economics. It's a vote yea or nay for the chemical and petrochemical industry and the future existence of our degrading ecology and environment. It's the insurance that our children will be able to eat for generations to come.

The advancement of food production over the ages has afforded incredible freedom. Today in this country only 2 percent of the population grows 98 percent of the food. The great arts and sciences of our society have flourished by the grace of this liberty. Herein is the conundrum plaguing the modern era: The very inventions and developments that make our lives easier are pathologically evolving and advancing to detrimental ends.

Food and agricultural technology is having devastating effects. Our insatiable need for bigger, better, faster food is destroying our environment and seriously jeopardizing our food supply. The year 1999 marked the first year in a hundred that the United States did not export grain.

Modern commercial food is an insult to our bodies, the economy, and the future of our land. It is polluting our water, raping our soil, and deteriorating the quality of the food we eat.

Organic and Commercial Agriculture

The ploughshare may well have destroyed more options for future generations than the sword . . .

So destructive has the agricultural revolution been that, geologically speaking, it surely stands as the most significant and explosive event to appear on the face of the earth, changing the earth even faster than the origin of life.

—WES JACKSON, *NEW ROOTS FOR AGRICULTURE*
UNIVERSITY OF NEBRASKA PRESS, 1985

Mankind is gaining 120,000 mouths each day and losing 20 million acres of food producing land each year. . . . We are in the throes of an apparently irreversible reduction of the surface of cultivatable land. The area of such lands has decreased by an estimated 20% in the last 100 years. Of the 40 billion acres remaining, at least 20 million disappear irretrievably each year. . . . Man, the destroyer, having wiped out hundreds of animal species, is well embarked on a course which threatens his own kind with extinction.

—*SURVIVAL INTO THE 21ST CENTURY*, VIKTORAS KULVINSKAS, MS,
© 1975, OMANGOD PRESS, WETHERSFIELD, CT.

A Brief History of Agriculture

More than half of America's world neighbors live quietly, supported by sustainable farming. Small farms support the community. It is not an easy life. Nor does it compensate for the crushing political and economical strife in so many of these societies. There is no easy answer. The pressures of new cash economies and overtaxing diminishing resources breed a new concept of poverty where before there may have been enough to go around.

For thousands of years, a balance between hands and earth existed. We must feed and rest the earth in order to be fed in return. Traditionally, seeds and knowledge are passed from generation to generation as heirlooms. For ages, seeds have adapted to and thrived in particular regions, grown resistant to local elements and pests, and produced food that is esteemed for taste and variety along with superior nutritional value. Until the modern era, the responsibility to feed the children and the people remained in the community. It requires a tenacious management of resources and hands for a fair exchange with the earth.

Many things have changed in the last half century. Farms have become factories in America. The spirit of conquest has turned to the land. War was applied to the soil. We turned swords into ploughshares.

Commercial farming is a direct by-product of World War II. Before 1940, little or no toxic chemicals were used as agricultural fertilizer or pesticide. The post-war chemical industry decided that food production was a great way to earn peace-time dollars. Nitrate reserves left over from ammunition factories were called "fertilizer" and sold to farmers. Nerve gas was sprayed and used for pest control. Tank technology was applied to tractors. And so began the conquest of commercial farming in America.

In 1940, there were more than 6 million family farms in America, averaging 175 acres per farm. By the end of the twentieth century, commercial farming left less than one third of those farms remaining with each farm on average tripling in size. The number of people working on farms has fallen more than 70 percent in the last seventy years. Less than 2 percent of the population today produces the food for the nation. Thousands of family farms have been absorbed by conglomerate corporations and massive federally subsidized farms. In modern mono-cropping style, by 1990, American farmers owed banks more than $200 billion. At that time, this was more than Brazil and Mexico owed the United States combined.

Farming has become grossly displaced, and the repercussions are unquantifiable. A growing population and needy lifestyles have put more and more pressure on farms to produce more and more food. To meet these demands, scientists have revolutionized agriculture in the last half century. Use of hybrid seeds, mechanical labor, and heavy chemicals enables high volumes of food to be produced from vast single-crop fields. Mono-crops are a disaster for land that requires rotation and variety for pest control and to keep the soil rich in nutrients and minerals. Pesticides and synthetic fertilizers have replaced cooperative planting, natural pest resistance, and vital soil.

Today, fields and orchards are manufactured for mass production. More than one third of all the produce grown in America comes from just 20,000 square miles of semiarid desert in the Central Valley of California, specifically the Sacramento and San Joaquin valleys. Such heavy dependence on such a small pool of resources is destined for destruction.

Factory farming is an industrial feat. Food is grown to literally accommodate the shape of the machinery. Land is leveled with lasers so monster machines can process large pieces of land in one swoop, and the precious topsoil blows away in the wind. Synthetic fertilizers, poison gas, fumigants, and broad-spectrum insecticides are used to regulate the food products as they grow.

The earth cannot bear this abuse. Should this continue, the topsoil will erode, the water will drain, and the soil will exhaust. No farms, no food.

Treating Soil Like Dirt

Soil is some of the most precious matter on earth. Soil is the very medium that sustains all plants and vegetation. All living things depend on healthy soil for food. Humans depend on food for life.

Topsoil can be as shallow as an inch deep or as deep as several yards depending on geology and geography. The composition of soil greatly varies around the world and primarily consists of (1) disintegrated rock and decomposed organic, plant, and animal matter, (2) water, (3) anaerobic bacteria and microorganisms, (4) inorganic minerals, and (5) earthworms and insects. Fertile soil is a complex living material with an incredible, resilient capacity to support and sustain life when treated with respect.

> More than 50 percent of soybeans, 35 percent of corn, and 65 percent of canola grown in the United States are GMO foods. Three quarters of the world's crops of soybeans, corn, and canola are grown in the United States.

Modern commercial agriculture is irreparably depleting the nutrients in our soil. No nutrients in the soil means no nutrients in the food.

The current abusive methods of farming encourage growing mono-crops rather than sustainable crop rotation. Monoculture employs growing the same crops again and again on the same piece of land, sucking all of the nutrients from the soil and returning nothing back to the earth. With these methods, heavy chemical fertilizers are required to force the crops to grow. Crop diversity for natural pest control is ignored in favor of heavy application of insecticides, herbicides, fungicides, and rodenticides. The result is brittle, barren soil that must be treated with increasingly aggressive prescriptions of chemicals to keep the land productive.

These offensive modern practices completely exhaust fertile land in less than forty years. With all of our intelligence and ingenuity, there are more productive, responsible alternatives to the insanity of borrowing from our children's future.

There are tried-and-true methods that have been used for thousands of years to sustain the soil and the bloom of abundant produce. In China, sustainable agricultural has been practiced for thousands of years. The Chinese are feeding more than 1 billion people, about 20 percent of the world population, on less than 7 percent of the earth's arable land. Even today, sound organic farming keeps land viable and rich even after twenty centuries of continual use. It is possible.

What Commercial Farming Is Doing to Our Land

Topsoil

America has lost more than 75 percent of its topsoil through commercial farming. The national average is more than 8 tons per acre lost every year (which is enough topsoil to cover the state of Connecticut). If all of the topsoil lost in America alone from wind and water erosion were loaded onto freight cars, it would encircle the earth twenty-four times. It takes 200 to 1,000 years to create just one inch of topsoil. No modern technology can build topsoil more quickly than that.

Water

Six times the annual flow of the Mississippi River is extracted from America's rivers, streams, and underground aquifers every year. Seventy percent of that water is for agriculture and flesh farming (cattle, hogs, and chickens). Incompetent transport wastes almost 80 percent of that volume through leaks, hemorrhages, and evaporation. The precious water never even reaches the farms.

It takes more than 2 million gallons of water per acre annually to grow alfalfa in the dry Central Valley of California. Water is pumped more than 600 feet to the surface to supply the crop, drawing from precious "fossil water" that will never be replenished. It is absolutely unsustainable.

Another common technique is to pump billions of gallons of water from rivers and transport it to distant, naturally arid land for irrigation to farm (Palm Springs, California, or Las Vegas anyone?). Over-pumping rivers draws salt from the bays and deposits it onto fertile cropland. The result of this unsustainable practice is threatening to kill precious, fertile delta farmland. No farms, no food.

Land Clearing

More than 400,000 acres of rice and straw are burned in Sacramento Valley, California, every year. Since burning requires very little labor, it is a cheap way to clear fields. The typical practice of burning uses aircrafts that douse the land with napalm and set it ablaze. The chemical residue settles into the earth and poisons the air. The loss of organic minerals and materials is gargantuan and irreplaceable. The pollution is staggering. It is estimated by

> The best compost for the land is the wise master's feet and hands.
> —ROBERT HERRICK (1591–1674)

the University of California at Davis that this practice alone results in 7,000 tons of hydrocarbons and 58,000 tons of carbon monoxide entering the atmosphere every year. These are gases. Gases are light, so 7,000 to 58,000 tons is a serious amount of weight for such light stuff. The description of a "cheap" way to clear fields is clearly questionable. What expense will our children pay?

Fertilizers and Pesticides

More than 800 million pounds of toxic chemicals are used as pesticides each year on American farmland. More than 54 million tons of synthetic chemical fertilizer are used each year. Ironically, the percentage of crops lost to pests has increased about 20 percent in the last fifty years.

California alone uses hundreds of millions of pounds of toxic pesticides each year for commercial farming. From 1991 to 1995, there was a 31 percent increase in use of pesticides. In those four years alone, 161 million pounds rose to 212 million pounds. This was not spread across more farming acres but was concentrated more intensely on the same amount or even less acreage. In the same time frame, carcinogenic chemicals used as pesticides rose 129 percent to more than 23 million pounds per year. Toxic nerve poison legally deemed acceptable as pesticides rose 52 percent to more than 9 million pounds. Restricted chemical use for pesticides rose 34 percent to more than 48 million pounds per year. Frightening.

Strawberries and grapes are some of the most popular and common fruits, and are especially favored by kids. It is staggering to know that strawberries are doused with more than 300 million pounds of toxic chemical pesticides each year and grapes with 59 million pounds of toxic chemical pesticides. Sixty-five pesticides are registered for use on strawberries alone. Jam or jelly anyone?

Every day more than an estimated 1 million children consume unsafe levels of chemicals from commercially grown food. Childhood cancer kills more children under age fifteen than anything else in this country. One plus one equals . . .

The Environmental Protection Agency (EPA), the Food and Drug Administration (FDA), and the World Health Organization (WHO) are responsible for monitoring the food and water supply in America. These parent councils clearly recognize the dangers of chemicals and pesticides used in modern farming yet take no action to rectify the growing situation. These poisons are known carcinogens, substances that cause cancer, cause birth defects and sterility, and destroy the nervous system. Many

According to a 1993 Consumer Report:

· 71 percent of those surveyed were concerned about pesticides in food.
· 82 percent of those surveyed would buy only organic food if it was available.
· 84 percent of those surveyed believed the government should force farmers to use fewer chemicals in farming.

insecticides spawn directly from the technology of nerve gas perfected in World War II. How is this legal?

The EPA considers toxic chemicals acceptable within certain limits for agricultural use. Between 1982 and 1985, pesticide residue was found on 48 percent of all food tested by the FDA (that was more than fifteen years ago). It was considered "safe." The frightening relativity is that the FDA samples about only 1 percent of the food supply. Their current technology can detect less than half of almost 700 pesticides, herbicides, and fungicides acceptable to use, let alone chemicals in dangerous combinations.

> Several government reports conclude that 60–90% of all types of cancer in the U.S. are related to environmental factors ranging from food preservatives and additives to toxic chemical substances.
>
> —DOUGLAS M. COSTLE, FORMER DIRECTOR OF THE EPA

In America, we have the wheel of fortune of "Regulations." Many chemicals have been banned from use, including DDT, hexachloro, dieldrin, aldrin, chloradane, and chlorobenzilate. However, these banned toxic chemicals are still manufactured. They are exported to developing agricultural countries, especially Mexico and South America, where there are no regulations. Food is grown with no consumer or worker protection and exported right back to America. More than half of America's supply of commercial winter produce is from Mexico.

Poisoning Our Farmers and Their Families

Farmers are primary candidates for agricultural chemical poisoning. Cases of acute toxicity from exposure to chemicals and pesticides are painfully common among farmers and their families. Authorities suggest that more than 300,000 farmers have symptoms of pesticide-related illness.

While the EPA estimates that there are detectable chemicals in the fat tissue of *every* American, children in agricultural areas are hit the hardest. With developing immune and nervous systems, children are unjust victims of toxins at the hands of companies and organizations that should be ashamed of themselves.

Genetically Modified Organisms and Our Food

There is a growing concern about the impact that genetically modified organisms (GMO) and genetically engineered (GE) foods have on *health* and on *the environment,* not to mention their *social* and *economic effects.*

Impact on Health

It is likely that the long-term effects of GMO and GE foods will take years for scientists to detect.

Some GMO and GE foods are likely to aggravate and inflate food allergies. When genes from one species are spliced into another, the body cannot register or process the mutated combination properly. This genetic smorgasbord is dangerous, especially to sensitive persons. (This is a good point for a lawsuit.)

Most GMO foods are designed with antibiotic-resistant genes and are exposed to antibiotics, which can then be passed on to the bacteria in our bodies. This dangerous practice breeds super antibiotic-resistant strains of bacteria.

A 1999 study by the Scotland-based Rowett Institute found that GMO potatoes enlarge the endocrine glands and shrink the vital organs of lab rats. Predictably, this was later dismissed as faulty and inaccurate by industry standards.

In 1989, a GMO brand of L-tryptophan, a common dietary supplement, killed thirty-seven Americans and afflicted more than 5,000 others with a debilitating and potentially fatal neuromuscular condition before it was recalled from the public market.

> Since the 1940s, pesticide use has increased 10-fold, but crop losses to insects have doubled.
> —NATIONAL RESOURCES DEFENSE COUNCIL

A recent study by the United Kingdom's Economic and Social Research Council found that GE hybrid seeds, unlike their natural predecessors, do not take up minerals, such as iron and zinc, from the soil.

GMO food is an experiment, and we are all the guinea pigs.

Environmental Consequences

Bio-toxins spliced into GMO crops are now damaging beneficial insects. Ladybugs and lacewings, which eat the pests targeted by bio-toxins, are being poisoned themselves. Honeybees, which are essential for pollination, are also threatened. These bio-toxins can linger in the soil, a threat to agroecology for generations to come.

Bt corn (designed and marketed by Monsanto and Pioneer, bred to poison corn-eating insects) contains a bio-toxin that can spread through wind-borne pollen into pollen eaten by monarch butterflies. The monarch breeding ground dangerously corresponds with the U.S. corn belt, and the results are grievous. There is also a debate that wind-borne pollen from GMO crops will infest non-GMO crops nearby. There are no parameters to protect bio-toxins from spreading like the plague.

Social and Economic Effects

As natural seeds that have been grown for generations are replaced by GMO foods and "miracle seeds," farmers are caught in a cycle of dependency. The corporate seeds are designed with a "terminator gene" and cannot be replanted from the previous season's crop. The farmers are forced back year after year to buy seeds rather than reap the cycle of self-sustaining, biotic communities that have been maintained for millennia.

Three companies control 20 percent of the world's seed supply: Pioneer (now owned by DuPont), Monsanto (now owned by Pharmacia, formerly know as Upjohn), and Norvartis (the spawn of the merger of Sandoz and Ciba-Geigy). A monopoly of anything as precious as seed resources is a formula for catastrophe.

Irradiation

Irradiation is a dangerous practice designed to extend the shelf life of food by exposure to radiation from nuclear waste. This sounds like a surreal nightmare, but it is a common practice for meat, grains, herbs, spices, and some produce. While irradiation will kill food-borne pathogens such as *E. coli* and *Salmonella,* it will not eradicate all pathogens. Irradiation can only help to control contamination once it has occurred, but it cannot prevent it.

Irradiated food is exposed to dangerously high levels of radiation from Cobalt-60, Cesium-137, X-rays, and high-energy electron beams for one to two minutes in a concrete chamber. The levels of radiation involved are between 5,000 and 4 million rads (a standard measure for radiation doses). By comparison, a chest X-ray gives off no more than 1 rad. Irradiation is also called "ionizing radiation" because it produces energy waves strong enough to dislodge electrons from atoms and molecules, converting them to electrically charged particles called ions.

Support of irradiation practice is based on misleading studies. Bona-fide studies do show that the effects of irradiation include tumor growths, kidney damage, genetic and chromosome damage, and a spray of other complications.

Irradiated foods are shown to be depleted of minerals and vitamins, including A, C, E, K, B_1, B_2, B_3, B_6, and folic acid. They may also contain URPs (unique radi-

> The greatest danger of [chemical agriculture] pollution may well be that we shall tolerate levels of it so low as to have no acute nuisance value, but sufficiently high, nevertheless, to cause delayed disease and spoil the quality of life.
>
> —RENE DUBOIS, ENVIRONMENTAL SCIENTIST

The "Poverty & Hunger" report published by the World Bank concludes that there is no shortage of food on the planet, but that hunger is a problem of distribution, economics, and politics.

olytic products), dangerous chemical substances. Irradiation also creates free radicals, known culprits for cellular and tissue damage leading to premature aging.

How Can You Tell if Food Has Been Irradiated?

The FDA is supposed to protect and inform consumers of food safety, including irradiation. The FDA's Modernization Act of 1997 (FDAMA) has compromised the consumer's ability to identify irradiated food. Irradiated foods are supposed to be labeled as such by the FDAMA amendment in Section 306. This amendment requires that labels disclosing irradiated food be printed in the same size type as listed ingredients in packaged foods. However, any food that is not "entirely" irradiated does not have to be listed or printed as such. This leaves a broad margin of uncertainty. For instance, a package of soup that contains irradiated ingredients such as herbs does not have to provide this information on the label. With this haphazard system, there is very little security of thorough disclosure. The safest approach is to trust certified-organic food and ingredients.

Beware of foods identified as "cold-pasteurized" or "treated with irradiation pasteurization," as they are likely to have been irradiated.

Reduce Your Risk of Pesticides

1. Buy organically grown produce whenever possible!
2. Wash all produce! Although pesticides infiltrate fruits and vegetables through and through, concentrated pesticides on the skin can be washed away. A few drops of apple cider vinegar in a bowl of water are helpful for rinsing or scrubbing vegetables and fruit. Use a soft brush to clean tough fruits and vegetables.
3. Peel produce if it is not organic. Certain fruits and vegetables can be peeled to remove pesticides on the skin and to avoid waxes, which cannot be washed off. Unfortunately, peeling produce removes the vitamins and minerals in and under the skins. Peel inorganic produce such as apples, cucumbers, carrots, beets, peaches, plums, nectarines, pears, eggplant, parsnips, potatoes, turnips, yams, and squash.

Goliaths Against Davids

While small-scale farmers are being forced into economic impossibility by escalating land and production costs and are being undermined by government-subsidized mono-crops, a handful of corporate conglomerates is raking in millions and billions of dollars. Most of the following corporations are in the agriculture and petrochemical industry and are heavily invested in GMO food production:

Monsanto	Rhone-Poulenc Rorer
Dow Chemical	Avery Dennison
DuPont	Rohm and Haas
Chevron	American Cynamid
Shell	Philip Morris
Uniroyal	Nestlé
Vulcan	PepsiCo
Union Carbide	Coca-Cola
Stauffer Chemical	Anheuser-Busch

Don't Panic if It's Organic

The parameters of "organically grown food" do not accept irradiation as an acceptable process. In a vegetarian diet, dried spices and herbs are the most likely foods to have been exposed to irradiation. Be sure to buy "non-irradiated" spices and dried herbs. If it is organic, no need to panic.

Organically Grown Food

Organically grown food must meet accepted parameters in order to be labeled as such. Organic farming requires the responsible maintenance of healthy, fertile soil. Soil must be rested and fed through natural methods and without the use of chemical fertilizers, pesticides, fungicides, herbicides, and rodenticides.

The California Food Act of 1990 set a uniform standard for organic food production and handling. In 1991, Congress passed the Organic Foods Production Act as part of a national

The Delaney Amendment

The Delaney Amendment is found in Section 409 of the Federal Food, Drug and Cosmetic Act. It states:

> No additive shall be deemed safe if it is found to induce cancer when ingested by man or animal.

Under this amendment, if an additive is deemed unsafe, it cannot be legally used. Pesticides and agrochemicals that are known carcinogens that were approved prior to the Delaney Amendment continue to be used without discretion.

The EPA published findings in the report "Unfinished Business: A Comparative Assessment of Environmental Problems" that ranked pesticide residues in food as the number three cancer risk today.

—"The World Bank's Strategy for Reducing Poverty and Hunger:
a Report to the Development Community"

farm bill. There are many states that have independent certifications. Until the day that organic foods can be identified by one single, unified seal, be sure to only trust "organic" food that has a certified label.

The basic margins of organically grown food involve maintaining soil fertility through natural fortification and crop rotation. The following statements provide a loose estimate of what "certified organic" means:

1. Certified organic production must be in accordance with the uniform standards continuously for at least thirty-six months.
2. Soil enrichment must be obtained through (a) organic matter that has not been chemically fortified, (b) natural rock products that have not been mined or processed with synthetic chemicals, (c) beneficial bacteria and algae that are not chemically fortified, and (d) earthworms.
3. Crops and fields must be rotated on an annual basis. The same crop cannot be grown in the same field for more than one year. Crop rotation ensures that "heavy feeding"

crops like corn and soy do not deplete nutrients from the soil. Orchard trees, maple trees, and crops that take more than one year to mature are exempt.

4. Insect control is acceptable only by means of (a) predatory insects, (b) insect-disease cultures, (c) attractants, like beneficial insects, and (d) rotenone, pyrethrum, ryania, or sabadilla (certifiably safe herbicides).

5. Weed control can be pursued only by (a) crop rotation, (b) mechanical or hand-cultivation techniques, like weed whacking or good old-fashioned weeding, or (c) cutting of weed patches. Weeds cannot be controlled by chemicals.

6. Fungus and bacteria can be controlled only with products acceptable for soil enrichment.

7. Rodents can be controlled only by means of the rodent's natural enemies, natural repellent techniques, or traps.

8. Drying of food can be done only by means of natural field drying through bin aeration or artificial methods that do not exceed temperatures of 160°F.

9. If fumigation is necessary, only diatomaceous earth can be used. Diatomaceous earth is composed of soil that is like microscopic volcanic glass. The shards are so small and sharp that they cut the skeletons of bugs to smithereens.

10. All food must comply with FDA and state standards.

3

Enzymes:
The Spark of Life

What Are Enzymes?

Enzymes are the universal "spark of life." The word *enzyme* comes from the Greek root *enzymos,* which means "to cause change." Enzymes are responsible for every metabolic action in the body. From blinking an eye to secreting saliva, from the beating of the heart to digesting nutrients, enzymes are the champions that make it all happen. They are the catalysts that enable cells to work and chemical reactions to happen without themselves being consumed in the process. Enzymes are ancient and modern magic.

Enzymes are energized protein molecules made up of specific protein structures called *apoenzymes.* Enzymes work with cofactors, such as vitamins and minerals, to spark biochemical reactions. It is the energy created by the enzymes that produces biochemical reactions, which is the magic that orchestrates a trillion cells to cooperatively function. These actions and reactions regulate the body's diverse processes and are an essential part of larger processes like digestion. Without this "spark of life" of enzymes, life would simply cease to exist.

Specific enzymes are tailored for specific means and needs. There are thousands of different enzymes in the body, each with a precise encoded function. There are enzymes for digestion; cellular function and energy; repairing tissue, organs, and cells; utilizing and decoding nutrients; concentrating iron in the blood; coagulating blood; eliminating carbon dioxide from the lungs; detoxifying waste from the kidneys, colon, and liver; and a relatively infinite number of cooperative interactions that enable the miraculous process of life to happen.

Diplomatic Enzymes

Enzymes are the catalysts that spark the complex process of assimilation and digestion. Enzymes decode food. They delegate proper use of nutrition and translate how to turn chewed-up salad into vibrant body matter.

Imagine a delicious bunch of carrots. Each carrot is complete with the enzymes it needs for the nutrients to be digested, metabolized, and assimilated. In its natural state, it is at the peak of nutrition. It has precious vitamin A, iron, vitamin C, and superoxide dismutase and is choke with minerals.

Imagine those carrots steamed to mush, boiled into a purée for soup, stir-fried in cooked oil, or cooked into a carrot cake with processed flour and cooked oil. Enzymes are destroyed by these processes in varying degrees. The nutrients, which are also very heat-sensitive, are also degraded. When the cooked carrots are eaten, the body must produce enzymes to deal with the deficient food. Twice as much work is required to get half as much yield. Bad deal.

Steaming vegetables is a tricky example. It is possible to steam vegetables moderately so that the inside is barely cooked and the nutrients are only mildly affected. Moderate steaming helps to break down some of the fibrous cellulose that makes "tough" vegetables difficult to digest for a weakened system. This is especially true for the *Brassica* family, which includes broccoli, cabbage, cauliflower, and kale. Flash-cooking (for example, steaming or blanching broccoli for just a minute until it turns bright green) will not degrade the nutrition completely and may make the vegetable more digestible for some.

Optimally functioning digestive systems should be able to digest, assimilate, and eliminate raw vegetables smoothly. It is a diplomatic dance to determine what formula will be easier for your body in the case of "tough" vegetables: eating "tough" veggies in their raw state with digestive difficulty; or lightly steaming "tough" veggies to make them easier to digest at the expense of losing some enzymes and nutrients. Each of us will come to the table with a different system. The most gentle approach is to be open to your body's process to meet your system's needs most fruitfully and easily. The wisdom of the body will reveal its process if we trust it enough to listen and feel.

There are more degraded examples of foods deficient in enzymes and nutrients. These include any food cooked in oil, fried food, refined carbohydrates and flours such as breads and pastries, processed and cooked proteins, and any denatured, frozen, or pasteurized food.

There are three major categories of enzymes: digestive enzymes, food enzymes, and metabolic enzymes.

Digestive Enzymes

Digestive enzymes enable the breakdown of food so the body and blood can use nutrients. Enzymes are needed to assimilate a stalk of broccoli into tissue, blood, and organs.

Digestive enzymes are secreted along the intestinal tract, in pancreatic and intestinal juices, and in saliva. These digestive enzymes are designed to be suited for different foods. For example, broccoli requires digestive enzymes different from those required by mangoes, almonds, quinoa, or garbanzo beans.

Amylase

Amylase is secreted in saliva and pancreatic and intestinal juices. This enzyme is designed to break down sugars and carbohydrates.

There are three kinds of amylase tailored for different kinds of sugar: maltase, sucrase, and lactase. Maltase breaks down malt sugar from grains and carbohydrates. Sucrase breaks down cane sugar. And lactase breaks down milk sugar (lactose). More than half of the population of the world does not produce the lactase enzyme, which results in lactose intolerance, meaning they are "allergic" to dairy and are literally unable to digest milk and milk products. This overwhelming statistic suggests that dairy is entirely overconsumed (especially in America) and has an inappropriate role in many people's diets. Lactose intolerance is broadly symptomized by sluggish metabolism, congestion, skin problems, indigestion, bloating, low energy, and diarrhea.

Lipase

Lipase is necessary for digesting fat and is found in stomach and pancreatic juices. Lipase is also found in raw, unrefined fat in foods such as fresh nuts and seeds and quality pressed oils.

Protease

Protease breaks down protein and is found in stomach, pancreatic, and intestinal juices.

Food Enzymes

Enzymes are essential and irreplaceable for breaking down food in order to make nutrients available to the body. Our bodies demand a constant supply of enzymes for biochemical reactions. Digestion is just one of the processes that requires enzymes. Processed and cooked foods are devoid of enzymes and require an excessive draw of energy from the body for digestion. It takes a significant amount of energy for our bodies to produce enzymes to digest food that is lacking enzymes due to cooking, processing, and refining. Enzymes *are* available in unrefined, live food. Ergo, a choice is presented as to how you want to use the energy produced by your body. Eating balanced, raw, and living food requires a minimal expenditure of energy to assimilate and digest to *receive* energy. More energy for less effort. Good deal.

Eating cooked, processed, and refined food is a drain on the body because an inordinate amount of energy is required just to produce the enzymes needed to break down the foods versus using the energy to replenish, repair, and maintain tissue, blood, and organs. It's 3 P.M.: Do you know where your energy is?

Metabolic Enzymes

Metabolic enzymes are present in every cell of the body. They are responsible for energy production and detoxification. Metabolic enzymes are responsible for building blood, tissue, and organs from protein, carbohydrates, and fats. Every tissue of the body has metabolic enzymes tailored to specific needs. Metabolic enzymes decode and translate crude energy from food into usable energy for the body.

Superoxide Dismutase (SOD)

Superoxide dismutase (SOD) is a metabolic enzyme found in every cell in the body. SOD is considered to be an antioxidant. Antioxidants keep cell degeneration and destruction in check by neutralizing free radicals. A free radical is a destructive, "imbalanced" atom or group of atoms missing an electron that wreaks havoc by stealing electrons from other atoms, setting off a vicious cycle of imbalanced atoms. (Free radicals are rampant in cooked oil, irradiated food, and environmental pollution.) SOD specifically combats a common free radical called superoxide and is effective at protecting the cells' precious mitochondria, which manufacture energy, and store genetic information (DNA) of the cells, enabling healthy maintenance and growth.

Dietary Sources of SOD
High dietary concentrations of SOD are found in all green plants, especially young cereal grasses such as wheatgrass and barley grass, sprouts, and broccoli.

Enzymes and Heat

Enzymes are extremely sensitive to heat. Enzymes are destroyed by temperatures in excess of 110°F. Raw, living food is the only food complete with naturally occurring enzymes. Food that has been cooked, processed, refined, or pasteurized is deficient in the enzymes necessary for digestion and absorption. This forces our bodies, which are busy with a trillion other cells, to bear the burden.

There is, of course, a world of difference between steaming broccoli and deep-frying a white potato, for example. There is a certain level of educated compromise in modern living. It is pompous to suggest that we all move to the countryside to grow and harvest all of our food, but everyone in America has reasonable access to fresh produce and good-quality oil. Finding a sound formula that feeds the body, mind, and spirit is the quest of a lifetime.

Finding Balance

Bringing all of this to light is not intended to encourage an alarmist attitude. Balance is the omnipotent reasoning. Mental health is directly related to physical health. Emotional well-being has a crucial influence on our internal environment. Our thoughts can be as polluting as anything. Setting realistic standards and safety nets to catch us when we fall is an honest sequence for success in the long run.

Cooked oil is a tricky one! It is everywhere. It is futile to beat ourselves up for not being able to hold lofty ideals at all times. Take care to be responsible. If any denatured food has seduced your senses, it is smart and restorative to dose yourself with digestive enzymes, available in capsules in most health food stores.

Be allowing. What is done day in and day out directs health. A bite here and there flanked by the wealth of enzyme-rich food will not register on the Richter scale of damage. Thoughts can be as acidic as food.

Forgive the body and it will be forgiving. The body seeks balance. Swinging is a fun rush, but it sure is exhausting to have to pump all the time. Given time and a loving environment, the body will find homeostasis and good health naturally.

Abundant Wealth of Enzymes

There are foods that have enzymes above and beyond the call of their own digestive duty. Any food eaten with these generous models is extended the benefits of easy digestion.

Sprouts are the most abundant source of all. Sprouts are still growing when we eat them. Sprouts are peaking in nutrition and have more enzymes than they require to be broken down from such a simplified state. The protein is available in the simpler form of amino acids and the carbohydrates and starches as simple sugars. Sprouts are clean, easy enzyme-rich fuel. (See Chapter 16 for more on sprouts.)

Papaya and *pineapple* are also especially abundant in enzymes. Papaya contains *papain,* a proteolytic enzyme especially plentiful in the younger, green papaya.

Similarly, pineapple contains *bromelain,* also a proteolytic enzyme. Bromelain can be found in more abundance in younger pineapples and is concentrated in the fibrous core. Proteolytic enzymes digest proteins and are known for their anti-inflammatory properties.

Lipase is found abundantly in live fatty foods such as avocado and raw seeds and nuts. Cooked and processed fatty foods that are not rich in enzymes require the pancreas to secrete lipase-rich juices to deal with them. Pancreatic juices in the digestive tract create an alkaline environment, which is troublesome for digesting fats. By nature, fats require an acidic medium to be digested. When fatty foods are rich in lipase, they are properly attended to in the stomach, a naturally more acidic environment. Ergo, unrefined, live fats are more easily and efficiently digested and make for healthy cells.

Good fat rids the body of old fat. Live, lipase-rich fatty food helps to metabolize stored fat deposits. This is a diet that actually works. Eating good fat burns the stored fat. Beautiful deal.

Enzyme Supplements

A diet generous in raw and living foods provides more than enough enzymatic needs for the body. Raw and living foods transform degenerated tissues and weakened digestive systems that have been taxed by a refined and processed diet.

People with weakened conditions and digestive sensitivities, and especially the elderly, can benefit from taking enzyme supplements with food for optimum digestion. The body rejoices when extra enzymes are taken with an excessive meal or with heavy, cooked foods. It is a safety net for situations when compromising foods are eaten. Taking the responsibility to help digestion when poor food choices are made is much better than feeling heavy, tortured, and guilty after a meal. Enzyme supplements are synthesized digestive enzymes usually available as capsules in most health food stores. The potency of each brand will vary. Take care to look at the ingredients and the potency rather than just at the price tag. A dynamic support system is key for health and longevity.

4

Transitioning to Health

Each of us comes to the table with a different formula, body, background, habits, and needs. There are many elements and textures of living and habits, which result in a very individual state of health. Genetic predisposition, geographic locale, stress levels, family, and profession are just a few variables that greatly affect our health and well-being. With a few guidelines and suggestions, transforming mediocre and even poor health into more vibrant living can be an easy transition.

We are, each of us, in a state of evolution and growth. Our cells are rapidly regenerating and building new tissue, skin, organs, hair, bone, and blood. Change is the only constant. This is your chance. Setting realistic goals for healthier habits, rejuvenation, and restoration is proof positive for success and peace of body, mind, and spirit.

Immediate Considerations

1. Drink Plenty of Fresh Water

Our bodies are made up of about 70 percent water. Flushing the body with fresh water and staying hydrated are simple solutions for improved energy, clear skin, and balanced blood sugar.

A full glass of water (16 ounces) should be taken every two hours. The goal is to drink at least 1 ounce of fresh water for every 2 pounds of body weight every day. For most of us, this will be a significant increase in fluid, which might require extra trips to the bathroom at first.

If this feels like too much, cut back a little, but keep in mind that staying hydrated is a key element for systemic health.

Squeeze some fresh lemon or orange juice in the water for a touch of flavor and organic minerals. A nice glass water bottle is also a pleasurable incentive to drink from.

P.S. Juice and tea do not flush the body as well as clean, fresh water.

2. Balance Acid-Alkaline Conditions First Thing in the Morning

Upon rising in the morning, drink 16 ounces of room temperature water mixed with the juice of half a lemon or 1 to 2 tablespoons of raw apple cider vinegar. The balanced acidity of the lemon juice or apple cider vinegar establishes the right stability and balance in the stomach for the day. It gets the digestive juices flowing and all systems raring to go!

Also, a tonic of 1 tablespoon of apple cider vinegar in 8 to 10 ounces of water a half hour before a meal stabilizes the stomach by providing ideal acid-alkaline conditions for digestion.

3. Go Organic!

Organically grown food has a wealth of health to offer the body and the planet. Organically grown food has more nutrition and no harmful chemicals, pesticides, waxes, or residues. Pesticides have been directly linked to immune system and nervous system damage. Clean input is a clear message of health to the body, down to a cellular level, for high-quality integrity.

4. Eat Fresh Food with Every Meal and Snack

Eating fresh food with every meal and snack is a healthy trend for a lifetime of health. Including fresh fruit with breakfast or with a smoothie, for example, is a healthy welcome for every day. Complementing lunch or dinner with a fresh salad is a just improvement to any meal. Pile fresh vegetables, avocado slices, and sprouts on a sandwich. Have a fresh juice, a power smoothie, or a piece of fruit as a snack. Have fruit with or for dessert. Find fresh food you love and eat it to your heart's desire.

5. Exclude or Reduce Eating Dairy Products

Taking this step will have immediate results. Dairy coats the intestines with mucus. Eliminating dairy products will clear up the intestines and allow intestinal tissue to rejuvenate with renewed function. Digestion, assimilation, and elimination will become more efficient and easier. Energy, respiration, and cardiovascular health will improve without the clogging nature of dairy. Skin problems clear up, and many people shed unwanted pounds.

A good-quality olive oil replaces butter effortlessly. There are many tasty and improved dairy alternatives on the market today. The flavor and texture of soy, rice, almond, and oat alternatives are a bit different, but with newfound health, there is nothing to miss.

6. Exclude or Reduce Eating Fried Food, Fast Food, and Processed Food

These foods are detrimental to our health. Replacing these "habits" with real food and nourishment takes some willpower at first, but the rewards come quickly. Avoiding fried and processed food does the body good. This service will be repaid in increased energy, efficient digestion and elimination, clear skin, and a loss of unwanted pounds. It is more fun and easy to concentrate on the benefits than on feeling deprived. Find healthy, fresh foods you love and then enjoy them with a clear mind.

Choose steamed or baked vegetables over sautéed or fried food. Begin to prioritize whole foods over processed food. Choose whole grains over pasta and bread for real nutrition. Exercise simple, intelligent choices, such as choosing brown rice over white rice. Choose whole beans and tempeh over tofu. The more fresh, whole, and less refined and processed, the better.

7. Find Wheat-Free Alternatives

Wheat is a common culprit for sluggish digestion and allergies. Spelt, kamut, quinoa, corn, oats, and rye are much more intelligent and nutritious alternatives.

Choosing sprouted bread, wheat-free bread, and naturally leavened bread is the first step toward freedom from the loaf. There are some really delicious and satisfying varieties of wheat-free alternatives on the market that make choosing health a pleasure.

8. Take a Look at Oils

Where and how oil stands in the diet has a significant impact on health. Fresh, organic oil that has not been refined or cooked nourishes the body down to every last cell. The health of every cell membrane relies on essential fatty acids from healthy oil. Cooked and processed oil is harmful to the body's health on a broad level and is rampant with free radicals, which cause damage on a cellular level.

Eating fresh, healthy oils such as olive oil, flax oil, avocados, and raw seeds and nuts and eliminating processed and cooked oils will dramatically improve systemic health. Skin will be more supple and beautiful, digestion and overall energy will improve, hair and nail growth will be strong and dapper, and extra pounds will be easily shed.

Drizzle olive oil over fresh or steamed vegetables rather than sautéing the vegetables in oil. Replace all hydrogenated oil, such as margarine, which contains trans-fats, with tasty alternatives. Take a good look at salad dressings: Blend a fresh salad dressing or simply use good olive oil, vinegar, salt, and herbs instead of pasteurized salad dressing with unhealthy oils. Avoid canola oil, peanut oil, cottonseed oil, and any hydrogenated oil. Choose raw nuts and seeds over roasted varieties.

9. Take a Look at Sugars

Refined sugar offers to the body nothing more than sugar imbalances and energy crashes. There are many alternatives that will satisfy any sweet tooth (even a sugar junkie). Choosing organic, evaporated cane juice, maple syrup, or raw honey over white sugar is a delicious gift for health. White sugar is detrimental to the blood sugar and leeches nutrients from the body. Avoid corn syrup and high-fructose corn syrup for the sake of blood sugar balance and for avoiding energy crashes. Artificial sweeteners such as Nutrasweet (aspartame) are toxic and can be easily replaced by Stevia, a naturally sweet herb available in liquid or powder. (See Chapter 10 for more information on Stevia.)

10. Take Enzymes If You Indulge

During a time of transition, having a safety net is always a good idea. If a situation arises that seduces your better sense of health, take care to prepare for some damage control. Taking digestive enzyme supplements is an easy way to help curtail the effects of an overindulgent meal, too much late-night snacking, or a temporary slip into poor food choices. The digestive enzymes will be a great aid for easier digestion and moving on. While it is best not to live in crisis management, a backup plan is always helpful in tough situations.

11. Be Mindful of Emotions and Sensations Surrounding Eating

Part of the stride toward health and well-being is getting to know ourselves and our systems. Recognizing patterns and habits is the first step to freedom. It is worthwhile to consider cravings, desires, longings, and vices before falling prey and victim to old habits. Emotional turbulence and dependency on food are common aliments in this overfed, undernourished society.

Peace with food is possible. Eating should be a satisfying and joyful experience that nourishes the body. We give ourselves such a hard time! Relaxing into our process is a piece of freedom and liberation. Nothing worthwhile changes overnight. Learn forgiveness and how to be non-judgmental—these are the fresh air of relief.

Transitions to Consider in Three to Six Weeks

1. Begin to Exercise

Get your blood pumping by doing something you enjoy, such as yoga, walking, swimming, bicycling, or dancing. Do some exercise every day, even if it is as simple as parking at the far end of the parking lot for a longer walk or stretching first thing in the morning or before bed. Take up an active exercise that gets you sweating and feeling good at least three times per week for an hour.

Deep breathing increases the oxygen supply to the blood, which helps it to carry nutrients throughout the body to regenerate tissue, blood, organs, and skin. The skin is the body's largest organ. It is designed to eliminate toxins through sweat. Sweating feels great and can be a healthy approach to dealing with and relieving stress. Let the stress come out with some sweat, and the joyful benefits will come!

Getting out in the sun and fresh air is also great. Sunshine is great for the body, mind, and spirit (and enables us to assimilate certain vitamins).

Exercise is a key to vitality. Waking up the body with exercise will improve regeneration and rejuvenation on every level. Exercise also naturally releases endorphins in the brain, making everything brighter and more inspiring. It takes some willpower to begin an exercise program, but once you have a routine, even healthy habits are hard to give up.

2. Eat Only Whole Foods

Eat only natural, whole foods and as much organically grown food as possible. Choose as much fresh, raw food as possible and choose whole foods, such as steamed vegetables, whole grains, and beans. A diet consisting of 50 percent fresh, raw food is a healthy goal to meet. Go from there. Find a reasonable comfort level and keep pursuing whole, healthy goals.

3. Find Health Food Stores, Farmers' Markets, and Natural Foods Co-Ops

Getting acquainted with a good supply of fresh produce and quality food makes stocking the pantry easier and more fun. Find catalogs or search the Internet for high-quality and specialty products that might not be available in local stores. Fresh food can be purchased by mail from Diamond Organics 888-ORGANIC (674-2642).

4. Reevaluate the Pantry

A spring cleaning of the pantry to do away with canned food, junk food, processed food, and foods of the past peels away the old to make room for a well-stocked pantry with delicious, healthy choices. Donate unopened packages to a food drive or local shelter.

A pantry that is chock-full of good choices and condiments makes preparing good food much easier.

5. Begin Sprouting!

Sprouting is a dynamic world of texture and flavor. From simply soaking nuts and seeds to sprouting delicate alfalfa sprouts and hearty beans and grains, sprouting will open up another level of high-integrity nutrition. Sprouts are some of the most nutritious foods on the planet and help us get in touch with the life force in food and the process of growing.

Steaming sprouted beans and grains is another step toward fresh, whole foods. Sprouted long-grain wild rice is a savory, nutty base for many delicious dishes. Sprouted beans make fantastic hummus. Sprouted grains are easy to make into crackers, bread, and cookies. Soaking seeds and nuts in fresh water to add to any dish or as a snack make these protein-packed morsels more digestible, nutritious, and fresh to enjoy anytime.

Sprouting is as simple as getting a few large glass jars, some screen, and rubber bands. A dish rack near the sink will work to drain the sprouts. A few minutes a day of soaking and rinsing will create a whole new level of vitality in the diet. (See Chapter 16 for easy sprouting instructions and guidelines.)

6. Start Drinking Fresh Juice

Sample freshly made vegetable and fruit juices from a juice bar. Ask the counter person what he or she recommends for a novice juice drinker. Try drinking fresh juice at least three times a week. Fresh juice makes a great energy snack in the afternoon. Start the day with fresh juice once or twice a week for a vital, light breakfast.

Shop around for a new or used juicer for affordable home juicing. Look in culinary stores, health food stores, and on the Internet. The price of the juicer will pay itself off for years to come.

7. Eat as Much Fresh, Raw Food as Possible

Try eating only raw foods for one or two meals a day. Then try a whole day of eating only raw food to see how it fits. Choose only fresh, raw snacks such as fruit and soaked nuts or seeds. There are more and more choices in health food stores of raw, living energy bars, crackers, and snacks. Find a satisfying comfort level and work from there. There is no rush or need to feel deprived. Health is contagious and will grow with you.

8. Start Experimenting with New Recipes

Try new recipes that fit into your time schedule and resources. Making delicious food in your kitchen is a step toward freedom. Find tried and true, favorite flavors and work from there. Expand the horizons of your palate and creativity with new recipes. There are hundreds here in this book alone (and more where they came from!).

Experiment with seaweed and miso. Introduce cultured and fermented food to your palate. Use new herbs and spices, and the culinary genius in you may emerge.

9. Consider Day-to-Day Health Maintenance and a Detoxification Program

Even with a busy schedule, it is possible to cleanse the system. Simply eating well is a mammoth step toward rejuvenation and vitality. There are herbs, juices, supplements, and programs that can help aid and quicken the process of becoming fit, healthy, and well.

A program to regenerate the colon and intestines is a great place to start. Introducing a fiber supplement to your diet in the morning or evening will help sweep your intestinal tract of old, built-up matter that you are ready to lose. This will improve digestion and assimilation and strengthen the muscles of the colon. A mild, herbal laxative can help remove old toxins and rid the intestines of waste.

Taking probiotics, such as *L. acidophilus*, to populate the intestines with healthy bacteria is a big step toward proper digestion and assimilation of nutrients and food.

Consider drinking only juice one day every week. Choose a day, such as a Sunday, when you have the freedom to rest and relax. The digestive tract will have a chance to rest so the body can heal other areas that need attention. Getting comfortable and familiar with fasting once a week will prepare your body for a longer program.

Consider a longer cleansing program or fasting when you are ready. I highly recommend the Ejuva Program for an effective, responsible cleanse when the time is right. (See the Resource Guide for information.)

10. Start Reading More About Health, Nutrition, and Well-Being

Personal knowledge is the essence of freedom itself. The more we learn, the easier it is to diagnose our personal conditions. There is a lot of information available on health, diet, and nutrition. Don't buy everything you hear; there is a lot of rubbish amid the genius. The more you read, the easier it is to make clear, educated decisions about your own personal health.

11. Create a Good System for Your Household

1. Create a working schedule to keep the kitchen and pantry stocked with all of the right yummies.
2. Stock up on bulk foods such as nuts, seeds, grains, and beans. It will save money and resources.
3. Use a free day to make a supply of dehydrated breads, cookies, chips, and snacks.
4. Figure out a good schedule for soaking and sprouting food to have on hand for the week.
5. Plant an herb garden in your yard or in a window box.

Monthly or Bi-monthly

1. Make a variety of dehydrated flat breads, crackers, chips, cookies, and snacks. It is easier to do this with a concentrated effort and enjoy the harvest for a few weeks. The delicious benefits are worth the effort.
2. As you get into cultured and fermented foods, make a batch of dynamic kimchi or sauerkraut. One batch will keep fresh and tasty for a few weeks.

Weekly

1. Make a batch or two of seed and nut cheese to use throughout the week. Leave the seed and nut cheese plain, to be seasoned for different recipes.
2. Sprout seeds and grains for fresh, young delicacies such as sunflower sprouts, buckwheat lettuce, and wheatgrass or barley grass.

Bi-weekly

Figure out a schedule for soaking nuts, seeds, grains, and beans to have on hand for a variety of flavors and textures. It is easy to eat well when the goods are at your fingertips. Try sprouting beans and grains one day a week and nuts and seeds another day. Keep the rotation fresh and try new varieties.

Soaked almonds and long-grain wild rice are two things I always have on hand. They store well in the fridge for more than a week, provided they are covered with fresh water that is changed every two to three days. Soaked almonds are great for paté or a creamy dressing anytime. Wild rice is a satisfying, nutty base for any delicious meal.

When to Eat

Finding comfortable eating habits is a personal rhythm. Most of us are creatures of habit and perform best with a regular plan of events. In a time of transition, getting a handle on eating habits and good schedule can make or break the enjoyment of getting in touch with health.

Eating three big meals a day may not suit everyone. Many people do better with several smaller meals throughout the day. Eating small, regular meals helps maintain a good level of energy, boosts the metabolism, and discourages gorging on too much food at once.

It is best to eat only when you are really hungry and the stomach is empty and all of the food from the previous meal is digested. A sincere sense of hunger makes eating much more enjoyable. Eating out of habit or boredom is just that and offers diminishing returns for health.

Resting or reading for 20 to 30 minutes after a meal encourages vital digestion and premium assimilation of nutrients. Mothers everywhere ruled that there should be no swimming for a half hour after eating. This pervasive childhood rule is based on the fact that digestion requires a premium amount of energy. Mom did not want the muscles in your little legs to cramp in the pool because your body was busy digesting lunch. While few of us have the liberty for a swim after lunch, the same truth can be applied to engage proper digestion. Take a rest; this is a time for your body to feed and grow—no need to distract a brilliant, life-giving process. It is a great time to read, write in a journal, write a letter to an old friend, or call your mom and thank her for her multifarious wisdom that was not lost on you as a child; it just took a little time to sink in.

Similarly, to give digestion the energy it is worth, it is best not to eat when you are very tired, very cold or overheated, or after strenuous physical exercise or labor. Drink a large glass of water or a cup of herbal tea instead and wait until the apex has passed and true hunger is present. Presenting the body with food when it is prepared for it and not in a state of stress will return the favor of vital digestion and good energy for living.

Eating late at night or very early in the morning is taxing and stressful to the body and digestive system. Eating late at night sets up food to lay stagnant in the body. Sleep is a precious time for the body to recoup and wander the dreamworld without demands for digestion. Little energy is returned for this extra stress. More than likely, food eaten less than two hours before sleep does not get properly digested and leads to fitful rest, systemic imbalance, and weight gain. A piece of fruit or herbal tea is a soothing evening snack that will not interrupt a healthy cycle of good digestion and fine rest.

Eating very early or first thing in the morning also yields diminishing returns. Morning is a precious time for the body to be clear and balanced. Drinking fresh water with lemon or a splash of apple cider vinegar is a great morning tonic to set balance in the stomach and clear the scene. A good standard to meet is to evacuate the colon of the previous day's food before starting the process again. Early morning yoga, stretching, or a brisk walk sets a salutary tone for the day. A light breakfast of juice, fruit, miso soup, or a smoothie is a gentle welcome way to begin the day.

Part Two

The Raw Foods Pantry

5

The Essentials:
Fresh Produce

Any seasoned chef or lover of good food will agree that fine, fresh produce is an essential foundation for fine food.

Good, fresh produce is widely available almost everywhere, year-round. There are more varieties of common foods than days in the year, though certain specialties take some scouting to find and others are available fresh only in certain seasons. With a touch of resourceful creativity, produce that is generally available can easily make up for some of the more rare delicacies.

This section is presented in groups of botanical and culinary families and is an encyclopedia of information, providing the names and descriptions of an ample variety of fresh foods. The Essentials reaches from fruits and vegetables to spices and herbs; staple sundries from seeds and nuts to grains and beans; and culinary essentials and condiments, like oils, sugars, vinegar, miso, salts, and seasonings.

Allium Genus

Onions, garlic, leeks, chives, and shallots are all part of the lily family and the *Allium* genus, which has more than 325 members. There are many wild varieties, including the onion grass I used to pull up to smell when I was a kid living in the Northeast. All types in the *Allium* genus are characterized by a strong, pungent smell, which is caused by volatile acids under the skin.

Onions

Onions are underground bulbs that are related to the lily. There is archaeological and historical evidence that onions have been eaten for thousands of years. It is thought that onions originated in the Middle East and spread worldwide because they are easy to cultivate and they store well for a relatively long time.

There are many types of onions with varying potencies. Onions contribute a savory flavor to just about any dish. They're so delicious and nutritious. Onions grown in warmer climates are milder and sweeter than varieties from cooler regions. The sweet and mild varieties are best for raw food. To relax the bite of a raw onion, rinse minced onion under cold water.

Pungent Onions

RED ONIONS

Red onions are also called Italian onions. They have beautiful ruby skin with blushing red layers and a mild, sweet flavor. They are good in salads and in marinated dishes.

WHITE ONIONS

White onions have pearly-white skin and come in a variety of shapes and sizes. Their flavor and strength vary. Small white onions are generally the tastiest.

How to Cut an Onion Without Crying

I have heard many wild claims for how to keep the tears at bay while cutting onions. I have tried them all with varying degrees of success (like trying to cure hiccups). I do not mind the tears, as long as no other fluids get involved (sniff, sniff).

One suggestion that I have found to be quite effective is to slice onions under running water, although logistically it does not work out to chop onions under running water because they wash down the drain. Another suggestion, which some chefs swear by, is to bite a chopstick while cutting the onions. This unusual technique is to encourage breathing through your mouth, so the volatile oils of the onion do not sneak up your nose and irritate the mucous membranes and make your eyes and nose run. Otherwise, I find good ventilation to be a simple and effective solution.

YELLOW ONIONS

Yellow onions are one of the most common varieties of onions in the market. They have golden-brown skin and are very pungent. They're best pickled or well marinated.

Sweet Onions

MAUI ONIONS

Maui onions are grown in Hawaii—my home turf! The gentle, warm climate all year makes Maui onions one of the sweetest and most sought-after onions. They have pale-golden skin and are more squat than round. They're deliciously sweet, mild, and juicy. Maui onions are reasonably available in specialty stores and can be ordered by mail. Vidalia onions are a good substitute in their absence.

SPANISH ONIONS

Spanish onions are large, pale, copper onions. They are grown in warm regions and are among the mildest onions cultivated. With their delicate, sweet flavor, Spanish onions are ideal raw or marinated.

VIDALIA ONIONS

Named for Vidalia, Georgia, where they were originally grown, Vidalia onions are fairly large and round with pale-yellow skin and layers. These special onions favor a warm climate and are widely available in the summer, though more and more commonly throughout the year.

Shallots

Shallots are not onions, but a close kin. Small and slender, shallots have longer necks and golden-to-copper skin. They grow in small clusters and can be used in most places where onion is called for, though raw shallots have a stronger flavor than mild onions, and the quantity should be adjusted to taste.

Shallots are favored on sauces as they have very little fiber and dissolve easily into liquids. Because of their small size, they are convenient for recipes calling for only a small amount of pungent onion.

Garlic

Garlic is celebrated in cuisine all over the world. It is one of the oldest cultivated foods. The first known cultivation of garlic dates back to 3200 B.C. in Egypt. Garlic has tremendous therapeutic properties. It is known to improve circulation, lower blood pressure, and increase the absorption of vitamins and minerals. Raw garlic has powerful antibiotic properties. The ancient Romans used it to treat eczema and snake bites.

Store garlic in a cool, dry place. If the air is too damp, the bulbs will sprout. If it is too warm, they will disintegrate. Do not store garlic in the refrigerator. A brown paper bag in the pantry is just right.

When a garlic clove is split lengthwise, you'll see a pale-green shoot in the center. This is the part of the garlic that causes some people digestive difficulties. For best results, remove the shoot and carry on!

> Garlic breath can be chased away by chewing on parsley or cardamom seeds. Otherwise, make sure your friends and your honey-love eat plenty of garlic with you!

Elephant Garlic

Elephant garlic is a larger variety of garlic. Elephant garlic bulbs are about three times the size of traditional garlic, but they have a much milder flavor.

Traditional Garlic

Garlic bulbs should be tight, smooth, and plump with dry, papery skin. As a general rule, the smaller the garlic bulb, the stronger the flavor. Avoid bulbs that are beginning to sprout.

Leeks and Aboveground Onions

Green Onions

Green onions are also known as scallions or spring onions. They are harvested young while their aboveground shoots are still delicate and green. These slender stalks are favored for their mild, delicate oniony flavor. They are excellent sliced raw in salads and as a topping for soups.

Leeks

Leeks look like giant green onions, or scallions, with a mild bulb and a thick white stalk giving way to darker green leaves. They are about 10 inches long and 1 inch in diameter. It is important to wash leeks well, as grit gets lodged between the layers of skin and leaves. The smaller the leek, the more tender it will be. Like those of green onions, or scallions, the flavor and aroma of leeks are more delicate with sweet overtones and milder than those of most onions, and therefore favored to be used raw. They're excellent sliced thin and marinated or dehydrated into dried rings to top a salad.

Chives

Chives are delicate, wispy, hollow, green stalks—often considered an herb. Chives produce beautiful, edible, purple, puffy flowers that bloom in the summer. With their mild and delicate onionlike flavor, they are ideal to use raw, chopped and sprinkled on soups and salads.

Garlic Chives

Also known as Chinese chives, these are similar to regular chives with tall, wispy, hollow stems and similar edible purple flowers. Garlic chives have a mild garlicky flavor.

Crucifers

There are more than 380 genera and 3,000 species in the *Brassica* genus, of which crucifers are a part. Most grow in heads. *Brassica* members are high in sulfur and contain the chemical hydrogen sulfide, which gives the vegetables their distinctive smell.

Broccoli

The word *broccoli* comes from an Italian word meaning "cabbage sprout." A deep emerald green, sometimes tinged with purple, broccoli has tight clusters of tiny buds that sit on edible stems. It's very high in vitamin C, folic acid, calcium, riboflavin, and iron, and is available year-round. Look for broccoli with uniform color, perky buds, and fresh leaves.

Broccoli Rabe

Also called rapini, broccoli rabe is a leafy green vegetable with six- to nine-inch stalks; long, thin leaves; and scattered clusters of buds similar to broccoli. It has a pungent, bitter flavor.

Broccoflower

A cross between broccoli and cauliflower, this vegetable looks like a pale-green cauliflower and has a very mild flavor.

Broccolini

A cross between broccoli and Chinese kale, broccolini is bright green with crunchy, long, slender stalks and a bouquet of tiny buds, like small heads of broccoli. It has a subtle flavor with peppery undertones.

Brussels Sprouts

Brussels sprouts have been cultivated as far back as the Middle Ages in Flanders, which is now Belgium, hence the name after the city Brussels. Brussels sprouts grow in many rows on a single long stalk and resemble tiny cabbage heads; hence the name "sprouts." Germans call Brussels sprouts *rosenkohl,* meaning "rose cabbage," because they resemble rosebuds.

Cabbage

The word *cabbage* comes from the French word *caboche,* a colloquial term for "head." Cabbage comes in many shapes, colors, and textures, all of which grow in loose or compact heads. Valued as a good source of nutrition, cabbage has been depended upon for ages as it grows most of the year, even in cold climates, and stores well.

Cabbage is a great source of fiber and vitamin C. It is one of the few land vegetables that contains iodine. It also contains a healthy amount of vitamin E and calcium, which is about 33 percent more abundant in the outer leaves than the inner leaves.

Cabbage is also a good source of the healthy bacteria *L. acidophilus.* It is fermented into sauerkraut and kimchi in many cultures. (See Chapter 17 for more information.)

Loose Cabbage Heads

NAPA CABBAGE

Also called Chinese cabbage, this variety has a long head with a crisp, white, ribbed stalk and tender, crinkled, pale-green leaves. It is shaped like a thick head of celery. It has a pleasantly crunchy texture and mild flavor. This is my favorite of all cabbage.

SAVOY CABBAGE

This is a variety of white or green cabbage with beautifully textured crimped, curly leaves and a fairly tight, round head. Tender leaves and a mild flavor make Savoy cabbage a delicacy.

Tight Cabbage Heads

GREEN CABBAGE

This is one of the most common varieties of cabbage. It grows with tightly compacted heads and smooth, bright- to pale-green outer leaves and pale to white inner leaves.

PURPLE CABBAGE

This variety of cabbage is a beautiful reddish-purple with smooth leaves and a very tight, compact head. The head is commonly round, although some heads can be oval and pointed.

WHITE CABBAGE

Sometimes called Dutch cabbage, white cabbage is quite like green cabbage, only with very pale-green to white outer leaves. It is commonly found in round heads, although some heads can be oval and pointed.

Cauliflower

Cauliflower is thought to be originally from China and taken thereafter to the Middle East. By the twelfth century, it was grown in Spain and taken to England. Annually, China grows 1 million tons of cauliflower, and India grows 750,000 tons. Its name comes from the Latin words *caulis,* meaning "stalk," and *floris,* meaning "flower." Mark Twain claimed that "cauliflower is nothing but cabbage with a college education."

Cauliflower is composed of bunches of tiny florets on clusters of stalks. Most heads are white and some are tinged green or purple. The entire head and stalk are edible. It is high in vitamins A and C and rich in potassium, iron, and zinc.

Broccoli Romanesco

From northern Italy, broccoli Romanesco is also called summer cauliflower. It is a type of cauliflower with a unique appearance. It looks like a decorative cross between broccoli and cauliflower. Like cauliflower, Romanesco has a tight, compact head of florets attached to a cluster of stalks. But this pretty, pale-green vegetable rises into a pyramid in spiraling minaret-like cones, like a fractal, instead of the round head of a cauliflower. It has a mild, delicate flavor and is available only briefly in the fall.

Collard Greens

A staple of Southern cooking, collard greens do not form a head, but grow in a loose rosette at the top of a tall, fibrous stem. Collards have generous, flat, dark-green leaves with a pale stalk and veins and taste like a cross between kale and cabbage.

Kale

Kale is thought to be one of the first cultivated *Brassica* vegetables, and has been grown for more than 2,000 years. It is grown from its wild cousin, colewort, which still grows along the coasts of western Europe.

Kale prefers cold climates to develop its subtle sweetness and high nutrient content. It is high in calcium, iron, folic acid, vitamin C, and vitamin A. It comes in many colors and shapes and can usually be identified by dark, frilly leaves arranged in a loose bouquetlike formation. From deep green and emerald green to lavender and purple, the best kale is found in the winter months, although it is available year-round.

Curly Kale

Curly kale is the most popular kale variety in the market. It grows in a loose head with a strong, fibrous stalk. It has crimped, curly, bright-green or dark-purple leaves. It is beautiful and high in nutrients.

Dinosaur Kale/Black Kale

This variety has long, crinkled, dark-green, almost black leaves with straight edges. It has a strong flavor with bitter and spicy undertones.

Purple Kale

This variety has beautiful lavender to bright-purple flat leaves with curly, decorative ends. The purple hue lends a beautiful color to many dishes.

Asian Crucifers

Many Asian greens are from the *Brassica* genus. There are many more varieties of Asian greens than there are American names for them. Some are mild, and others are quite spicy. Asian markets often have a great variety, although be sure to buy organic, as greens grown outside of the United States are not subject to the same standards that regulate chemicals in agriculture.

Bok Choy (Pak Choy)

Related to Chinese cabbage and also called Chinese celery, bok choy has white to pale-green, thick, juicy stalks and tender, smooth, oval, green leaves. They resemble a bunch of wide-stalked celery with generous leaves. Bok choy has a lovely mild flavor.

Mustard Greens

Mustard greens are Asian greens that are commonly grown in the United States. They have deep- to pale-green, slightly puckered leaves with a fiery mustard bite. Younger leaves are more mild and delicate.

Tat Soi

Also called spoon mustard, tat soi has dark-green, spoon-shaped leaves and thick, crunchy, white stalks. It has a mild mustardy flavor.

Cucumbers, Melons, and Squashes (Vine Fruits)

These are the fruit of vine plants. These vines grow heartily on the ground and produce a generous amount of fruits. All flowers of this family are edible.

Cucumbers

Cucumbers are long, green, smooth-skinned vine fruit with pale to white, watery, crisp flesh. Most varieties have delicate edible seeds that run the length of the center of the fruit. Cucumbers should be firm from top to bottom and keep well in the refrigerator sealed in a plastic bag.

Cucumbers contain erepsis, a proteolytic enzyme that breaks down protein and soothes the intestines. This enzyme is accompanied by a bitter flavor in some varieties of cucumbers.

The delicate, neutral flavor is best with simple dressing and seasoning. Cucumbers are the traditional choice for pickles, as the flesh absorbs the flavor of vinegar and spices well.

Be sure to buy organic cucumbers. Commercial cucumbers are heavily treated with pesticides and are typically waxed to give them a glossy finish. If you are in doubt about its origins, peel the skin off the cucumberr. Using a citrus zester to "peel" an organic cucumber gives an attractive striped effect when sliced.

Cucumbers are known to beautify facial skin and soothe puffy eyes. Try putting a slice of chilled cucumber over each eye for 10 minutes. Cucumbers also sooth burns, especially sunburned skin.

Baby Cucumber
This is a young, immature cucumber with thin skin and immature seeds. It is delicate and crunchy.

English Cucumbers
This is a long variety of cucumber with thin skin and fewer seeds. It is delicate and crunchy.

Gherkin
This is a small cucumber with bumpy, almost warty skin and a crunchy texture. Gherkins are commonly pickled.

Kirby
This is another small variety of cucumber with smoother skin. Kirbys are also commonly pickled.

Melons

Melons are among the most delicious gifts of vine fruits. They are juicy fruits of summer vines, varying in shape, skin, and flesh color. The wide varieties of melons have different degrees of intoxicating sweetness.

There is an old rule that states "eat melons alone, or leave them alone!" Melons digest simply and quickly without interference from other foods, including other fruits. A melon for breakfast is one of the most luscious pleasures I know.

There are hundreds of varieties of melons, many of which do not have common names. They are best found fresh in markets and farmers' markets in the peak of summer.

Cantaloupe
This is a round, medium-sized variety of melon with a dull yellow-beige, netted skin and blush to bright-orange flesh. Cantaloupe is very fragrant and so sweet.

Charantais
This is a small, round variety of melon with smooth, pale-green skin with dark stripes and sweet orange flesh. It's one of the choicest melons when available.

Galia Melon
This is a small, broad, oval-shaped variety of melon with netted skin that appears to "stretch out" when ripe. The flesh is pale yellow, super sweet, and juicy.

Honeydew
This is a round, medium to large variety of melon with smooth, pale-green to yellow skin and pale-green, juicy flesh. It's the sweetest of all melons.

Icebox Melon
This is a rounder variety of melon with a light-green rind. It has red, crunchy, juicy, sweet flesh.

Muskmelon
This is an oval, medium to large variety of melon with thick, smooth, ribbed skin and pale-green to pink, juicy flesh. Very sweet.

How to Pick a Good Melon

Choosing a good melon is an art. Some varieties, like cantaloupe, are very fragrant when ripe. Most should gently yield to the pressure of thumbs at the base.

My mother has a gift for choosing melons, especially cantaloupes (which she lovingly calls "'loupes"). I hope that this is a genetic gift from dominant genes. Every summer, I study her while she studies the melons. I watch her when she's not looking to catch her in secret conversation with the melons. I asked her to school me and I think it is rubbing off. She, of course, has always been one of my best teachers, especially with fine food.

From my mom to you, here are things to look for when choosing a good "'loupe":

- First of all, be mindful. (You can't be thinking twenty other things while looking for your "'loupe.")
- Look for uniform skin and color. Avoid "dents" and green coloration. The surface should look generally symmetrical and pleasing.
- Heavier melons tend to have more flesh and less seeds. Feel the heft of the fruit for uniform weight and for overall quality.
- The stem under pressure needs to be a little "giving." (Hard equals unripe and crunchy. Too soft equals overripe and mushy.)
- When good, a melon gives off a very distinctive essence—very sweet. Your mind starts to associate this with some of the fruit's other properties, such as color, taste, and texture. It's sort of like sniffing a favorite perfume, only this is edible and the experience is partly visual.

Ah, mama mia . . . I only hope to be as good as you someday.

Ogen Melon

This is a small, round variety of melon. One ogen melon is just enough for one person. It has thin, pale skin with green stripes and juicy, pale-green to cream-colored flesh. It's one of the choicest melons when available.

Orange Honeydew

This round, medium to large variety of melon has smooth, pale-green to yellow skin similar in appearance to a common honeydew. The flesh is blush to bright orange and very juicy. It is one of the sweetest melons.

Picnic Melon

This is the largest variety of melon—and it's fit for a crowd. It has an oblong shape with dark-green skin and generally has juicy, crisp, red flesh, although it may sometimes be orange or blush in color.

Rock Melon

This is a small, oval variety of melon with beige skin. It seems that the rougher the skin, the sweeter the melon. It has orange-yellow, fragrant flesh.

Seedless Watermelon

This is a hybrid variety of melon, bred to yield very few immature seeds or no seeds at all. Seedless fruit is generally much less nutritious, including a lower mineral content, than seeded varieties.

Watermelon

This is a larger, refreshing variety of melon that usually has crimson-red flesh. A perfect summer food, it is made of up to 96 percent water. The juice helps flush and balance the kidneys. Watermelons should have taut skin and should sound firm to knocking knuckles. (I have been known to live on watermelon and spirulina for much of the summer, feeling the best I ever have.)

Yellow Watermelon

This is a round, novel variety of melon with blush to bright-yellow flesh. It has pale- to bright-green skin with dark stripes. It's very crunchy and sweet.

Summer Squash

Summer squashes have a delicate vegetal flavor. This means that the aroma and flavor are quite mild with gentle vegetable tones rather than sweet tones like a fruit. Alone, summer squashes are quite bland and welcome and soak up any good seasoning, marinade, or sauce. Generous yields are harvested throughout the summer. Squash is native to the Americas, though eaten widely throughout the world.

Pattypan Squash

These are small, squat squashes with a slightly firmer texture than zucchini and a similar mild flavor. They are scallop-edged and delicate, with thin, pale-green to bright-yellow skin.

Spaghetti Squash (Spaghetti Marrow)

This is a long, thick squash with smooth, pale-yellow skin. It is much firmer than other marrows. Spaghetti squash is named for the texture of the cooked stringy flesh that resembles spaghetti.

Summer Crookneck Squash

This is a pale- to bright-yellow summer squash with firm flesh and a flavor similar to zucchini. It has a thin tapered neck and mildly bumpy skin.

Yellow Zucchini (Yellow Summer Squash)

Yellow zucchini is a summer squash with thin, bright-yellow skin. It tends to be straighter with firmer flesh than green zucchini and has a similar mild, welcoming flavor.

Zucchini (Summer Squash)

The word *zucchini* comes from the Italian word *zucca,* meaning "gourd." Zucchini is actually an immature marrow, which is a much larger version of a summer squash. It is a popular and versatile variety of summer squash that is available year-round. It has a thin, dark-green skin and firm, pale flesh. Younger zucchini have delicate marrow flesh and smaller and less detectable seeds. Immature (baby) zucchini have no seeds at all.

Winter Squash

Pumpkins and winter squash are fruits of a generous vine indigenous to America, harvested in the fall and into early winter. There are literally hundreds of varieties, all of which generally have a thick, hard skin to temper colder weather, which sweetens their mild, firm flesh.

Winter squash tends to be slightly starchy and is traditionally baked with spices and seasonings. To prepare raw winter squash, the meat can be sliced thinly and soaked in water or marinated with lemon juice to leech out excess starch. A happy medium is to lightly steam the flesh for soups and satisfying savory dishes.

The seeds of winter squashes are incredibly nutritious and abundant in protein and healthy oils. Pumpkin seeds are commonly toasted with salt, although any squash seed can be used. Cooking seeds and nuts is not highly recommended, as the precious oils and nutrients are detrimentally altered by heat. Squash and pumpkin seeds can be blended with water and strained to produce a milk that makes an excellent base for soups.

Acorn Squash

This is a medium-sized, heart-shaped variety of winter squash with a beautiful, fluted, dark-green to orange skin. It has bright- to pale-yellow, slightly stringy flesh and a mild flavor. It is traditionally baked with maple syrup and spices but is delicious steamed as well.

Butternut Squash

This large, long-necked winter squash with smooth, pale-orange to beige skin has brilliant orange, smooth, rich flesh. It is excellent in soup.

Delicata Squash

This is a smaller, pretty squash with smoothly ribbed, yellow skin, flecked with orange and green. It has very sweet yellow-orange flesh—sweet enough to use raw.

Kabocha

Also called Japanese pumpkin, this attractive medium to large squash has thick, bright-green skin and bright-orange, smooth, dense, sweet flesh.

Pumpkin

This is one of the most popular winter varieties suited for the late fall festivities of Halloween and Thanksgiving. It has wide, ribbed, bright-orange skin and a sweet, honey-flavored flesh that works well in sweets and savory dishes.

Fruits

Apple

There are more than 7,000 varieties of apples, of which only a handful are available in American markets. Apples are members of the rose family. Originally grown in Kazakhstan, apples were among the first known cultivated fruits in America. Many varieties faced extinction during Prohibition, as they were commonly pressed into hard cider and were therefore considered contraband. Bah!

Johnny Appleseed (John Chapman) actually did spread bushels of seeds and seedlings throughout North America from which many domestic varieties have been developed. Apples do not fruit true to seed, meaning that if the seeds of a fruit were planted, the tree that grew from the seeds would bear fruit quite different from the fruit the seeds came from. Every apple seed will grow a new, genetically mixed strain and must be grafted to maintain direct genetic lines. They have grown a long way from the tart nature of wild apples, such as crab apples, to sweet, succulent modern varieties.

Apple trees bear fruit in North America from late summer through the fall. They store well and are available year-round in the market. Apples float because they are 25 percent air and bruise easily because they are 25 percent water.

Apples are high in malic acid and tartaric acid, both of which inhibit the growth of bacteria and yeast in the digestive tract. Apples are also a rich source of pectin, a beneficial fiber, shown to remove cholesterol and toxic metal and radiation residue from the system.

Apples are best stored in a cool place. To keep fresh, store in a plastic bag in the crisper compartment of the refrigerator where the humidity is high.

Braeburn Apple

This medium-sized, taller variety of apple has yellow to green to pale-red skin. It has dense, crispy flesh, and a sweet-tart flavor. It is available to some degree year-round.

Crimson Apple

This is a very small apple—you can easily hold four in one hand. They have pale-red skin, which is sometimes speckled with yellow. Sweet and crunchy, crimson apples are perfect for kids. They are available in specialty markets.

Fuji Apple

One of my favorite types of apple, these are medium to large and round with deep- to pale-red skin. They are crispy, juicy, and very sweet. Increasingly popular, Fuji apples are widely available year-round.

Gala Apple

This is a medium to small, round apple with pale-red skin and pale-yellow speckles. It has a mild, sweet flavor. Gala apples are moderately available year-round.

Golden Delicious Apple

This is a medium to large, tall, round apple with golden skin. They are crunchy and very sweet and juicy. Avoid soft and mealy apples—the Delicious varieties are prone to become mealy and soft more easily than other varieties. Golden Delicious apples are very common and are available year-round.

Granny Smith Apple

Granny Smith apples are medium to large, round apples with pale to rich-green skin. They are lower in sugar than most varieties, making them somewhat tart. They were discovered in Australia in 1868 by Mary Ann Smith. Virtually indestructible, they are widely available year-round.

Jona Gold Apple

This is a larger, round apple with golden to red skin. Jona apples are dense, crisp, tart, and sweet, and are moderately available year-round.

McIntosh Apple

This is a medium, squat, round apple with firm deep-red to green skin, soft flesh, and a tart flavor. They are available seasonally.

Pippin Apple

This is a medium to small, squat and round variety of apple. It has pale-green to yellow skin and is very crispy with a sweet-tart flavor. It is available seasonally mostly in the northeast states.

Red Delicious Apple

One of America's most common varieties, Red Delicious is a medium to large, taller variety of apple with deep-red skin. It is crunchy, sweet, and juicy. Avoid soft or mealy apples. They are available year-round. (I was reminded of how very good Red Delicious apples are on the Riviera in Italy, which, strangely enough, sported the best and freshest I've ever had.)

Spartan Apple

This is a medium, squat variety of apple with red to green skin and a tart flavor. It is available only in season, usually at farmers' markets or apple orchards.

Apricot

The apricot originated in China more than 4,000 years ago, though today California produces more than 90 percent of the world's crop. They were named "moons of the faithful" by Confucius, who ascribed his knowledge to the apricot tree. They are a primary food of the Hunzas, a Himalayan tribe known for unusual longevity, whose members commonly live to be more than 100 years old.

The inner pit, or kernel, of the apricot is valued for its medicinal and antioxidant properties. The kernels are often pressed for their quality monounsaturated oil. Apricots are high in copper and cobalt and are commonly used in the treatment of anemia.

Asian Pear

Asian pears are the oldest known cultivated pears. A Chinese gold-prospector first introduced the fruit to the States in the mid-1800s. They are also known as apple-pears because they have the firm crunch of an apple and the juicy sweetness of a pear.

Asian pears are best when firm and sweet smelling. Their thin skin varies from pale yellow and smooth to bronze and lightly textured. The fruit matures from July to October.

Korean Apple-Pear

This very large variety of Asian pear has lightly textured bronze skin and is firm, crunchy, and sweet.

Shinko Apple-Pear

This larger variety of Asian pear has yellow-green skin and is very sweet and crunchy.

20th Century (Nijisseiki) Apple-Pear

These are medium-sized Asian pears with golden-yellow, smooth skin. They are very juicy, sweet, and crunchy.

Avocado

Avocados date back to 8000 B.C. in Mexico and Central America. There are hundreds of varieties of avocados. Like apples, they do not fruit true to seed (see page 60). Living in Hawaii, I see as many varieties of avocados as there are shades of green. Commercially available varieties are grafted from mother trees to maintain pure genetic lines. Hass and Sharwil are common varieties, valued for their rich, buttery texture and small seed.

Avocados are like fruit butter. They are satisfying fatty fruits, rich in easily digestible mono-unsaturated fat (80 percent) and potassium. Their protein makeup is similar to mother's milk, and they are known to beautify the skin.

Avocados do not ripen on the tree and are harvested while still hard. They soften as they ripen. A ripe avocado should be soft, but firm to the gentle squeeze. It takes several days to a week to ripen a hard avocado, so any good chef must plan ahead. However, there are a few ways to quicken the ripening process:

- Pop the stem off the top of the avocado.
- Place the avocado in a brown paper bag and put it in a warm place—for example, on top of the refrigerator or in or on a gas oven with a pilot light. (Make sure the oven is off!)

- Place the avocado in a brown paper bag along with other ripening fruit, especially bananas, which will help it ripen more quickly.
- An old-school trick is to bury an unwrapped avocado in flour or rice.

Once an avocado is ripe, it can be stored in the refrigerator for a few days.

Alligator Pear Avocado

This is a large, light-colored, smooth-skinned variety of avocado with a large pit and a very mild, sweet, fruity flavor. The flesh is more watery and less fatty than that of the avocados most of us are familiar with. Alligator pears are a common variety found in Florida.

Cocktail Avocado

This small delicacy is no bigger than a plum. It has textured medium-green skin and a little pit. It's available in specialty markets.

Fuerte Avocado

This is a medium-sized, smooth-skinned avocado. Like the alligator pear, fuerte varieties have flesh that tends to be lighter and less fatty in texture than typical avocados. They are generally available in California and Florida, though I have seen them regularly in New York and other parts of the country in stores that have a good variety of produce.

Haas Avocado

This is a delicious smaller, textured, dark-skinned variety of avocado with a small seed. It is very creamy and rich. It is the most commonly cultivated avocado and is widely available.

Sharwil Avocado

This medium to large variety of avocado has textured rich-green skin and a small seed. It is buttery rich and creamy. It's widely available.

Banana

There are more than 300 varieties, of which only a few are commonly available. Bananas are a starchy fruit. The starch converts to a much simpler sugar as it ripens. Ripe bananas are much more digestible and nutritious than unripe ones. Golden-yellow skin with speckles of brown is a perfect indication of ripeness.

A rack of bananas grows to hang from one thick, juicy stalk. The rack ripens slowly and is harvested while still green and cut into bunches or "hands."

It is essential that you buy organic bananas. Most commercially grown bananas are grown outside of the United States where there are little to no regulations on pesticides. The bananas are harvested green and "gassed" to ripen. Yuck. Fortunately, organically grown bananas are widely available for a reasonable price.

Bananas should not be refrigerated, as the skin will brown and the flesh will get soggy. Too many ripe bananas? Try peeling any extra bananas and freezing them for a frozen feast of fresh sorbet or a smoothie.

Apple Banana

This medium to small variety of banana has slightly squared seams. It has a lighter flavor—sweet with a mild tang. It's very popular in Hawaii.

Bluefield Banana

This variety is generous in size and sweetness. It has rich yellow skin and very creamy and rich white flesh. It is moderately available.

Chinese Banana

This thin, long, golden variety of banana is prized for its sweetness, delicate flavor, and smooth flesh. They can be found in Hawaii and specialty stores.

Cuban Red Banana

This stout variety of banana with golden-red skin has a semisweet, starchy flavor. It's available in specialty markets.

Ice Cream Banana

A large variety with frosty, pale skin, this banana has square seams and a creamy, vanilla flavor. They can be found in some specialty stores in the United States.

Ladyfinger Banana

This is a small delicacy—its bunches are only several inches long. It has a creamy, sweet flavor. It is available in specialty markets.

Plantain

A plantain is a large, broad, green-skinned banana. It is very starchy and dry with 18 percent less moisture than other bananas. It is commonly used in cooking, particularly in Caribbean and Southern cuisine, but it can be marinated and used raw in dishes or dehydrated into chips. It is available in specialty and ethnic markets.

Williams Banana

The most commonly available banana in the market, it is medium-sized and yellow-skinned and has a sweet flavor.

Berries

Berries are one of the most colorful and succulent treats, celebrated by children and fine-food connoisseurs alike. Wild berries have been eaten since the dawn of time in the Americas and cultivated for thousands of years. Favored for dynamic sweet-and-sour flavor and brilliant color, most berries have a very high content of vitamin C. They are rich in pectin, an insoluble fiber that helps them gel and acts as a gentle intestinal sweep. All berries, especially blueberries, are an excellent source of antioxidants, keeping skin and tissues healthy and beautiful. Imagine, these delectable morsels are also so good for the body.

The best berries are available fresh during summer months, though common berries like strawberries and raspberries are available fresh year-round. Berries taste best fresh from harvest, before they have been refrigerated. Organic frozen berries can be used to replace fresh berries in many recipes. Frozen berries will last for months when stored in an airtight bag and are always a good treat to have on hand to whip into a nut cream or for fresh fruit sorbet.

Blackberry

This is a large, deep purple, heavily seeded berry with a sweet-tart flavor. Native to North and South America, it has been used medicinally for more than 2,000 years. The blackberry is a member of the rose family, and there are more than twenty-four species. The most common varieties on the market are the Albino and the Dewberry. It fruits from June through July.

Blueberry

This is a smooth, round, indigo-skinned berry with very small seeds. Native Americans called this berry "Starberry" for the five-pointed mark where the berry meets the stem. It fruits from May through October. Americans consume more than 200 million pounds of blueberries each year—more than 90 percent of the world's crop.

Boysenberry

This is a glossy, dry, plump, reddish-purple berry resembling an elongated maroon blackberry. It's a hybrid cross between a blackberry and a loganberry or raspberry. In the 1920s, a farmer named Rudolf Boysen grew this variety. Mrs. Cordelia Knott relocated some of these bushes to the famous Knott Farms, which is still a popular name brand for jellies and jams.

Cranberry

Cranberries are one of only three native fruits in North America. Native Americans called this variety a "cranberry," as it was believed to resemble the head of a sand crane. They are round, crimson red to maroon in color, and tangy tart in flavor. They are best grown in a bog. Cranberries are very high in vitamin C. A good, fresh cranberry will actually bounce.

Currant

Currants are firm, small, and shiny berries, of which there are several varieties.

BLACK CURRANT

Black currants have dark purplish-brown skin. These fairly common berries are favored for their sweetness.

PINK CURRANT

This rare variety has a colorless skin over a pale-pink flesh. It's both mildly sweet and tart.

RED CURRANT

A red currant is crimson red. Its tart flavor is good for juice and jelly. It is the most common type of currant.

WHITE CURRANT

White currants have transparent skin over pale-white flesh. These rare berries are also both mildly sweet and tart.

Mulberry

These are elongated berries with a deep-maroon to purple color. They are sweet and succulent.

Raspberry

This large, delicate, sweet, juicy berry is a member of the rose family and has been cultivated for more than 2,000 years. Raspberries range in color from delicate bronze to pale-pink to brilliant red to deep purple. It fruits from June to July.

Strawberry

One of the first fruits of the year, beginning as early as February and peaking in April through June, strawberries have been celebrated as a fruit of fertility. Common strawberries are bright red, though some varieties are pale-pink and even orange. They vary in size from a Ping-Pong ball to a thimble, but the smaller berries are often more flavorful. Strawberries are a member of the rose family and range in flavor from sweet to tart. Tiny, wild strawberries of France, called *fraises de bois,* are prized for exquisite sweetness and flavor. In a single season, if laid end to end, California's strawberry crop would encircle the globe fifteen times.

Breadfruit

This large, starchy fruit is a staple in Polynesia. The size of a small football, it has pale-green, small-sectioned skin, and is golden when mature. Generous breadfruit trees grow up to sixty feet tall. A white sap, which is used for glue, rises to the stem when the fruit is picked. The fruit has firm, pale flesh, and young fruit is cooked as a starch like potato or taro. It softens and sweetens as it ripens. It has a strange sweet-and-sour flavor with a pungent smell. It fruits from May through December.

Carambola

The crosscut of this bright-yellow fruit looks like a five-pointed star, hence its more familiar name, "star fruit." This sweet, juicy, citrus-flavored subtropical fruit is originally from Sri Lanka and Southeast Asia.

Cherimoya

Mark Twain called the cherimoya (also known as a sugar apple) "deliciousness itself." This medium- to large-sectioned, green-skinned fruit has creamy vanilla-colored flesh that kind of tastes like a combination of mango, vanilla, banana, pineapple, and coconut.

Cherimoyas originated in the Andes Mountains at elevations up to 6,000 feet. They were highly prized by Incan emperors. They were planted in California in 1871. Cherimoyas are the third most commonly grown subtropical fruit. There are several types.

Atemoya
This is a hybrid "moya." This variety is smaller in size than other cherimoyas with few seeds and distinctly sectioned skin. It is green to golden in color and very sweet.

Rollinia Deliciosa
This variety of cherimoya is pale golden with firm flesh. It has a lemon-custardlike flavor.

Soursop
Soursop has a smoother skin than other cherimoyas with spines and fibrous, chewy flesh. It has a sour-pineapplelike flavor.

Sweetsop
This very sweet variety of cherimoya has many seeds.

Cherry

Originally, cherries hailed from Asia Minor. Cherry pits that date back to the Stone Age were found in Switzerland. Ancient Greeks used cherries to treat epilepsy. The trees fruit during a very short season—June through July. Cherries with a fresh green stem last longer. There are many varieties of cherries, both sweet and tart.

Bing Cherry
Red to mahogany in color, these cherries are sweet, juicy, and crisp. They have a smaller seed. They are the common cherries that most Americans eat.

Rainier Cherry
This larger variety is pale red to golden in color. It's very crisp and sweet.

Surinam Cherry
These subtropical cherries are bright crimson in color with dimpled stripes. They have a sweet-tart flavor.

Citrus Fruits

Citrus is a generous and favorite family of fruits, varying in flavor from super sweet to tangy and sour. Known for their wealth of vitamin C, these fruits made possible long sea voyages to the New World by preventing scurvy, a disease caused by severe deficiency of vitamin C.

The skin of citrus fruits is where the essential oils and concentrated vitamin C are contained. The "zest," the shaved outer peel, is a beautiful garnish and a flavorful delicacy. The flesh is found in wedged sections of juice suspended in small cells. The white pith that holds the fruit together is high in valuable bioflavonoids.

Citrus seeds are very bitter and harbor very potent natural antibiotic properties. Citrus seed extract is commercially available and is used to inhibit microbes, parasites, and bacteria. I always have a bottle with me, especially when traveling abroad.

Grapefruit
This large fruit is sweet-sour to sour in flavor with yellow to pink skin. Sprinkle a little salt on your grapefruit to make it taste sweeter!

PINK GRAPEFRUIT

This grapefruit has blush-colored flesh and yellow skin. It's sour and sweet.

RUBY RED GRAPEFRUIT

This grapefruit has bright pink to red flesh. It's prized for its sweetness.

Kumquat

No bigger than a half-dollar, this fruit is bright orange, has an edible peel, and is sour and sweet.

Lemon

This fruit has yellow flesh and skin. The citric acid content of lemons is four to five times higher than that of oranges and three times higher than that of grapefruit, giving it quite a sour flavor.

The lemon is a natural preservative and is used as an alternative to vinegars in many recipes. It's a natural antiseptic and antimicrobial and removes foul odors. Lemons have been used as a very effective cleaner and underarm deodorant (yes, it is true!) for ages. Lemons make a good scrub for a cutting board to remove garlic and onion flavors.

Adding a dash of fresh lemon juice to drinking water renders the water much more hydrating and tasty, as it increases the production of fluids in the body. Ahh!

Lime

A close cousin of the lemon, the lime has green flesh and skin. It is sour and astringent with sweet undertones. It complements most flavors without intruding. Limes can substitute for lemons in most cases. Lime trees are generally grown with fewer chemicals than lemon trees. They tend to be less prone to fungus and insect infestation. This is partially because limes are not as hybridized and are closer to wild fruit than most commercial citrus. Their relationship to elements and pests is less compromised.

Orange

Oranges are the most popular of all citrus fruits. Oranges originated in the fertile area of the Tigris and Euphrates rivers and had been cultivated in Iraq long before the Middle Ages.

Orange trees take more than five years to fruit and then can produce up to 1,000 pounds of fruit in one season for another fifty years. Generous. They are very high in vitamin C.

BLOOD ORANGE

This delicacy has blood-red flesh and dark-orange to mahogany skin.

MANDARIN ORANGE

This small, squat, easy-to-peel orange is from China and is prized for its sweetness. There are three types.

Clementine. Cultivated mainly in Spain and North Africa, clementines are a type of mandarin orange with a thin skin and a deep orange flesh. They are usually seedless. Available in good produce stores.

Dancy. The dancy is a type of Mandarin orange that is quite small, deep orange in color, and very juicy.

Tangerine. Tangerines are originally from Asia, but are named after the Moroccan city, Tangier. They are small, squat, very sweet, and very easy to peel because of their loose skin. There are three varieties.

HONEY TANGERINE. This type of tangerine is paler orange in color and very sweet and juicy.

ROBINSON TANGERINE. This is a larger tangerine variety. It is a vibrant orange-red and is very sweet and juicy.

SATSUMA TANGERINE. This variety of tangerine has a tighter skin than the others and is very juicy and sweet to tangy in flavor.

NAVEL ORANGE

This common variety is very round with very orange skin. The bottom looks like a belly button, or "navel."

VALENCIA ORANGE

This is the most common orange variety. It has a tight skin and is excellent for juicing.

Pomelo

This is a huge, unsymmetrical fruit that is closely related to the grapefruit. The pomelo has thick yellow to green skin and drier, sweet, yellow to blush flesh.

Tangelo

Tangelos are a brilliant cross between an orange, pomelo, and tangerine, they're the size of a generous orange with an outward belly button, where the fruit meets the stem. It has a smoother skin and is very, very juicy and sweet. It's the best for juicing. Americans consume more than 80,000 tons of tangelos a year.

HONEYBELL TANGELO

Honeybell tangelos are large and bell-shaped with deep-orange, smooth skin.

MINNEOLA TANGELO

This variety is medium to large and oval to round with light- to deep-orange, smooth skin. It's very juicy.

ORLANDO TANGELO

This variety is large and round with deep-orange to red, smooth skin.

Coconut

If you knew you were going to be stranded on a deserted island with only one thing, you should choose the coconut. The coconut palm and fruit are versatile resources used for food, drink, clothing, shelter, and a myriad of domestic needs.

The king of tropical fruit, coconuts bear meat and water that change as the fruit matures. The younger nut, or green coconut, has an electrolyte-rich elixir known as "coconut water." This is not to be confused with "coconut milk," which is pressed from mature coconut meat or a combination of meat and water. There is a tremendous amount of nutrients in young coconut water. The water of a young coconut feeds the coconut "seed" for many months while it prepares to grow into a tree. Young coconuts have a slippery, soft meat that can be easily removed with a spoon. Hence called "spoon meat" or "jelly meat," with low fat and highly available protein.

Young coconuts, also called Thai coconuts, husked down to a smooth, stout cylinder and wrapped in plastic, are reasonably available in ethnic markets. These plastic-wrapped Thai coconuts are a far cry from the delight of a fresh coconut straight from the tree, but nevertheless are an oasis of hydration and nutrients when away from the islands.

As the coconut matures, the nutrients of the water feed the maturing meat, and the meat becomes thicker and denser. Mature coconut meat has naturally saturated fat. A plant-based diet including coconut meat is not a threat to cholesterol levels. In fact, the oil from coconuts contains lauric acid, which may be helpful in breaking down fatty deposits in the body.

Coconuts are available year-round.

Date

Dates are the oldest known fruit. There are more than 400 varieties. They are originally from the Middle East, and they thrive in desert conditions. They were imported to the States from

French Morocco in the 1920s. Dates have the highest natural sugar content of any fruit. They are very rich in vitamins A and B_1 and magnesium and phosphorus. Mature date palm trees will produce up to 300 pounds of fruit in one season. They fruit from July through October.

Bahari Date

This is a small, firm date that has a pale-brown color and a mild flavor.

Black Sphinx Date

The black sphinx date is a deep-brown, very soft variety of date grown in Arizona. It has a low impact on blood sugar levels.

Deglet Noor Date

This date has semisoft to firm flesh. It is the most popular variety of dates.

HONEY DEGLET DATE

This is a small, very soft variety of the deglet noor date and is light in color and very sweet.

Halawy Date

This is a soft variety of date with thick flesh.

Medjool Date

The medjool is a semisoft, large date. It has a dark-caramel color and a smooth, sweet flavor.

Thoory Date

This date has firm skin and is very dry.

Zahidi Date

This is a small, soft date that has a light-caramel color and is very sweet.

Durian

The durian has endured a love-hate relationship with many people, even in parts of the world where it is indigenous. Some varieties reek like strongly matured cheese, and many people find the odor offensive. Considered a delicacy, the large, dull-green, spiky fruit of an evergreen tree yields a yellow, rich, delicious, custardlike flesh. High in protein, it's certainly worth the experience. It's native to Indonesia, where it is highly prized and considered an aphrodisiac. Durians are generally available in Asian markets.

Fig

The fig is a prize from the Mediterranean from more than 5,000 years ago and was a favorite of Cleopatra. So valuable to the Greeks, figs were once illegal to export. There are more than 600 varieties in shades of purple, green, white, and red. Figs have more potassium than bananas and more calcium than milk.

Fig flowers grow inside the fruit. If allowed to mature completely on the tree, the ends will split open into a blossom. However, birds generally eat the fruit before this spectacle can be enjoyed. Most commonly enjoyed as a dried fruit, figs are high in minerals and are a good source of fiber.

Black Mission Fig

This is a deep-purple variety of fig that is very sweet. They are commonly found dried in the market.

Calimyrna Fig

This blond variety of fig is golden to green in color and makes a very sweet delicacy.

Grapes

Grapes are one of the oldest and most cherished fruits. Egyptian pharaohs adored grapes. These precious fruits were used as currency in the Mediterranean. In the 1700s, Franciscan monks carried grape seeds north from Mexico to cultivate them in California for sacramental wine.

In the 1800s, choice grape vines were brought to California from the most revered lines in France. Soon after, a grape-fungus epidemic killed most of the original vines in France. Fortunately, the California crop was able to revitalize and restore the original vineyards in France.

The skin and seeds of grapes contain precious medicinal compounds. Resveratrol in grape skins is known to fight cancer. The seeds contain the flavonoids known as OPCs (oligomeric proanthocyanins), which are also contained in pycnogenol. OPCs are very powerful antioxidants and precious essential fatty oils that beautify skin and hair. The frostlike appearance of grapes is called "bloom" and actually serves to protect the fruit. Many modern varieties are hybridized to be grown seedless, but these hybrid forms are lacking valuable nutrients and minerals. Grapes with seeds are the best pick.

The best varieties I have had are old vineyard varieties in Europe with family names. The market in the states offers a few standard varieties. The best fruit grows from June to November.

Champagne Grapes

This is a very tiny, purple, seedless variety. They're a beautiful delicacy, but are hard to eat because they're so small!

Concord Grapes

These grapes are dark purple to black and usually contain seeds. They are very sweet and are commonly used for juice.

Flame Seedless Grapes

These crunchy grapes are sweet and tart, and crimson to red in color.

Red Globe Grapes

Red and juicy, this is a large-sized variety of grapes.

Thompson Seedless Green Grapes

This variety is pale green, slightly oblong, crisp, and sweet.

Guava

There are more than 150 varieties of this subtropical fruit. During harvest, many trees have to be picked as many as thirty-five times as the fruit matures at different stages. The guava is one of the few tropical fruits with pectin, a natural gelling agent. Hence, it is popular to use guava in jams and jellies. Generally heavily laden with seeds, the guava has a sweet-tart flavor. It has five times more vitamin C than an orange.

Common Guava

The common guava is yellow-skinned with blush to pink flesh. It's soft to squeeze when ripe. It has many seeds and a sweet-tart flavor.

Pineapple Guava

Also known as frejol guava, this variety is larger than common guava and oblong with green skin and white flesh. It has a flavor reminiscent of sweet and sour pineapple. It's crisp like a pear with small edible seeds.

Strawberry Guava

The size of a quarter or half-dollar, this variety has red skin, pink to red flesh, and many seeds. It's sweet and tart.

Jackfruit

This is the world's largest tree fruit. (We once weighed one in at 96 pounds in my restaurant.) Much of the fruit is inedible. The elastic membranes around the seeds are the favored part. It is said that Wrigley's Juicy Fruit chewing gum was fashioned after the flavor of the jackfruit.

Kiwi

Primarily grown in New Zealand, the kiwi may be named for the national bird of New Zealand, whose feathers are the same perky green as the flesh of a common kiwi. Considered one of the most balanced and well-rounded nutritional fruits, the kiwi fruits from a vine. This fruit, whose flesh is flecked with many tiny black seeds, has been cultivated for more than 700 years in China. There are more than 400 varieties, but only a few are available in the market. It grows well in a climate that gets a chill.

Golden Kiwi

This variety of kiwi has smoother, beige to brown skin covering its golden flesh.

New Zealand Hayward Kiwi

This is the most common variety of kiwi available. It has beige to brown, fuzzy, thin skin and green flesh. It has a sweet-tart flavor.

Longan (also known as Dragon's Eyes)

Closely related to the lychee, this is a smaller fruit with an easily peeled, smooth, brown skin, and translucent, sweet, musky, fragrant flesh surrounding one smooth round, inedible seed. Native to China and Thailand, it is grown in clusters on ornamental trees.

Lychee

The first recorded book written about fruit in A.D. 1056 was written about the lychee. The size of a huge grape with a rough and tough red, bumpy skin, lychees grow in clusters on leafy, brittle trees that fruit for up to 100 years. They have translucent flesh, with one smooth, slippery, inedible seed per fruit. Delicious and fragrant with the sweet taste of honeydew melon, they are difficult to pick because the branches of the lychee tree are very brittle and break easily.

Mango

Found in Burma and Asia more than 6,000 years ago, mango is the world's most popular fruit. In India, it is considered the "food of the gods." There is little more intoxicating than the smell of a sweet, ripe mango. Botanically related to poison oak, the sap from freshly picked mango inflicts some unfortunates (myself included) with "mango rash," similar to the miserable rash associated with poison ivy and poison oak. Bah, humbug!

Common Mango
This variety of mango is small with green to yellow skin. The flesh is stringy and sweet.

Golden Glow Mango
This variety of mango has green to golden skin and sweet and tart, pale-golden flesh.

Haden Mango
This is the variety of mango found commonly in the market. It has an oval shape; red, gold, and green blush skin; and yellow, fibrous flesh. It's very sweet.

Keitt Mango
This is the largest variety of mango. It has yellow-green to rose skin and buttery, pale-yellow flesh. It's very fragrant and sweet, but doesn't contain much fiber.

Kent Mango
This variety of mango has a large, irregular, oval shape; orange-yellow to red-blush skin; and yellow-orange, sweet flesh. It's juicy but doesn't contain much fiber.

Pyree (also spelled Piree) Mango
These mangoes are some of the most sought-after, especially in Hawaii. They are oblong with yellow-green to blush skin. The golden-yellow flesh is buttery smooth and has a superior, sweet, fragrant flavor.

Thai Mango
This long, flatter variety of mango has yellow skin and is stringy and sweet. Available in the market.

Nectarine

Nectarines are closely related to peaches with smooth, yellow-orange to rosy skin. They are generally sweeter and keep longer than a traditional peach. Their name comes from the Hellenic word meaning "nectar of the gods."

Papaya

The papaya tree is a single-stemmed herbaceous tropical tree—so fast-growing that it can grow from seeds into a tree that bears fruit in only nine months. It's native to tropical America. Columbus called the papaya the "fruit of the angels." Its size varies from palm-size to more than a foot long. Its flesh has a golden-yellow to orange-rose color and varies in sweetness. Its pepper-flavored black seeds are used to season salad dressing and, in large doses, as an antiparasitic medicine.

Papaya is an abundant source of papain, a proteolytic enzyme that breaks down protein.

Babaco Papaya

This is the largest papaya variety. It has a fluted shape, green to golden skin, and yellow-orange flesh. It has a hollow center with little to no seeds. It's mildly sweet, like a bland melon. This variety is common in Mexico.

Green Papaya

This variety is very firm with white flesh, undeveloped white seeds, and a bland flavor. It is very high in the enzyme papain and is commonly used in Asian-style salads and slaws.

Solo Papaya

This variety of papaya is pear-shaped and has yellow skin with yellow to orange flesh. It is named "solo" because it is the perfect one-person snack.

Strawberry Papaya

This is the sweetest, choicest variety of papaya. It's grown mostly in Hawaii. It has an oblong shape and golden to orange skin covering dark rosy-pink flesh. Very sweet and aromatic, it's the best!

Passion Fruit (Liliko'i)

The prolific fruit of a tropical vine, the passion fruit is named for the wild and exotic flower with sedative properties. Ripe fruits are yellow or purple with a hard, shiny skin that wrinkles as it ripens. The sweet and tart, pulpy flesh is sharply aromatic and laden with crunchy, edible seeds. It's very high in vitamin C.

Peach

Peaches have been cultivated for more than 4,000 years in China. Today, the peach crop in America exceeds that of the rest of the world combined. Peaches are America's third favorite fruit. There are more than 300 varieties of peaches, which fall into two categories—clingstone and freestone—in reference to how easily the flesh pulls away from the pit. Most peaches have yellow to rosy flesh. White peaches are rarer and more exceptional in flavor. All have fuzzy skin from yellow-orange to rose.

Due to the delicate nature of a peach, they are picked when hard but mature. Allow to ripen at room temperature, free from the weight of a pile.

Peach juice makes a wonderful cosmetic moisturizer. The peach kernel, inside the pit, shares similar characteristics with its close relative, the almond and the apricot kernel, although it is not as widely available.

Pear

Pears are members of the rose family. There are more than 3,000 varieties. One of the oldest cultivated fruits, they were first planted in the United States in 1620. A ripe pear should yield just slightly a light squeeze near the stem. Pears are best bought unripe and allowed to ripen at room temperature. To ripen pears quickly, put them in a paper bag with an apple. To keep a cut pear from turning brown, brush with lemon juice.

Pears are said to have an enzyme that promotes relaxation.

Bartlett Pear
This is a bell-shaped variety of pear with pale-green to golden, smooth skin. It's soft when ripe and juicy. This is a summer fruit.

Bosc Pear
The bosc pear is crisp and has a long neck and brown to yellow, slightly rough skin.

D'Anjou Pear
The D'Anjou pear has an oval shape and pale-green, smooth skin. It's soft when ripe and juicy. This is a winter fruit.

Persimmon

Also known as Sharon fruit or kaki, the persimmon has smooth, bright-orange skin. It's fragrant when ripe. It's sweeter in cold temperatures (store ripe fruit in fridge). Unripe fruits are tannic, and make your mouth feel very dry and puckered, astringent, and inedible.

There are more than 2,000 varieties of persimmon, some of which have been cultivated for centuries. Persimmon wood is one of the hardest woods in the world and is used to make golf clubs.

Fuyu Persimmon
This is a flat persimmon variety, like a squat tomato. It is deep-orange and firm and crunchy, even when ripe. It is not as astringent as other varieties are when they are unripe.

Hachiya Persimmon
This is a larger variety of persimmon with a pointed base. The flesh is incredibly juicy and succulent and has a brilliant orange color. It is very astringent and inedible when unripe.

Physalis Fruit

A round orange fruit the size of a cherry, this fruit is also known as a cape gooseberry. A pretty papery husk like a lantern adorns this sweet, sharp fruit.

Pineapple

Pineapples are a universal symbol of hospitality. They have fragrant, tangy to sweet, golden-yellow to white flesh with a rough skin pieced together like a mosaic of hexagons and a spiky crown. Pineapples are a relative of the bromeliad family of flowers. They take eighteen to twenty-two months to mature. Pineapples must be picked ripe, as the fruit's starch does not convert to sugar after it is harvested. For even distribution of sugar, store pineapples upside down.

Pineapples are rich in bromelain, an enzyme that digests protein, most concentrated in the core of the fruit.

Red Spanish Pineapple
This variety of pineapple is cultivated primarily in the Caribbean.

Smooth Cayenne Pineapple
This is the most popular and available variety of pineapple. It is grown in Hawaii.

Household Uses for Pineapple

Use the acid in pineapple skins as a natural whitener for clothing: Soak pineapple skins in a bucket of water overnight. Remove the skins and soak the clothes for several hours in the water. Wring out the clothes and put through the rinse cycle of the washing machine (compliments of an old Hawaiian auntie on Maui).

For a sensual cuticle softener, mix together 2 tablespoons of fresh pineapple juice and 1 tablespoon of apple cider vinegar. Soak nails in the mixture for a half hour.

Sugar Loaf Pineapple
This sweet, low-acid variety of pineapple is popular in Mexico.

White Pineapple
This is a white, low-acid, choice variety of pineapple.

Plum

There are more than 2,000 varieties of plums. They are originally from the Caucasus Mountains in Asia. California boasts 90 percent of the country's harvest. Plums have an unusual characteristic of increasing their content of delicious sugars after the fruit is picked. Like pears, plums are best bought firm and given a chance to ripen at room temperature.

European Varieties of Plum
European varieties have blue to purple skins, are smaller than other plums, and are sweet. They are often dried into prunes.

Japanese Varieties of Plum
Japanese varieties have golden-yellow to green skins. They are larger than other plums with a sweet-tart flavor.

Pomegranate

It is claimed that pomegranates have been cultivated since prehistoric times. Originally from tropical Asia, pomegranates have been cultivated in the Mediterranean for ages. An ancient symbol of prosperity and fertility, each pomegranate has up to 800 edible seeds surrounded by a crimson, cellular kernel of sweet-tart juice and white pithy membrane. The skin should be scarlet to rosy, shiny and smooth.

Pomegranate juice is known to stimulate digestion and irreversibly stain everything. A beloved friend, Eddie-I, taught me an elegant technique to savor all of the succulent juice of a pomegranate without opening it and making a mess. Begin by gently pressing through the skin to break the cells of juice of the flesh. The fruit will begin to soften as it is broken inside. Be gentle not to break the skin. When it is thoroughly juiced inside, bite a small hole in the skin, plant your lips, tilt your head back, and nurse the juice out. Absolutely divine.

Sweet Pomegranate
This variety is green to red blush with pink juice.

Wonderful Pomegranate
This is the most common variety of pomegranate. It has deep-red to purple skin and crimson flesh.

Prickly Pear

The juicy fruit of a prickly pear, also called a cactus pear or panini, is actually a huge berry, with many small edible seeds. Its green-golden to red-purple flesh is similar to the flesh of a firm watermelon. It's very refreshing and hydrating.

Picking a prickly pear is a complicated ordeal due to the thousands of microscopic spiny thorns. It is necessary to wear rose-pruning gloves and to stand upwind while picking.

Rambutan

A close relative of the lychee, this tropical fruit is growing in popularity. It was named from the Malay word for "hair of the head," in reference to the soft, spiny, red tendrils covering its firm shell. It has sweet, white, translucent flesh that sticks to its one seed. It is similar to the lychee in flavor, like a fragrant honeydew melon. The rambutan is native to Southeast Asia and is available mid-summer through early winter.

Sapote

The sapote family of fruits is one of the most succulent and prized of fruit varieties. The flavor and textures are unusual and delectable. From the size of an egg to a small football, with texture from custard and cream to velvet avocado and that like caramelized flan, these fruits are worth scouting out. This diverse family is native to Mexico and Central America, and popular varieties are widely grown in California today.

Black Sapote

Black sapotes, also called chocolate-pudding fruit, have deep-brown, creamy flesh that resembles chocolate pudding. They are sweet with a hint of vanillalike flavor. The skin is smooth and dark green.

Canastelle Sapote

A velvety delicacy, canastelle is deep orange with a dry, creamy flesh. Known also as eggfruit because its color and consistency resemble that of cooked egg yolk (also known as yellow sapote), it has a flavor similar to pumpkin cheesecake—very rich and decadent.

Originally from pre-Columbian civilizations of Central and South America, it's available in ethnic markets. Not to be missed.

Mamey Sapote

This large, oval-shaped fruit is pinkish-brown with slightly rough skin that feels like a cross between sandpaper and peach fuzz. The flavor of its rich, orange-pink flesh is a cross between a sweet avocado and a creamy sweet potato. Prized as an aphrodisiac, it's native to Central America and celebrated in Mexico, South America, and the Caribbean. It's available in the United States in ethnic stores. This is a summer fruit.

Orange Sapote

This is a round fruit with smooth green to orange skin. Its flesh is similar to the mamey sapote—creamy and rich with magnificent flavor and a texture that is similar to a flan. Very exotic.

Sapodilla Sapote

This smaller, oval fruit, also known as chicle, has an unassuming brown, potatolike-textured skin, golden-brown flesh, and a honey-caramel-maple-syruplike flavor. It's tannic and astringent when unripe, making the mouth feel very dry and puckered.

The white sap of the chicle fruit was used by pre-Columbian Native Americans as chewing gum. Modern-day health industrialists are bringing back its popularity.

White Sapote (Vanilla Sapote)

This variety's smooth green skin yellows when ripe. It has creamy, yellow flesh and a sweet, creamy vanillalike flavor. Currently cultivated in California, it's available from May to August.

Lettuces and Greens

Lettuce

Butter Lettuce

Butter lettuces grow in tender loose heads of bright- to pale-green leaves. The leaves softly fold in. Lightly crunchy and delicate, this is the most tender of all lettuces. This variety is generally available.

BIBB LETTUCE

Similar to Boston lettuce, Bibb lettuce has slightly ruffled, delicate light-green leaves gathered in a loose head with a crunchy center.

BOSTON LETTUCE

Tender and crunchy, these are loose heads with flat green leaves gathered to a crunchy pale-green center. Delicious.

Crisphead Lettuce

Crisphead lettuces are crunchy and crispy. Most varieties are very juicy with a mild flavor and are considered more of a culinary treat than iceberg lettuce. They have bright- to pale-green leaves in tight, crunchy heads. They are high in silica.

Green Leaf Lettuce

This variety is similar to red leaf lettuce, but with bright- to pale-green, curly leaves. Again, the ruffled leaves are delicate and soft and the stem is juicy and crispy.

Green Oak Leaf Lettuce

This variety of lettuce has delicate, frilly, tapering, bright- to pale-green leaves, a loose head, and a crisp, pale stem.

Iceberg Lettuce

This is a pale-green, tight head of lettuce with a mild flavor. It's good for shredding. Organic varieties are excellent.

Loose Leaf Lettuce

Loose leaf lettuces do not grow in heads, but in a loosely bunched arrangement of leaves. These lettuces produce a succession of leaves in which the outer leaves can be continuously harvested without taking the whole plant from the garden.

Loose leaf lettuce is beautifully ornamental with curly-edged leaves. They are generally delicate leaves, ranging in color from deep purple and red to bright and pale green. These varieties are easy to find in markets.

Red Leaf Lettuce

A delicate arrangement of long, reddish-purple, curly-edged leaves, the ruffled leaves are soft and the pale-green stem is juicy and crispy. These are sweet and tasty.

Red Oak Leaf Lettuce

This variety of lettuce has frilly, delicate, reddish-purple leaves, a loose head, and a crisp stem.

Romaine Lettuce

This is a long, tight, crispy head of lettuce with bright-green leaves fading to pale yellow near the center. This lettuce is a classic in Caesar salad. It is juicy and mild in flavor.

Chicory Greens

In the late eighteenth century, certain varieties of chicory were grown in Europe for the root, which is dried and added to coffee. During that time, a Belgian man named M. Brezier discovered that the leaves could be eaten, though he mysteriously kept this culinary delight a secret. After his death, it became a popular vegetable in Belgium and soon in much of Europe.

Chicory is a flavorful family with diverse textures, tastes, and appearances. Chicory greens are sometimes mild, although they tend to be spicy and bitter. They are rich in silica and fiber and make a gorgeous addition to any salad.

Chicory

Chicory is also called "curly endive." It has narrow, twisted leaves in a frilly, loose head. Dark-green leaves fade to pale green and white near the center of the head. Chicory is pleasantly bitter. The inner leaves are the most tender.

Endive

A type of chicory with delicate, crisp, cup-shaped, smooth leaves. Grown in the dark to keep a pale-green and yellow to white leaf color, escarole is mildly flavored for the chicory family. It's delicate, crunchy, and delicious.

Escarole

Escarole has fairly broad leaves for the chicory family, resembling the loose heads and leaves of butterhead lettuce. Dark-green edges fade to pale-green stems near the center. Good escarole has a nutty flavor, although some may be quite bitter.

Frisée

Tightly curled and very decorative, frisée has small, tender, delicate, lacy leaves. Pale-green leaf ends fade to a white center arranged in a loose, wild head. Frisée is mildly bitter.

Mizuna

Feathery light-green leaves fade to pale yellow near the center of mizuna's loose, frilly head. It is mildly peppery, and the center leaves are more delicate.

Radicchio

Radicchio is also called "Italian chicory." It has reddish-purple leaves with white ribs wrapped in a tight head. Radicchio is favored for its beautiful vibrant color. It is pleasantly bitter.

Deep Greens

Beet Greens

Beet greens are too often neglected for the more popular deep-red-purple root part of the beet plant. Beet greens are deep green with crimson-purple veins and have a strong, earthy flavor. Baby beet greens are delicate and delicious, and make great additions to salads.

Chard

Chard is a member of the beet family. Chard does not grow an edible root but produces broad, generous, deep-green, ruffled leaves with a juicy stem, not unlike celery. The stem is favored for the bright variety of color, from deep crimson to canary yellow and pale cream.

Chard has a strong, earthy flavor. It is best marinated. It also makes an excellent wrap for paté, for an effect similar to stuffed grape leaves (dolma).

Growing Baby Beet Greens

It is easy to grow baby beet greens on your windowsill. Simply cut off a half inch of the beet top. Place in a shallow bowl or on a plate with a lip and fill with a half inch of water. Leave it on the windowsill in indirect sunlight. Add water to keep the water level at a half inch as necessary. Beet leaves will sprout and grow in a few days. This is a wonderful way to grow greens in cold climates.

Sorrel

Sorrel looks a lot like spinach with broad, smooth, deep-green leaves on leggy stems. It has a distinct and lovely zesty lemon flavor. It is used more often as an herb than as a green. Sorrel is one of my favorites.

Spinach

Spinach has a loose head of dark-green leaves with leggy, fibrous stems. The flat varieties are tastier and more tender. The older, crinkly varieties are tougher and more bitter. Baby spinach is a tender, delicate treat.

Spinach is very high in iron and chlorophyll and rich in vitamin A. It also has an exceptionally high calcium content, which is neutralized by its high oxalic acid content. Oxalic acid is known to "block" the absorption of calcium. Steaming or marinating spinach in lemon may reduce the oxalic acid content, making calcium more available in the body. Spinach has a mild, earthy flavor. It's great with lemon, garlic, good-quality olive oil, and sun-dried sea salt.

Spicy and Bitter Greens

Bitter greens are some of the most nutritious and neglected foods. Many bitter greens can be wild harvested and are considered wild plants or weeds. Be certain that these greens are organic and have not been treated with chemicals or pesticides.

Traditionally, bitters are used to strengthen the appetite and digestion. Bitter foods strengthen the peristaltic action of the colon, which is necessary for good digestion and elimination. Bitters are also generally very good for the liver. These greens have a very strong flavor and are best as a peppery addition to many salads and dishes.

Arugula

Originally from Italy, arugula has dark-green leaves that resemble elongated oak leaves. Arugula has a very spicy flavor. Young leaves are more tender and tasty. Older leaves are spicier and can be bitter.

Dandelion

Considered a weed in most suburban lawns, dandelion is one of the most nutritious greens and is excellent for the liver. Dandelion can be wild harvested, although it is important to harvest organic greens. Many lawns are treated with chemicals, which are unadvisable on any level. Tender leaves are best. Dandelion has a rich, sharp, bitter flavor.

Watercress

Watercress grows in small bunches in freshwater streams with many small green leaves and tender, leggy stems. It can easily be wild harvested and makes a great, spicy addition to salads or an accompaniment or garnish. It has a peppery flavor and is tender and delicious.

Mushrooms

Botanically, mushrooms are somewhere outside of the plant kingdom. Long associated with magic and the supernatural, there are more kinds of mushrooms than there are days in the year.

Picking wild mushrooms is not safe unless you are well educated and confident about identifying edible varieties. Many are delicious and nutritious, but many are deadly and poisonous.

It is recommended to marinate or cook mushrooms to neutralize potential toxins. Mushrooms can also be marinated with lemon juice or vinegar to counterbalance toxins. The fleshy meat of mushrooms absorbs flavor and savors marinades superbly. Mushrooms have a high water content, which is released when they are cooked or marinated, and, in turn, the flesh absorbs the marinade and seasonings in its place.

Because of their high water content, mushrooms should not be washed with water but wiped clean with a dry towel or paper towel instead.

Many mushrooms are known to boost immune response to cancer and viral infections.

Cultivated Mushrooms

Cultivated mushrooms are grown in controlled conditions. Be certain to buy organic varieties. They are mild in flavor and are widely available.

Button Mushrooms (White Mushrooms)

These small white mushrooms are the most common mushroom available. Mild in flavor, they are often served raw in salads. They have smooth caps and pink to beige gills that darken as they mature.

Crimini Mushrooms

Crimini mushrooms are cultivated baby portobello mushrooms. They are small with a fairly thick stem and a darker, pale-brown cap. They have a stronger flavor and a meatier texture than button mushrooms.

Field Mushrooms and Wild Mushrooms

Field mushrooms are cultivated varieties of wild mushrooms. Connoisseurs claim that wild mushrooms are the only mushrooms with flavor. Wild varieties can be found in farmers' markets and specialty stores in the autumn, when mushrooms are in season.

Chanterelle Mushrooms

This is a frilly, trumpet-shaped, delicate variety of mushroom. They are cream to vivid yellow in color and have a slightly fruity flavor. They are firm and almost rubbery in texture. They have a gorgeous color and shape and a magnificent flavor.

Enokitake Mushrooms

This is another Japanese mushroom prized for its delicacy. They grow in clusters of snowy-white, pin-sized caps. They have a sweet, fruity flavor.

Dried Mushrooms

Most wild mushrooms are available dried. To reconstitute dried mushrooms, soak them in warm water for 20 to 30 minutes. Dried mushrooms are nutritious and delicious, having a stronger flavor than the fresh varieties, but, as with any dried food, such as dried herbs, dried mushrooms do not have quite the same delicate texture, flavor, or nutritional value as fresh mushrooms.

Morel Mushrooms

Morels are some of the finest edible fungi of all. Cone-shaped with a crinkled, spongy cap and hollow in the center, they are the first wild mushrooms of the year available in the market.

Oyster Mushrooms

An ear-shaped mushroom with pale-brown to yellow color. Oyster mushrooms are widely cultivated, though the wild variety grows on rotting wood. They have a delicious flavor and texture.

Porcini Mushrooms (Italy)/Ceps or Cèpes Mushrooms (France)

This mushroom variety is one of the finest. They are golden, meaty, bun-shaped mushrooms with a spongy material instead of gills on the underside of the cap. They have a fine suede texture and a delicious buttery flavor.

They are widely available in the autumn in Europe and can be found dried in specialty markets in the United States.

Portobello Mushrooms

These are large, broad-capped mushrooms with a wonderful meaty texture. Because of the generous flesh, portobellos are favored for grilling.

Shiitake Mushrooms

These Japanese mushrooms grow on trees or logs. In Japanese, *take* means "fungus" and *shii* is what they call the "hardwood tree" from which the mushrooms are harvested. They have a meaty flavor and savory texture, and are widely available fresh and dried. They are known to induce an immune response against cancer and viruses.

Nightshade Vegetables

Most nightshade vegetables, such as tomatoes, are actually fruits—except for potatoes, which are considered a root vegetable. Nightshade vegetables are botanically classified together because they share many of the same alkaloids and because they grow at night. Some of these alkaloids, such as solanine, are toxic and cause problems for people who have very sensitive systems. Sensitivity can result in indigestion or aggravation of arthritic conditions. Extreme reactions such as headaches and vomiting are rare. Some people experience an elated feeling after eating nightshades, which sometimes accompanies an inability to focus mentally. Some traditions and schools recommend that nightshade vegetables not be eaten at all because of these toxic alkaloids. As with the success of many approaches, all things in moderation offers a happy medium.

Many of the strong components of nightshade vegetables are concentrated in the skins. Negative effects can be reduced by peeling the skins of tomatoes and peppers.

There are other members of the nightshade family called *deadly nightshades,* like the beautiful and fragrant belladonna flower. These plants are very toxic but have been used medicinally for ages.

Bell Peppers

Bell peppers (also called sweet peppers) and chili peppers are members of the *Capsicum* genus and come in a wide variety of colors. Although bell and chili peppers are distinctly different in taste—bell peppers have a sweet flavor, while chili peppers are hot and spicy—they share the same name, "pepper," given by conquistadors during Columbus's time who found bell peppers in America while searching for the spices and hot peppers of the Orient. Instead of the spices of the Far East, Columbus found maize, potatoes, peppers, and tomatoes. Natives of the Americas seasoned their food with ground peppers. Because of the similar, bright spectrum of color of chili peppers and bell peppers, the name "pepper" was given to both and stuck.

Bell peppers have glossy, taut, crisp skin. Choice specimens should not be wrinkly or soft. The flesh is crisp and juicy and full of flavor. Bell peppers are a very good source of vitamin C and silica.

Avoid Chemicals and Pesticides

It is essential to use only organic tomatoes and peppers. Both have a very thin skin and are subject to an incredible onslaught of chemicals and pesticides in commercial cultivation.

The EPA and the National Academy of Sciences studied commercially grown food that has the greatest estimated risk of causing cancer because of the high levels of toxic chemical residue and carcinogenic agricultural chemicals. In order of risk, the most dangerous commercially grown foods are tomatoes, beef, potatoes, oranges, lettuce, apples, peaches, pork, wheat, soybeans, beans, carrots, chicken, corn, and grapes.

Green Bell Peppers

Green bell peppers have a mild, slightly sweet flavor. This variety has pale- to deep-green skin and flesh. Most green peppers are actually immature red bell peppers that have been picked young, before color and flavor have a chance to develop.

Orange and Yellow Bell Peppers

Orange and yellow bell peppers taste quite a bit like red bell peppers, although they are usually a touch less sweet. They have brilliant yellow or orange skin and flesh.

Purple Bell Peppers

Purple bell peppers have a similar mild flavor to green peppers. Their dramatic color fades to green if the peppers are cooked.

Red Bell Peppers

Red bell peppers are a brilliant bright red to crimson red and are very sweet.

Chili Peppers

Chili peppers come in every shape, size, and degree of spiciness. There are more than 200 varieties of chili peppers, all members of the *Capsicum* genus. The substance in chilies that makes them hot and spicy is a volatile oil called capsaicin. The amount of spiciness varies from plant to plant and depends on growing conditions. The more the plant has to struggle to survive in terms of light, water, and soil, the more capsaicin is produced and the hotter the chili.

The capsaicin in chili peppers is concentrated in the pith and seeds (about 80 percent). To make chilies milder, remove the pith, veins, and seeds before using. The tip of the chili is also milder than up near the stem.

Chili peppers range in size from a quarter inch to twelve inches. The general rule is, the larger the chili, the more mild the flavor; the smaller the chili, the hotter the heat. The color varies from green and yellow to red and purple, and the shape varies from long and narrow to globular and plump.

Regardless of size and shape, fresh chili peppers should have even, taut skin, free of blemishes. Many chilies are slightly wrinkled, even when fresh. Fresh chilies can be stored in the refrigerator for several days. Dried chilies will keep for two to three years.

Anaheim Chili Peppers

Named for the Californian city Anaheim, this chili pepper is also known as a chili Colorado. A larger, long chili pepper with a pointed end, it's about six inches long and two and a half inches thick. They have smooth bright-red or dark-green skin and a mild, sweet taste. The red varieties are riper with a more developed sweetness.

Cayenne Chili Peppers

Cayenne chili pepper is one of the most popular chili peppers. Usually found dried and ground, the fresh cayenne pepper is a medium-sized, long and thin, bright-red pepper. Very spicy.

Habanero Peppers

Habanero means "from Havana." One of the hottest of all chili peppers, the habanero pepper is red when fully ripe. There are also yellow and orange varieties. Unripe habaneros are dark to pale green. These peppers are squat and round and are thirty to fifty times hotter than jalapeño peppers. Very hot.

Hungarian Sweet Chili Peppers

Hungarian chili peppers are the peppers used to make the spice paprika. Elongated peppers, they are five to six inches long and two to two and a half inches thick. They are deep crimson red, sweet, and hot. Some varieties are sweeter and others are hotter.

Jalapeño Peppers

Jalapeño peppers are also very popular chili peppers. These peppers are medium in size with a rounded point. They start green and mature red. They can be mild to quite spicy.

Serrano Chili Peppers

This is a small pepper with quite a kick. One to two inches long and a half to three-quarter inches thick, it is deep green to scarlet red in color. The red varieties have a touch of sweetness along with the clean, biting heat. This is one of the hotter peppers.

Thai Chili Peppers

Also called birdseye chili, this is a very small bright-red pepper—about one and a half inches long and a quarter inch thick. Three serrano chilies are equivalent to one Thai chili. It has a swift and lingering fiery heat.

Eggplant

The eggplant is technically a berry. They range from two to twelve inches long with a tough, smooth, glossy skin that is typically deep purple. White, yellow, and striped varieties are available.

Eggplant has a very mild, slightly bitter flavor. The texture is spongy and soaks up and absorbs flavor very well.

Common Eggplant

This eggplant is oblong and smooth and has dark-purple skin. Pale flesh contains many small seeds.

Japanese Eggplant

This is a longer variety of eggplant with purple or striated skin.

Tomatoes

Tomatoes are one of the most popular vegetables celebrated in many cuisines around the world. Gorgeous colors and a succulent texture are accompanied by a wealth of vitamins and phytonutrients.

Tomatoes are native to western South America and have been widely cultivated in all of South America and Mexico since before the sixteenth century (when the Spanish invaded). Cortés sent golden tomatoes back to Spain to be cultivated. English horticulturists began to grow tomatoes in the sixteenth century mainly for decorative ornament. It was not until the first red tomatoes arrived in Italy in the eighteenth century by two Jesuit priests that tomatoes began to enjoy favor in cuisine. By the mid-nineteenth century, tomatoes were cultivated and eaten extensively all over the world.

Sun-Dried Tomatoes

Sun-dried tomatoes have a rich and delicious flavor. They have been cut and dried in the sun or dehydrated. The result is an intensely flavored, sweet, dark-red dried tomato. Sun-dried tomatoes can be bought dry or packed in oil.

Sun-dried tomatoes can be softened and rehydrated by soaking them in water. The water from soaking can be used in dressings and soups. Do not use dried tomatoes that have been treated with sulfites to maintain a bright color. Any type of tomato can be used to make sun-dried tomatoes. Tomatoes with fewer seeds are favored because they have more meat and yield better results.

Homegrown tomatoes are without a doubt the best. Tomatoes that have been allowed to ripen on the vine are succulent and sweet. Many tomatoes in the store are picked before they are ripe to keep fresh. Store-bought tomatoes should have uniform color and taut skin. The green top should be fresh and perky. Under-ripe tomatoes can be ripened in a paper bag. Tomatoes should not be refrigerated, as they lose flavor in the chill.

Beefsteak Tomatoes

This is a very large variety of tomato. Deep red with ridges, they have a wonderful flavor and are very juicy.

Cherry Tomatoes

This is a very small and dainty variety of tomato that grows in clusters. They are commonly red, but are also available in yellow and orange. They are very sweet—like candy.

Common Tomatoes

Common tomatoes are the standard variety found in the market. Red and round, they should have uniform color and be firm and yield slightly to pressure. Vine-ripened are the sweetest variety.

Roma Tomatoes

Also called plum tomatoes, they have a strong tomato flavor. Their flesh is thick and has much fewer seeds than most varieties.

Yellow Tomatoes

Yellow tomatoes are similar in shape and characteristic to red tomatoes, but have a beautiful golden-yellow color.

Yellow Pear Tomatoes

Yellow pear tomatoes are about as small as cherry tomatoes, but have a tiny pearlike shape.

Root Vegetables and Tuber Roots

Root vegetables and tuber roots grow under the soil with a bouquet of leaves above ground to absorb energy from the sun by photosynthesis. Root vegetables are a grounding, hearty food and are rich in minerals. Generally starchy and filling, root vegetables have been valued through the ages as a staple food, because they grow and store well in winter months.

The term *root cellar* came from a time before refrigeration when root vegetables were stored in a cellar about six feet underground where the earth maintains an ambient temperature of about 50°F all year.

Beets

Beets have been eaten since Roman times and were valued for their sugar content. The beet is a firm, purple-red root with a sweet, earthy flavor. Beets are an excellent source of potassium, iron, calcium, and vitamin A. They make a brilliant dye for foods—even sweets. Smaller beets are more tender.

Chioggia Beets

Also called "candy cane," chioggia is a variety of beet with concentric rings of red and white, which are quite beautiful.

Golden Beets

This is a beautiful variety of beet with brilliant golden-colored flesh. Golden beets lose their color if they are exposed to air too long. They have a milder flavor and are not as high in minerals or vitamin A as with other beets, but they are beautiful.

Burdock

Burdock is one of the most nutritious foods for building healthy blood. Burdock has a long tapering root that grows many feet into the ground with rough, dark-brown skin and pale-white flesh. It has a sweet-bitter earthy flavor and a tender-crisp texture. Smaller pieces of burdock are more tender. Burdock makes an excellent addition to fresh vegetable juice.

Carrot

Carrots are one of the best known and favorite root vegetables. Carrots are actually a member of the parsley family.

Modern-day carrots have been quite hybridized from the original carrot, which was grown 2,000 years ago during the Middle Ages. The original carrot was purple or white, not the bright orange we are familiar with today.

Carrots have a tremendous amount of vitamin A, which aids good vision and night vision. They are also a good source of vitamins B_3 and E and potassium, calcium, iron, and zinc.

Celery Root

Celery root, also known as celeriac, is the root of the common celery stalk. It has firm white flesh and a knobby appearance. The taste is a cross between strong celery and parsley. It's great shredded in salads and soups.

Horseradish

Horseradish is a pungent, spicy root that grows in long, grouped clusters with rough brown skin and white flesh. It is often mixed with mustard or added to wasabi, a Japanese condiment that is served with sushi.

Jerusalem Artichoke

Jerusalem artichokes are related to the sunflower and have little to do with Jerusalem. The name is derived from the Italian word for sunflower, *girasole*. They are more appropriately called sunchokes. Indigenous to America and Canada, Jerusalem artichokes were cultivated by the native inhabitants long before the Europeans arrived. They are small, knobby tubers with white, crisp flesh and a distinct nutty flavor. They are excellent raw.

Jicama

Jicama is known as a Mexican potato. A firm, crispy, juicy root vegetable with smooth, pale-beige skin and sweet, white flesh. The flavor is a cross between an apple and a potato. They are excellent raw.

Parsnip

Parsnips are related to carrots and are similarly sweet with a distinct earthy flavor. They have a long body like a carrot, broadening at the top with cream to white flesh. Parsnips were very popular, especially in the winter months, before the potato was introduced. Grown in the fall and winter, parsnips develop a wonderful sweetness, favored in root vegetables, with the first frost. They are rich in calcium, iron, and potassium and are a decent source of vitamins A and C.

Radish

The word *radish* comes from the Latin word *radix,* meaning "root." The radish is the root of a plant in the mustard family. The flesh is firm and the flavor is peppery. The skin of radishes ranges from bright red to white, black, purple, and every shade in between.

Common Radish

The common radish is globular and oval-shaped with pink-red skin. The size of the common radish ranges from the size of a quarter to the size of a tomato.

Daikon Radish

This is a large white-skinned radish with a wonderful crunch and a mildly peppery flavor. Daikons can reach up to one and a half feet in length with a diameter several inches wide.

Watermelon Radish

This is an elongated medium-sized radish with bright-green skin. The flesh fades from the green skin to a brilliant pink-red to a white center, almost like the coloring of a watermelon.

Sweet Potato

Sweet potatoes are a starchy, sweet root vegetable native to tropical America. The skin ranges from white to purple-pink to reddish-brown. The flesh ranges from white to orange, and a special variety grown in Hawaii has brilliant purple flesh.

Turnip and Rutabaga

Turnips and rutabagas are actually members of the *Brassica* genus. They are not considered gourmet vegetables, but more of a food for fodder. They are a good source of calcium and potassium.

Yams

Yams have been a staple food in many parts of the tropical and subtropical world. Its rough skin is beige to brown, and the flesh is pale to bright orange and starchy sweet.

Sweet potatoes and yams are often confused, though they are from different species. Some dark-skinned varieties of sweet potatoes are incorrectly sold as yams. The flesh of pale sweet potatoes tends to be drier than that of real yams.

Yams can be found in many good produce markets and Latin American stores. They contain more sugar than sweet potatoes and are not as rich in vitamin A and C. Both sweet potatoes and yams like to be stored in a cool, dry place, but not in the refrigerator.

Shoots and Stems

Artichokes

Artichokes are one of the most beautiful and unusual vegetables. Artichokes are actually the large flower bud of an edible thistle that dates back before Roman times. Artichokes naturally contain a chemical called cynarin, which is known to affect and enhance the flavors of sweet things.

Artichokes are grown all over the world, although California almost exclusively produces the crop for the United States. In Italy, France, and Spain, artichokes are harvested while they are still young and the entire artichoke is delicate and edible. The heart of the artichoke is the part most commonly enjoyed.

Asparagus

Asparagus is one of the most delicious and finest vegetables available. It is part of the lily family and has a relatively short growing season. It grows green spears with tightly furled tips. The ancient Greeks enjoyed wild asparagus, and by Roman times, it was widely cultivated. Today, it is sought after all over the world. Asparagus is rich in vitamins A, B_2, and C, and is a great source of potassium, iron, and calcium. It has an indescribable taste and needs only the simplest of dressing for a divine dish.

Viola Asparagus
Viola is a purple variety of asparagus similar in appearance and flavor to green asparagus.

White Asparagus
White asparagus is packed in soil while growing to prevent the development of chlorophyll, which turns it green. Though quite rich in vitamins and minerals, like green asparagus, white spears are usually thicker and smoother than the green variety.

Celery

Prior to the sixteenth century, celery was used only medicinally. Today, it is one of the most popular vegetables. Celery grows in a bunch of ribs with delicate leaves that can be used as a seasoning. The outer stalks tend to be a more vibrant green, and the inner heart is pale green to pale yellow and deliciously tender. Choose bunches that are tight and firm.

Celery is very low in calories and rich in natural sodium, potassium, and calcium.

White Celery

White celery is grown with soil mounded around the stalk to prevent chlorophyll from developing and turning the stalks green. Like green asparagus, it is rich in sodium, potassium, and calcium.

Fennel Bulb

The root of the fennel plant is a broad, white, layered, bulbous root. It is delicately flavored and sweet like fennel. It is excellent shaved into salad. Its flavor complements apples and celery. Fennel has a balancing effect on blood sugar and is prized for its slimming qualities.

Hearts of Palm

Hearts of palm is the inner portion of the stem of a particular palm tree called the cabbage palm. Most palm trees, including coconut palms, have a heart, including coconut palms, but the whole tree must be sacrificed for this delicacy. The cabbage palm, however, grows like banana trees, shooting up new trees from a common root structure.

Hearts of palm are most commonly found canned, but fresh hearts of palm are preferred for their exceptional taste. Ivory colored and layered like marrow, they resemble thick white asparagus with a firm, smooth texture and a delicate flavor.

Water Chestnut

Water chestnut is a common name for several plants that grow similarly to rice, requiring plenty of water and warm temperatures. Indigenous to Southeast Asia, the roots are planted in the spring in paddy fields and flooded until harvest in the fall.

Fresh water chestnuts have rough dark-brown skin; crunchy, juicy flesh; and a mild, slightly sweet flavor. Water chestnuts are most commonly found canned.

6

Algae and Seaweed

Algae and seaweed make up a group of very simple and nutritious plants that grow in fresh water and ocean water. The simplicity of their nutritional matrix provides a bio-available source of protein, minerals, vitamins, and nutrients.

Microalgae

Microalgae, a single-celled plant, was the first life on the planet. The nucleic acid (RNA/DNA) codes of the ancient, primitive organism of spirulina reveal more than 3.5 billion years of life. These microalgae are spiral-shaped and are a brilliant emerald-blue-green. The cells are so small that they are measured in microns, millionths of a meter.

Microalgae are packed with nutrients. Because algae is so simple, they are extremely bioavailable, meaning our bodies can easily assimilate the nutrients and minerals.

Spirulina, chlorella, and wild blue-green algae *(Aphanizomenon flos-aquae)* microalgae are the highest sources of protein, provitamin A (beta-carotene), nucleic acids (RNA/DNA), and chlorophyll of any plant or animal food on the planet. "Some forms [of algae] are thought to contain every nutrient required by the human body" (P. Pitchford, *Healing with Whole Foods* [Berkeley, CA: North Atlantic Books, 1993]).

Algae and Cell Walls

The cell wall of microalgae has a unique structure not found anywhere else in the plant kingdom. Spirulina has an extremely digestible cell wall woven from complex and simple sugars and amino acids. When spirulina is ingested, this structure has been shown to fortify connective tissue and "teach" our tissue to be more resilient and elastic. Chlorella, on the other hand, has a very indigestible cell wall interlaced with compounds that are similar to bacteria. Accordingly, when chlorella is ingested, these cell walls seem to "teach" our cells how to be strong and resistant to invading bacteria and toxins.

Algae and Blood Sugar

Algae helps improve blood sugar imbalances, such as diabetes, hypoglycemia, and manic depression. The protein of algae is "predigested" and readily available to use, which results in the regulation of blood sugar levels.

Microalgae and Protein

Studies have shown that spirulina has three times more protein than beef and that it is four times more absorbable than beef protein.

Microalgae contain the essence of protein. Relatively unmatched, algae is abundant in essential amino acids, the building blocks of protein, and abundant amounts of nucleic acid (RNA/DNA). Nucleic acid is a precious and unusual characteristic found in food. It is the map that plans the combinations of amino acids that build the many different proteins that make up the trillion of cells in our bodies. A food that supplies the map and the material to make protein is monumental.

In the modern age, pollution, electricity, radiation, stress, and urban conditions have a negative impact on RNA/DNA and normal cellular regeneration. Damaged cells that regenerate unmonitored and uncontrollably are known as cancer. Microalgae are a simple whole-foods "supplement" that support and nourish our bodies with profoundly simple nutrition with billions of years of DNA and RNA to support a future of health.

Spirulina

Spirulina is a spiral-shaped, single-celled organism, rich in an unusual blue pigment called *phycocyanin*. Phycocyanin is a biliprotein known to enhance mental functioning by drawing together and arranging amino acids in the brain for neurotransmitter formation. It has also shown the capacity to inhibit the growth of cancer colonies in the body.

Spirulina contains the healthy unsaturated fatty acid gamma-linolenic acid (GLA), which supports prostaglandin, a hormonelike substance known to promote health and immunity.

Spirulina may be the most bioavavailable algae because the cell walls are made up of totally digestible nutrients. Most plants, seeds, and microalgae have cell walls made up of cellulose, an indigestible carbohydrate (sugar). The walls of spirulina are composed of complex sugars interlaced with amino acids, simple sugars, and protein, called mucopolysaccharides (MPs), which are easily digested.

MPs are accredited with fortifying body tissue, notably connective tissue, which has shown to make tissue more elastic and resilient.

Chlorella

Chlorella is another incredible algae, with a nutritional portfolio comparable to spirulina. Compared with spirulina, chlorella has less protein and only a fraction of the beta-carotene, but almost twice as much nucleic acid and chlorophyll.

The cell walls of chlorella are unusual and interesting. Unfortunately, the cell wall of chlorella is indigestible and is usually "broken" to increase the bioavailability. Breaking the cell wall is an expensive process done in a lab, which drives up the price and might compromise the integrity of the product. Although the cell wall might inhibit absorption, it has shown to be effective in binding with heavy metal, pesticides, PVCs (polyvinylchlorides), and other carcinogens to be safely carried out of the body.

These curious cell walls have a homeopathiclike approach to increasing immunity and protecting against cell mutation. The cell walls contain complex polysaccharides and other compounds similar to those found in bacteria. Instead of our cells being harmed by these compounds, the cells are strengthened and fortified. The tough cell wall may "teach" our cells to be strong against invading toxins, organisms, and bacteria. Interesting.

Chlorella does not contain the precious biliprotein phycocyanin, though it has more nucleic acid (RNA/DNA) than any other known food. The unique nature of chlorella's nucleic acid is known as the "chlorella growth factor" (CGF). First isolated in the 1950s, it is credited with being effective at improving growth patterns, especially in children and the elderly who are recovering from injury, disease, degeneration (including brain disorders such as Alzheimer's), and nerve disorders. The nucleic acid in our bodies naturally depletes with age and with exposure to urban conditions such as pollution and radiation. RNA and DNA are essential and are necessary for choreographing cellular regeneration, growth, and repair.

Wild Blue-Green Algae

Wild blue-green algae is a bitter wild microalgae that grows in only a few places in the world. Most blue-green algae in the United States comes from Klamath Lake in Oregon. Several companies harvest and package blue-green algae under closely monitored conditions, as this microalgae can transform into an extremely toxic plant under certain conditions.

Wild blue-green algae has shown to open and stimulate neural pathways and to enhance mental clarity. It enables many people to maintain focus and may be successful in treating disorders such as attention deficit disorder (ADD).

Its capacity to balance the nervous system is therapeutic for many who suffer from excessive stimulation and stress, drink too much coffee, and eat too much salt.

E3 Algae

E3 algae is a fresh blue-green algae available from a company called Earth's Essential Elements (see the Resource Guide for more information). It is the only algae sold in a fresh, liquid form wild harvested from the pristine upper part of Klamath Lake in Oregon, California.

Seaweed: Macroalgae

Seaweed grows all over the world, varying in nutrients, minerals, and fiber depending on ocean temperature, light exposure, depth of growth, and the tides. Seaweed grows in a large variety of colors, including reds, yellows, browns, greens, and purples, depending on the spectrum of light able to reach the depths where the fronds grow.

Sea vegetables have been valued and eaten for millennia all over the world. In Japan, seaweed is prized for its beautifying effects on hair and skin. Honored for regulating blood cholesterol, sea vegetables are also known to remove heavy metals and radioactive elements from the body. It also has natural antibiotic properties that have been shown to be effective against penicillin-resistant bacteria.

Many varieties of seaweed are available in health food stores and Asian markets. Seaweed is generally packaged dried. Seaweed is best stored in glass jars in a cool, dark, dry place, which will keep it fresh for months.

Most varieties of seaweed need to be soaked in water to soften and freshen them—except dulse, powdered kelp, and nori sheets. The remaining water is a valuable nutrient-rich elixir, excellent for soups, as a potassium broth, or to feed to plants.

The Incredible Nutrition of Seaweed

Ocean water contains all of the minerals and trace elements of blood. Seaweed vegetables supply all of these minerals and trace minerals needed for human health.

Seaweed is considered a macroalgae, because of the simple structure of its plant tissue. The generous nutritional portfolio of sea vegetables is considered to be very bioavailable, meaning it is very easy for our bodies to digest and assimilate the nutrients.

Seaweed is up to 38 percent protein. It is an excellent source of vitamins A, C, E, B_1, B_2, B_6, and precious B_{12}.

Seaweed also has a magnificent substance called ergosterol, which is converted to vitamin D in the body.

> The human fetus begins its development in a saline solution in the womb and is nourished and cleansed by blood that has almost the same composition as seawater. Seawater contains all of the minerals found in our blood. Dried unwashed seaweed will contain all of the minerals found in seawater. Certain types will, of course, be higher in some minerals than others.

Seaweed and Minerals

Seaweed has more minerals than any other food. Modern farming methods heavily feed from the soil resulting in drastic depletion of soil minerals and nutrients. The topsoil erodes and the minerals wash away. These minerals end up where all water is eventually found, in the sea. Seaweed can supply many missing nutrients and precious deficient trace minerals.

Sea vegetables contain ten to twenty times the mineral content of land vegetables. Seaweed is abundant in essential minerals, especially in calcium, iodine, and iron. Without a doubt, seaweed is one of the most nutritious foods on the planet.

Types of Seaweed

Agar-Agar (Gelidium)
Agar-agar, also called kanten in Japan, is classified with several other seaweeds in a family called agarophytes. Agarophytes grow 15 to 200 feet below the surface of the water in waving feathery fronds of red, brown, and purple up to 3 feet long.

Agar-agar packaged in the market is generally found in clear flakes, powders, or "bars." Traditionally, it is used as a gelling agent, although it is excellent in seaweed salads. One bar of agar-agar equals ¼ teaspoon powder or 3 tablespoons of light flakes. This amount will gel 2 cups of liquid.

Alaria *(Alaria marginata)*

Alaria is very similar to wakame. It grows in generous, delicate fronds. Alaria is rich in calcium and B vitamins. It is harvested on American coasts.

Arame

Arame is a member of the kelp family that grows in bouquetlike fronds, usually along with hijiki. Arame is a tough seaweed that grows in dark-brown fronds. It is typically cut into thin strips and sun-dried, steamed, or boiled to soften and then is dried again into thin black strings.

Dulse *(Palmaria palmata)*

Dulse is a reddish-purple North Atlantic sea vegetable that grows in flat, smooth, mitten-shaped fronds. It is harvested in the very Northeastern United States and Canada and has been harvested in Western Europe for thousands of years.

Dulse is very high in iron and protein and is rich in vitamin A, the B-complex vitamins, and chlorophyll. It has more soluble fiber than oat bran.

Hijiki

Hijiki is a member of the kelp family that grows in a bush of branches up to six feet tall. The fresh brown plants are harvested and dried in the sun, sometimes boiled and dried again until they are black.

Hijiki has the highest content of calcium of any seaweed. It is abundant in iron, iodine, vitamin B_2, and niacin (vitamin B_3). Hijiki is known to regulate blood sugar levels and to aid in weight loss.

Irish Moss *(Chondrus crispus)*

Irish moss grows in broad, forked, pale reddish-purple fans. Irish moss contains carrageenan, a widely used ingredient as a thickener in many packaged foods from soy milk to salad dressing and shampoo.

Irish moss is very high in sulfur (40 percent). It contains calcium chloride, which is known to be a beneficial tonic for the heart and to balance the endocrine system.

Kelp/Kombu *(Laminaria)*

Kelp is the largest of all sea vegetables, growing up to 1,500 feet long. Kombu is a type of kelp, which grows in cool waters. Kelp is considered to be a completely mineralized food and increases the digestibility and nutritional value of all food it is prepared with.

Nori *(Porphyra tenera)*

Nori is also called "laver" in Scotland and "sloke" in Ireland. Nori is most commonly sold in pressed sheets that are used for sushi rolls. Nori is a dark purple-green seaweed that grows in large hollow-tubed fronds. After harvest, nori is typically dried, shredded, and pressed into sheets.

Nori sheets can be found toasted or untoasted in health food stores and Asian markets.

It is 48 percent protein, the highest of all seaweed. Nori is abundant in vitamin A, thiamine (vitamin B_1), and niacin (vitamin B_3). The tender fiber of nori makes all of the precious nutrition in it very digestible.

Sea Lettuce *(Ulva lactuca)*

Sea lettuce is a delicate bright-green seaweed that grows in the warm waters of the Pacific. Sea lettuce is very high in calcium, silica, and B vitamins.

Silky Sea Palm *(Postelsia palmaeformis)*

Sea palm is a wonderful, unique, delicate frond that grows in Northern California. Sea palm is very rich in calcium and B vitamins.

Wakame *(Undaria pinnatifida)*

Wakame is a tender, olive-colored seaweed that grows in winged fronds, up to twenty inches long, in shallow water. Wakame is very high in calcium and is abundant in niacin (vitamin B_3) and thiamine (vitamin B_1).

7

Legumes and Beans

Legumes have a unique and complex nutritious portfolio. High in protein, legumes also have a good balance of carbohydrates and fat. The protein in beans helps to regulate sugar and water in the body and to manage metabolism. Legumes have precious B vitamins as well as potassium, calcium, and iron.

Digesting Beans

Some people have trouble digesting beans and suffer from gas, flatulence, and irritability. Trisaccharides, complex sugars, and enzyme inhibitors such as phytic acid are the common culprits in beans that cause gas. Soaking and sprouting beans activates enzymes and simplifies the starches and eliminates the enzyme inhibitors for easier digestion. (See Chapter 16 for more information on sprouting.)

Beans

Adzuki Bean

This is a small, dark-red legume that is high in protein, calcium, phosphorus, potassium, iron, and vitamin A. Adzuki beans are prized by Asian doctors for their medicinal value, especially in tonifying the kidneys.

Black-Eyed Pea

Originally from Africa, black-eyed peas, also called "cow peas" or "China beans," are popular in Southern cuisine and "soul food." Black-eyed peas can be eaten fresh from the pod.

Garbanzo Bean

Also known as the chick pea, this is a large, golden to pale-brown bean widely known as the staple ingredient in hummus, a Middle Eastern spread that also includes sesame tahini, lemon, and parsley.

Garbanzo beans contain more iron than any other legume and are a healthy source of unsaturated fat. They are high in potassium, calcium, and vitamin A.

Lentil

Lentils were one of the first known cultivated crops. In India, more than fifty varieties of different colors and sizes of lentils are cultivated. Green lentils, yellow lentils, red lentils, baby French lentils, and split lentils are some of the widely available varieties.

Lentils are a member of the pea family but are treated more like beans. They sprout and cook more quickly than most beans due to their smaller size and texture. They are high in calcium, magnesium, potassium, phosphorus, chlorine, sulfur, and vitamin A.

Mung Bean

Mung beans are a member of the kidney bean family, originally from India. Mung beans have a strong presence in traditional Chinese cuisine. Reputed to be very detoxifying, mung beans have a mild, sweet flavor.

Soybean

The soybean is the only bean that is a "complete" protein in and of itself. Originally from China, the soybean is the most versatile bean used for food and oil. Soybeans are 40 percent protein and 20 percent lecithin, an integral part of the membrane of every cell in the body and protective brain sheath. Lecithin is valued for breaking up old deposits of fat in the body.

When Henry Ford designed the first automobile, he intended to run the engine on soy oil. The diesel engine was also designed to run on soy and vegetable oil. Most tractors have diesel engines. The plan was for farmers to grow their own fuel. However, the oil industry, run by giant corporate conglomerates, snuffed the idea in favor of mining petroleum oil. Petroleum oil is made up of hydrocarbons, in essence, smashed vegetable matter that has been fermented for millions of years. Carbohydrates, from fresh vegetable matter, have a very similar molecular structure. There is very little difference in running an engine on hydrocarbons or carbohydrates. Our dependency on foreign oil continues to fuel a world war for control. Regardless of who controls the remaining fossil fuels such as oil, we have surpassed consuming more than half of all the world's known oil supplies.

Every diesel car will run on vegetable oil with 70 percent less emissions! Yes, this is true. Please read this paragraph again to marinate your brain in the beauty of possibility for our real future. Growing oil versus blood for oil. The choice is ours. For more information, please read *From the Fryer to the Fuel Tank*, by Joshua Tickell (Veggie Van Publications, 2000).

Legumes: Peas and Green Beans

Peas and green beans have been eaten since the beginning of time. There is archaeological evidence that peas were cultivated as long ago as 5700 B.C. Most peas are best fresh, straight from the pod. The harvest season for garden-fresh peas is relatively short; it lasts only several weeks in the early summer. Most markets do carry peas most of the year. Flash-frozen peas are an alternative when fresh varieties are waning or unavailable. Peas and green beans are good sources of complex carbohydrates, protein, and chlorophyll.

Most Digestible Beans	*Moderately Digestible Beans*	*Least Digestible Beans*
• Adzuki	• Black beans	• Black soybeans
• Lentils	• Kidney beans	• Soybeans
• Mung beans	• Lima beans	
• Peas	• Garbanzo beans	

Peas

English Peas

The English pea is the most common garden pea. It's best fresh, right from the pod. It is bright green and quite sweet. The pods are quite fibrous and not choice for eating.

Petits Pois

Petits pois are not immature peas, but a dwarf variety. Small, bright-green peas are taken from the shell. They are quite sweet and delicate. Fresh petits pois are rarely available in the market, but are quite easy to grow. Although they are readily available frozen, the frozen peas pale in comparison to the fresh ones.

Snow Peas

Snow peas are eaten whole—peas and pod together—a delicate bright-green pod with small, flattened peas inside. They are sweet with a quintessential pea flavor. They are available fresh in the market most or all of the year.

Sugar Snap Peas

Sugar snap peas are very plump with crisp, edible pods. They are bright green and perky and quite sweet. They "snap" when broken in half.

Green Beans

Fresh beans are a vegetable originally from the Americas, cultivated for thousands of years by indigenous people in the north and south of the continent. Some varieties are available fresh year-round in the market.

Serving Green Beans

- To keep green beans crisp before serving, plunge them in salty ice water.
- To remove the ends of green beans, gather them together in a bunch and chop off a quarter inch of the stem tops all at once. The pointy ends do not need to be cut off and add a nice visual accent to many dishes.

French Beans

French beans encompass many varieties, including haricot verts, snap beans, yellow wax beans, and bobby beans. Three to four inches long and slim, they should be crisp when fresh (firm enough to snap in half). They are best when young. They have a mild vegetal flavor.

Thai Beans

These beans are about six to eight inches long. Although they are flexible, they should be crisp enough to snap when broken.

8

Grains and Grasses

Grains are considered one of the most important staple foods throughout the world. Nutritionally, grains have a diverse portfolio of protein, carbohydrates, fiber, vitamins, and minerals. Most grains have the following four components:

1. The *hull* of a grain is its protective outer layer. Generally, the hull is inedible although it is valuable for sprouting grains into grasses, such as buckwheat.

2. The *bran* of grain contains the valuable fiber and B vitamins. Fiber is essential for digestive and intestinal health. Fiber adds bulk to food, aiding the timely manner of digestion from consumption to elimination. Moreover, fiber stabilizes blood sugar during digestion by regulating nutrients and sugar in the digestive tract.

3. The *germ* contains vitamins, minerals, protein, and the precious oils of a grain. Germ is an essential source of vitamin E, a nutritive antioxidant that protects cells and tissue from the damaging compounds called free radicals.

   Sprouting grains has shown to amplify the nutrition of the germ. A four-day wheat berry sprout has 30 percent more vitamin E than wheat at any other stage in its development or maturity, including whole wheat.

4. The *endosperm* or *gluten* of grains is the starchy kernel. This is where the complex carbohydrates reside. Grains with more gluten, such as wheat, are stickier and favored for breads. Much of the allergy to wheat is actually a symptom of intolerance to gluten. Generally, grains with less gluten are easier to digest and more nutritious.

Sprouting grains makes gluten more digestible. Growing grains into grasses almost eliminates the gluten found in whole grains.

Grains and Protein

Amino acids are the building blocks of protein. There are twenty-two amino acids. Healthy adults can produce fourteen, and children can produce eleven of the amino acids. There are eight "essential amino acids" that our bodies cannot produce. They are referred to as "essential" because they are essential to the assimilation and formation of protein. The protein in grains is generally deficient in one or two of the essential amino acids.

There are three ways to benefit from the protein in grains:

1. Soak and sprout grains. Studies show that sprouted grains have 10 percent more protein than a dry seed and that sprouting increases the essential amino acid lysine, which is necessary to "complete" protein, by 16 to 25 percent.
2. Grow grains into a grass, such as wheatgrass, barley grass, or buckwheat greens. Young grasses contain all of the essential amino acids necessary to build protein, as well as a wealth of chlorophyll, B vitamins, iron, and minerals.
3. Complement grains with fresh sprouts and greens (or, traditionally, beans). Most sprouts and fresh leafy greens contain all of the essential amino acids. Beans and grains are a traditional combination in almost every culture. Beans typically contain the essential amino acids that are commonly missing or unavailable in grains, making beans and grains a "complete" protein.

Grains and Carbohydrates

Carbohydrates are basically complex sugars. Saliva is the predominant catalyst that begins the digestion process. Ptyalin, an enzyme in saliva, breaks down carbohydrates into maltose, the more simple sugar. In the intestines, the enzyme maltase breaks down maltose into dextrose, a simple sugar. It is essential to chew carbohydrates and grains well because maltase can only act on maltose, which is produced by the salivary glands during the process of chewing.

Grains and Grasses
Amaranth

Amaranth is one of the smallest and most nutritious foods. Amaranth is not a true cereal grain, but a starchy seed that grows by the thousands in a tight head of a broad-leaf plant. Grown by the ancient Aztecs in South America and in the Himalayan regions of India, Nepal, China, and Tibet, amaranth is a hearty plant that can thrive in weak and poor soil and drought conditions.

Much of the high-protein complex is concentrated in the germ of amaranth. At 15 to 19 percent protein, amaranth surpasses most meat-based proteins. It is also rich in lysine and methonine, two essential amino acids necessary for the assimilation of protein but are rarely found in wheat and most other grains.

Amaranth has more calcium than milk and contains the cofactors magnesium and silicon, which are necessary to make calcium bioavailable.

Barley

Barley is one of the oldest cultivated cereal grains. It has been grown for more than 8,000 years to produce bread and beer.

Whole barley grains look like pale-golden wheatberries with a spilt in the middle and pointed ends. Pearled barley is a pearly-white color with a split in the middle and rounded ends.

Barley has two inedible outer hulls that are usually removed by machine. The remaining hull is very valuable. Aleurone is a precious layer that is removed to create "pearled barley." Whole barley, also called "sproutable barley," is far more nutritious than "pearled barley." Whole barley has twice the amount of calcium, three times the amount of iron, and 25 percent more protein and fiber than "pearled barley."

Whole barley can be used to grow barley grass. Similar to wheatgrass, barley grass is an outstanding source of chlorophyll, amino acids, enzymes, and vitamins. Popular in Japan, barley grass is dried into a powder that is used as a supplement and in healthy drinks. (See Chapter 16 for more information on sprouting.)

Buckwheat

Buckwheat is considered an alkaline grain. Buckwheat is not technically a cereal grain, but an edible fruit seed from a plant that resembles a bush rather than grass. Buckwheat has mildly mucilagenic properties, which makes it easy to digest and soothing to the digestive tract.

The bioflavonoid rutin, found in buckwheat, helps heal and support capillaries, reduce blood pressure, and stimulate circulation, especially to hands and feet. Rutin is also known to neutralize the effects of radiation and X-rays.

Whole buckwheat can be purchased several ways: whole and raw, dehydrated, and toasted. Whole, raw buckwheat groats are a pale beige. They are excellent to soak, sprout, and dehydrate. Dehydrated buckwheat makes delicious raw breakfast cereal, crunchy crackers, bread, and sweet treats. (See Chapter 18 for more information on dehydrated foods.) Toasted buckwheat, also called "kasha," is a darker reddish-brown and is more flavorful and fragrant than raw or dehydrated buckwheat.

Buckwheat can also be found in the dark, indigestible hull for growing buckwheat greens. Buckwheat greens are sprouted and planted in soil, like wheatgrass. These delicate, tasty greens are rich in chlorophyll, enzymes, and vitamins.

Corn

Corn is the traditional grain of the Native Americans. Today, it continues to be a staple starch in Central and South America. Fresh corn is a grain that can be used and enjoyed like a vegetable. Fresh corn has more enzymes and vitamins than dried corn, although is usually available only in warm months. Corn is low in the essential amino acids lysine and tryptophan, which are necessary for the assimilation of protein. To improve this deficiency, corn is best eaten with greens or beans.

Blue corn, indigenous to the lands of the Hopi and Navajo peoples in southwestern America, remains unhybridized and more nutritious than yellow and white varieties, with 21 percent more protein, 50 percent more iron, and twice the amount of manganese and potassium.

In America, corn is a highly exploited crop. Most commercial corn is genetically modified and hybridized for high yield and high sugar content. Very few native varieties are still grown. Select companies recognize the value of preserving and protecting original botanical genetic species and specialize in heirloom varieties.

Millet

Millet was widely cultivated in Mesopotamia as early as 3000 B.C. In China, millet has been farmed for more than 3,000 years. Evidence shows that millet was grown during the Stone Age in lake regions in Switzerland. However, millet was not considered an important grain outside the fertile valley until post-Roman times.

Millet is one of the few alkaline grains. It has a very rich protein and amino acid portfolio and is high in silicon, which is good for bones and connective tissue. Millet has incredible anti-fungal properties and is an excellent grain for those with an overgrowth of *Candida.*

Millet is gluten-free and has been traditionally used to strengthen weak digestion.

Oats

Oats are a gentle and nutritious grain. Very popular as a breakfast cereal, oats can be found in many forms, including oatmeal or rolled oats, steel-cut oats, and whole oat groats.

Whole oat groats have an unadulterated nutritional portfolio. Oats are high in silicon, which is essential for connective tissue health and to renew bones. They are also rich in phosphorus, which is necessary for brain and nerve development.

Quinoa

Originally grown in the South American Andes for thousands of years, quinoa is one of the most ancient and nutritious foods. The Incas called quinoa "the mother grain."

Quinoa is not actually a grain, but a starchy seed fruit that grows in clusters at the end of a stalk of an annual herb. Also known as "the lost grain of the Incas," quinoa has been cultivated in the mountains of Peru and Bolivia for more than 3,000 years. Quinoa was the primary staple of advanced Incan civilization until the 1500s, when Pizzaro, the Spanish conquistador, "discovered" this part of the New World. Thereafter (after Spanish settlement), quinoa production dwindled until it was "rediscovered" in the twentieth century and is enjoyed today as one of the most delicious and nutritious grains.

Quinoa is still primarily farmed in South America. Some quinoa is grown in the high altitudes of Colorado, but most attempts to grow it outside its indigenous environment have been fruitless.

There are hundreds of varieties of quinoa—from yellow and orange to red, pink, purple, and black. Quinoa is naturally covered with a bitter resinous substance called saponin. Saponin can be used to make soap and skin-care products but is inedible and must be removed by a labor-intensive washing process before quinoa is fit for human consumption.

Quinoa has the highest protein of any grain. Akin to amaranth, quinoa has a generous amino acid portfolio that includes the essential amino acid lysine. Likewise, quinoa is very high in calcium (more than milk) and contains the essential cofactors silicon and magnesium, which are necessary to assimilate calcium. Quinoa is very high in B vitamins, iron, phosphorus, and vitamin E.

Rye

Rye is a very hearty grain with a sweet-and-sour flavor. Traditionally made into sourdough breads, rye can also be sprouted and grown into grass.

Rye is extremely hearty and grows well in poor soil and thrives in cold climates as far north as the Arctic Circle.

During the Middle Ages, rye was the major staple consumed by the poor. Ergot is a fungus that infects cereal grasses, especially rye. It was responsible for the outbreak of "St. Anthony's Fire," a toxic and sometimes deadly condition that struck areas of high rye consumption during the Middle Ages. It is now understood that one of the chemicals in ergot is lysergic acid, the active ingredient in LSD-25. Modern cultivation and standards maintain safe control over rye production and processing to prevent ergot.

Rye is rich in fluorine, a rare nutrient that strengthens teeth and tooth enamel.

Rye grass can be grown much like wheatgrass and barley grass. Rich in chlorophyll, iron, B vitamins, vitamin E, amino acids, and enzymes, rye grass has a bitter flavor and cleansing properties.

Wheat

Wheat has been cultivated since the Stone Age (9000–6000 B.C.). There are two kinds of wheat: "emmer," which includes modern wheat, and "einkorn," which includes spelt and kamut. These ancient varieties (spelt and kamut) were difficult to remove by threshing (beating to separate out the grain) because the grain is covered by a tough sheath.

Wheat has three parts: bran, germ, and gluten. Wheat *bran* is the fiber, associated with cereal. Wheat *germ* is the part that contains all of the precious oils, such as vitamin E, and is destroyed in the milling process. Wheat *gluten* is valued for making bread fluffy and tasty. The gluten contains protein and vitamins and is also "gummy" and more difficult to digest.

By biblical times, the ancient cereals kamut and spelt had been replaced by durum wheat, a species with naked grains that were rich in gluten. Modern wheat has been hybridized to have an imbalanced amount of gluten. As with life, there is a tradeoff: more gluten, less fiber, and fewer nutrients in the germ.

Wheat is known to aggravate allergic reactions. This is often the case with flour that has been stored for too long and is rancid from oxidation. Allergy to wheat is often an allergy to "gluten." Sprouted wheat causes fewer allergic problems, and wheatgrass rarely causes any at all.

Wheat absorbs a broad range of nutrients, but requires rich soil from which it heavily feeds. Wheat has a decent nutritional portfolio that compares to the needs of the human body. However, modern wheat farming leaves the soil devoid of minerals, and wheat has been hybridized for taste rather than for nutrition. Modern wheat alternatives such as spelt and kamut are a healthier choice.

Kamut

Kamut is a variety of durum wheat that was grown in Egypt more than 5,000 years ago. But about 2,000 years ago, kamut began to be increasingly replaced by other modern, high-gluten strains. It was still grown consistently for thousands of years until the mid-1900s. After World War II, kamut faced extinction in the face of industrial mono-crops of hybridized, high-yield strains.

The story continues when a handful of kamut seeds were recovered from a burial crypt in the 1980s. The seeds were brought to America where kamut has been grown and continues to flourish in Montana.

Kamut is about twice the size of modern wheat with much less gluten. Although it shares many similarities with modern wheat, it is far less agitating (approximately two-thirds less agitating) to those with allergies to wheat and with gluten sensitivity.

Kamut is hearty and nutty tasting with a finer and more delicate texture than modern wheat.

Spelt

Spelt is an ancient grain originally from Southeast Asia that was brought to the Middle East more than 9,000 years ago and through Europe thereafter. Spiritual and mystical writings of St. Hildegard, a twelfth-century healer, recognize spelt as the grain best tolerated by the body for health.

Spelt has enjoyed a popular surge in American health food. Prior to several years ago, spelt was primarily fed to racehorses and livestock in lieu of oats.

Spelt grows in a very thick husk, which naturally protects it from insects and pollutants. Hence, it not usually treated with chemicals and pesticides, and is more likely to be "organically grown." Spelt is higher in protein and nutrients than modern wheat. The water-soluble fiber of spelt makes it easy to digest and assimilate. Spelt does contain gluten, but it is typically tolerated by those with gluten sensitivity.

Spelt has a tasty, nutty flavor, a generous supply of nutrients, and a versatile consistency. It is an excellent alternative to modern wheat.

Wild Rice

Wild rice is neither rice nor grain. It is actually the fruit seed of a tall aquatic grass indigenous to the Great Lakes and the northern United States and southern Canada.

Wild rice is known to have been harvested by Native Americans more than 10,000 years ago. Native Americans traditionally harvested wild rice by canoe in the wetlands of shallow ponds and lakes. The grass was bent into the canoe and thrashed with the paddles. The seeds were then sun-dried or parched to crack the hull and trampled.

Today, some wild rice is still wild harvested in natural wetlands, but most "wild" rice sold in stores is not wild at all. It is grown in commercial diked paddies from hybridized seeds with toxic agrochemicals and is mechanically harvested.

Wild rice has a satisfying nutty flavor and is rich in protein, iron, and B vitamins. It is excellent soaked and sprouted.

9

Nuts and Seeds

Nuts and seeds have concentrated nutrition in a small package. Rich in protein, vitamins, minerals, and healthy fats, nuts and seeds are some of the most nutritious foods in the world.

Soaking and Sprouting Nuts and Seeds

Nuts and seeds are the procreative essence of a plant. They are the source of all plant life. Imagine, in just one almond, there is the potential for an almond tree. All of that potential energy is stored in the nut, waiting to be awakened. Sprouting nuts and seeds awakens the energy, and, as the seed's cellular memory is roused to grow, the nutritional value increases.

Alfalfa

In Arabic, *al-fal-fa* means "the father of all foods." Arabs were the first to use alfalfa for food and to feed their racehorses. In America, alfalfa was considered food only fit for fodder until Dr. Ann Wigmore uncovered the incredible nutrition available in alfalfa sprouts.

Today, alfalfa is America's most popular sprout. So it's easy to find these small, juicy sprouts, power-packed with nutrition.

Alfalfa seeds have a tremendous life force. A mature alfalfa plant has roots that reach up to 100 feet into the earth.

Alfalfa sprouts have eight enzymes that help digest carbohydrates, protein, and fat. They are also extremely high in vitamins A, E, and D.

Almonds

Almonds are the only nuts that alkalinize the blood. One fifth of the weight of almonds is protein. Almonds are power-packed with potassium, calcium, magnesium, folic acid, riboflavin, fiber, phosphorus, and vitamin E. Almond oil is one of the best oils for the skin and is most nutritious. Almond butter is made by grinding almonds into a paste to achieve the consistency of peanut butter.

Almonds are grown primarily in California and Spain. Because of the popular demand for almonds, California almond growers annually lease bees to pollinate their trees to ensure generous production of almonds.

Protein: 18.6%
Fat: 54.2%

Brazil Nuts

Brazil nuts are from a giant tree in the Amazon in South America. Brazil nuts have a dark-brown triangular shell that is the hardest of all nut shells. They have rich, white flesh and are very high in potassium, phosphorus, sulfur, and selenium, a powerful antioxidant.

Protein: 14.3%
Fat: 66.9%

Broccoli

Sprouted broccoli seeds have enjoyed recent popularity. They contain many phytonutrients and antioxidants that are known to help heal and prevent cancers.

Cashews

The tropical evergreen cashew tree is related to poison ivy and poison sumac. Indigenous to Central and South America, cashews are primarily grown in India. The poisonous properties of the shell are leeched away by heating the cashew apple (the fruit of the cashew nut) until the outer shell bursts. There are sun-drying methods that do not involve high heat, but sun-dried cashews are difficult to find.

The inner shell is cracked to reveal a white, kidney-shaped nut that is very high in vitamin A, potassium, phosphorus, and magnesium.

Protein: 15%
Fat: 46%

Clover

Clover seeds are small seeds for sprouting with an incredible nutritional portfolio of amino acids, minerals, and vitamins.

Coconuts

Coconuts are the fruit of a tropical and subtropical palm. Prized for the nutrient-rich fresh coconut water, the meat is harvested at varying maturity and dried. The younger the coconut, the more nutrients in the water. As the coconut matures, the flesh thickens and hardens and assumes a higher fat content. Young coconut meat, called "spoon meat" or "jelly meat," is soft enough to be easily scooped out with a spoon and is a delicious, light delicacy.

Mature dried coconut
Protein: 3.5%
Fat: 64.9%

Flaxseeds

The seed of flax is rich in nutrients, healthy essential fatty acids, and soluble fiber. Mucilagenic, slippery, and slimy when moistened, flaxseed is very easy on the digestive system and acts as a mild laxative.

Flaxseeds are rich in lignans, hormonelike substances that are known to balance hormone levels in the body.

Flaxseed is pressed into flaxseed oil, which is valued for its beneficial essential fatty acid content, which includes omega-3, omega-6, and omega-9 fatty acids.

Protein: 22%
Fat: 45%

Hazelnuts (Filberts)

Hazelnuts are rich, grape-sized nuts with a reddish-brown skin and a creamy-white meat, delicious in sweet and savory foods. Hazelnuts grow wild in temperate climates around the world. They are high in potassium, phosphorus, sulfur, and calcium.

Protein: 12.6%
Fat: 62.4%

Hemp Seeds

Hemp seeds are delicious, small white seeds, like sesame, with a green filament. They have enjoyed a very scandalous presence in the United States. The hemp plant, which is grown for fuel, textiles, and fiber, is a botanical cousin to marijuana. Hemp, however, does not contain THC, the intoxicating chemical in marijuana.

Choose hemp seeds that have had the tough shell removed. Hemp seeds found in the shell have been sterilized, steamed, or toasted so that they cannot germinate and grow.

Hemp seeds are one of the most nutritious seeds. With a tremendous amount of protein, the oil in hemp seeds has an unparalleled essential fatty acid portfolio. In addition, hemp seeds have all of the essential amino acids.

Protein: 35%
Fat: 54.7%

Macadamia Nuts

Macadamia nuts are originally from Australia, but today, Hawaii is the world's largest grower. If you can believe it, the tree that produces macadamia nuts was originally grown as an ornamental tree.

The sweet, rich, white, marble-sized nut is housed in one of the toughest shells of all time. It is one of the most delicious nuts.

Protein: 7.8%
Fat: 71.6%

Pecans

The pecan is a member of the hickory family, native to America. Pecans are grown in temperate climates, primarily in Georgia. The meat looks somewhat like a walnut with a golden-brown skin and a buttery-rich kernel. They are high in potassium, phosphorus, and vitamin A.

Protein: 9.2%
Fat: 71.6%

Pine Nuts

Pine nuts are harvested from several varieties of pine trees. The nuts are actually from inside of the pinecone. The harvesting is very labor intensive, reflected in the exorbitant cost.

The Mediterranean, or Italia, pine nut is from the stone pine. It is torpedo-shaped, with a light, delicate flavor and is generally more expensive. The Chinese pine nut has a stronger flavor and a trianglular shape. Both varieties are very fatty and delicious.

Protein: 9.2%
Fat: 47.4%

Pistachios

The pistachio is native to the Mediterranean region. It has a characteristically green kernel and a sweet, mild flavor housed by a hard, tan shell that splits open when the nutmeat is mature.

Protein: 19.3%
Fat: 63.9%

Pumpkinseeds

Pumpkinseeds are medium-sized, dark-green seeds from a pumpkin squash. In the pumpkin, the seeds are housed in a white shell.

Delicious and abundant in healthy oils, fiber, phosphorus, and vitamin A, pumpkinseeds are a very effective antiparasitic, expelling intestinal parasites and worms.

Protein: 29%
Fat: 47.6%

Radish Seeds

Radish seeds are small like alfalfa seeds. They are good to sprout and have a spicy kick.

Sesame Seeds

Sesame seeds are the first recorded seasoning, dating back to 3000 B.C. in Assyria. They were brought to America by African slaves who called them benné seeds.

These tiny flat seeds are exceptionally high in calcium (100 grams of sesame contain 1,125 mg of calcium, while 1 pint of milk contains only 590 mg of calcium). They are also rich in phosphorus, potassium, magnesium, and vitamin A. Also available in black and various shades of brown, sesame seeds have a delightfully nutty and slightly sweet flavor.

Sesame seeds are commonly ground into a paste called tahini, which is used widely in Middle Eastern cuisine.

Protein: 18.6%
Fat: 49.1%

Sunflower Seeds

Sunflower seeds come from the glorious and showy sunflower, with bright-yellow petals and a generous face, which houses the seeds. Sunflowers are indigenous to America and were celebrated by Native Americans long before Europeans. Russia is now one of the largest producers.

The seeds have a black-and-white striped shell that must be removed before eating. Seeds in a shell can be used to grow sunflower greens (see Chapter 16).

Sunflower oil is very high in healthy polyunsaturated fat. It is also very high in potassium, phosphorus, silicon, calcium, and vitamin A.

Protein: 24%
Fat: 47.3%

Walnuts

Walnuts are the fruit of a walnut tree. There are two popular varieties: *English walnut,* also known as *Persian walnut,* and the *black walnut.* The English walnut has more fat and less protein than the black walnut. Both are delicious, however. They have thin golden skins and rich, buttery nutmeat. They are a good source of potassium, magnesium, vitamin A, and phosphorus.

Protein: 14.8%
Fat: 64%

10

Herbs,
Edible Flowers,
and Spices

Culinary herbs are the fragrant leaves of annual and perennial plants that complement and balance the flavor of many foods. Herbs can be purchased fresh or dried. Fresh herbs are much more fragrant and flavorful than dried herbs. Many fresh herbs are available year-round in the market. Look for herbs that are clean and fresh. Avoid wilted or browning herbs.

Fresh herbs will stay fresh in the refrigerator for up to a week if stored properly. Remove any wilted leaves, wrap the herbs in a barely wet paper towel, and store in an airtight plastic bag. Alternatively, the stems of a bouquet of fresh herbs can be placed in a tall glass with two inches of fresh cold water and stored in the refrigerator. The water should be changed every two days.

My mother taught me to freeze fresh herbs with water in ice-cube trays in the height of summer bounty for autumn and winter when fresh herbs are not as prolific. The ice cubes can be thawed a few at a time as fresh herbs are needed. Brilliant. Freezing the herbs with water preserves much of the fresh flavor and color of herbs, such as basil, parsley, oregano, marjoram, savory, rosemary, lemongrass, lavender, cilantro, and mint. The texture and flavor of herbs frozen with this technique are significantly more pronounced than drying herbs for storage.

To preserve fresh herbs in ice, loosely fill two-thirds of each compartment of a standard ice-cube tray with fresh herbs. Fill the tray with fresh water and freeze. To use the herbs, simply thaw a few cubes at a time. The herbs will keep fresh frozen for months in a prime state of suspended animation.

With a little exploration, this technique of freezing herbs in ice has a bouquet of possibilities. Adding colorful edible flowers such as pansies, calendula, rose petals, and delicate lemon or orange slices, pomegranate seeds, berries, and grapes awakens a world of color, flavor, and texture for simple delight and fine culinary art.

Growing Herbs and Edible Flowers

Growing a plot of fresh herbs and edible flowers in the yard or in planter boxes on the windowsill is an easy and rewarding project. Most herbs and edible flowers can be purchased at a nursery and transplanted to a prepared plot of soil or a flowerpot or window box. Buying herbs and flowers that are already growing saves a good amount of time and effort. Planting "starts" is much easier with quicker rewards than growing plants from seeds.

Fresh herbs are easy to grow. Herbs like parsley, cilantro, basil, oregano, savory, thyme, marjoram, and mint need very little attention. Rosemary is a heart herb that will grow into a generous bush over the years and can survive cool weather and mild winters without flinching.

Edible flowers are a delight for any yard, house, or apartment and lend a gorgeous addition to fine food. Flowers like pot marigolds, calendula, pansy flower, impatiens, roses, day lilies, and gardenia flowers are a visual feast for the senses and a make a lovely delicacy for culinary presentation.

Young herbs and flowers are available in gardening stores and most hardware stores. A flower pot or window box and good potting soil, some sun, and water are all that is needed for herbs and flowers to flourish just about anywhere. Check out a gardening book for caring for your plants tailored to your environment.

Herbs

Aloe Vera (*Aloe barbadensis*)

Aloe vera is a rosette of long, fleshy, tapering, green, spiny leaves. It is a succulent perennial of the lily family. It blooms a tubular yellow, orange, or red flower atop a tall stalk.

The inner, gooey flesh of the leaves is used medicinally and for particular nutritional uses. Aloe aids digestion. Just under the skin is a bitter yellow sap used as an effective laxative.

There are more than 300 varieties. They range in size from two to twenty feet tall. Native to Africa and Mediterranean regions, aloe vera has been used for more than 2,500 years.

Basil *(Ocimum basilicum)*

This annual prefers full sun to partial shade. It's a full, leafy herb with a bushy appearance and broad oval leaves. The French call basil *herbe royal* for its superior, complementary flavor. Basil is generously used in Italian and Mediterranean cuisine. Its traditional medicinal use is to relieve vomiting and nausea, especially morning sickness. Basil flowers in July and August. The many types of basil include the following:

- *Anise basil*—sweet anise flavor and fragrance. Smaller, broad green leaves.
- *Bush basil* (dwarf basil)—compact. Small, tight leaves.
- *Cinnamon basil*—cinnamon flavor and fragrance. Smaller, broad green leaves.
- *Lemon basil*—strong lemon fragrance. Smaller, tighter leaves.
- *Lettuce-leaf basil*—generous leaves. Traditional basil flavor. Excellent for salads.
- *Purple basil*—striking deep-purple leaves. Ornamental. Traditional basil flavor.

Cayenne *(Capsicum Annum)*

The fruit of a nightshade, cayenne is hot and spicy. It improves circulation and stimulates digestion. Extremely high in vitamin C and other strong antioxidants, it protects against free radicals (oxygen compounds that damage cell membranes and disturb metabolic pathways).

Cilantro/Coriander *(Coriandrum sativum)*

Coriander and cilantro come from the same annual plant. Favored worldwide, this plant has been cultivated for more than 3,000 years in China, the Mediterranean, and Egypt. Cilantro, also known as Chinese parsley, is a bright-green herb with fanning, flat, smooth, delicate leaves. Slender, erect, slightly grooved stems produce leaves, seeds, and tiny white flowers.

Coriander is the yellowish-brown seed produced by the plant. Best freshly ground, coriander has a sweet, woody flavor with a touch of bitterness. Coriander is celebrated in Asian and Middle Eastern cuisine.

Comfrey *(Symphytum officinale)*

Comfrey is a hardy, upright perennial plant with broad, sometimes fuzzy, dark-green leaves. Comfrey is a rare plant source for vitamin B_{12}.

The use of comfrey has been recorded as far back as 400 B.C. by the Greeks who used it to stop bleeding. Named from the Latin word *conferta,* meaning "to grow together," comfrey is a fast protein builder and helps the blood to coagulate. It is very effective when applied externally to wounds.

Dandelion *(Taraxacum officinale)*

This aster family perennial prefers full sun. Typically considered a weed, dandelion is one of the most nutritious greens. The French call it *dent de lion,* or "lion's tooth," for its jagged, dark-green, bitter leaves, which can be used in salads or juiced. The dried root and leaves are traditionally used as a rich coffee substitute.

As do most bitters, dandelion helps the liver secrete bile and stimulate digestion. Its use was first recorded in tenth-century Arabian medical texts and then later in sixteenth-century British apothecaries. European herbalists use dandelion to cure anemia, build blood, and aid digestion.

Dill *(Anethum graveolens)*

Named from the Norse word *dilla,* meaning "to lull," dill is sometimes used to induce sleep. Dill has a long, hollow stalk and feathery leaflets like a smaller version of fennel. With a distinctly sweet, sharp flavor, fresh dill stores well frozen.

Fennel *(Foeniculum officinale)*

This semi-hardy perennial is often cultivated as an annual. Fennel has a distinct flavor much like anise. The Greeks called fennel *marathon,* meaning "to grow thin," as it was valued for weight loss. Fennel grows from a bulbous root in branching green stems with wispy, feathery leaves and small yellow flowers. It is excellent for digestion and sweetening the breath.

Its traditional medicinal uses include arthritis, cramps, gastric ailments, exhaustion, low-immunity levels, poor memory, recovery from strokes, constipation, and obesity.

Green Tea

Green tea and black tea are from the same species of evergreen shrub. Different processing techniques result in the distinctive characteristics of different kinds of tea. Green tea is dried from the fresh tips and shoots. Black tea is from the denser, withering part of the plant that is rolled and dried. Oolong black tea is semifermented and dried. Green tea has a mild amount of caffeine; black teas have more concentrated amounts of caffeine.

Green tea has valuable phytonutrients, nutrient-rich compounds found in plants with health-giving properties. These phytonutrients, also called flavonoids, include catechin, epicatechin, and epigallocatechin. These phytonutrients have shown definitive results in sloughing off unwanted cholesterol deposits.

Effective antioxidants, also found in green tea, protect cells and scavenge free radicals, which damage tissue in our bodies. Studies show that antioxidant activity peaks 30 to 50 minutes after drinking green tea.

Green tea is an exotic addition to Asian marinades, especially to soak seaweed in.

Lemongrass *(Cymbopogon citratus)*

A perennial, tufted plant with long, green, sharp-edged leaves. When cut, lemongrass has a lovely, citrus-bouquet aroma, which is favored in Thai dishes. The flavor complements coconut and curried food. It's a subtle, culinary delight.

Licorice *(Glycyrrhiza)*

Licorice is an erect branching perennial plant with flowers resembling sweet pea. Licorice has a distinctly sweet flavor, aiding digestion and sweetening the breath. It measures fifty times sweeter than sugar, but contains no sugar. It is very balancing for blood sugar and the kidneys. Whole licorice root has been used for ages as a natural toothpaste because it whitens teeth.

Licorice is one of the oldest and most valued herbs. Hippocrates, Theophrastus, and Pliny all refer to licorice as a medicinal herb for health in their respective writings.

Marjoram *(Origanum marjorana)*

Marjoram is a perennial herb with a shallow root system and fuzzy, oval, pale-green leaves. There are several varieties of marjoram, all with a slightly spicy, herbaceous flavor, like a mild oregano.

Mint *(Mentha)*

There are more than twenty-five species of wild and cultivated mint. Mint has been recognized since the first century A.D. Mint is suspected to have originated in the Mediterranean region, although the truth remains a mystery.

It has a quintessential fresh, mint flavor. It is excellent with sweets and chocolates and in chilled teas and fruit juices.

American Apple Mint *(Mentha gentilis variegata)*

Also called golden apple mint, this variety has smooth, broad, pale gray-green-yellow variegated leaves. It has a delicate, fruity spearmint flavor.

Chocolate Mint *(Mentha piperita)*

This variety has small, smooth, dark-green leaves with a purple-red stem and veins. It has a deep, rich, mint flavor.

Curly Mint *(Mentha spicata)*

With wide, crinkled, dull-green leaves, curly mint makes a beautiful ornamental. It spreads quickly in a garden and grows up to two feet in height. It has a mild mint flavor.

Orange Mint *(Mentha citrata)*

With smooth, broad, dark leaves, edged with a touch of purple, this mint has a sweet, light, fruity mint flavor.

Peppermint *(Mentha piperita)*

Peppermint is also called "lamb mint." There are two types of peppermint: English black peppermint *(Mentha piperita vulgaris),* which has dark, smooth, green leaves and a strong biting mint flavor, and white peppermint *(Mentha piperita officinalis),* which has light-green, smooth leaves and a strong mint flavor.

Oregano *(Origanum vulgare)*

A close twin to marjoram, oregano is an aromatic, herbaceous perennial. Oregano grows small, oval leaves on erect, fuzzy, square stems. Oregano is used in cuisine all over the world in Mediterranean and South American cuisine. It has a strong, slightly spicy flavor that is often associated with Italian food.

Parsley *(Petroselinum crispum)*

Parsley is one of the most common and complementary herbs. A bright-green biennial, it is very high in chlorophyll, vitamin C, and vitamin K and strengthens collagen, which is essential for clotting blood. Used worldwide, it can often be found in French, Middle Eastern, Japanese, and Mexican food.

Traditionally used to treat jaundice and diseases of the bladder and kidneys, parsley is a purifier of the urinary system.

Curly Parsley

This is the familiar curly bunches of leaves that are often used as a garnish.

Italian Parsley

This variety of parsley has flat leaves with pointed tips that are similar in appearance to cilantro leaves or celery leaves. It has a stronger flavor than curly parsley.

Rosemary *(Rosmarinus officinalis)*

The Latin name for rosemary means "dew of the sea." Rosemary is a pungent and fragrant bush or shrub that resembles evergreen needles. Dainty lavender-colored flowers decorate the branches at times. It is an aromatic herb that complements thyme, oregano, and garlic.

Rosemary is known as a tonic for the liver and for cleansing the gallbladder. It also has soothing and calming properties. It has long been known to be good for the heart and to reduce blood pressure. Traditionally used for heart and liver disorders, high blood pressure, influenza, fatigue, digestive complaints, menstrual cramps, nervous disorders, and insomnia, this kind herb also has been used as a tonic for the hair and scalp for ages. It has been said that where rosemary grows of its own free will, there it is that the woman rules the house.

Thyme *(Thymus serpyllum* and *Thymus vulgaris)*

This herb has been traditionally used for digestive problems, fever, liver disorders, and fatigue.

Edible Flowers

Flowers are candy for the eyes. Edible flowers embody the essence of elegance and are a culinary delicacy. A sprinkling of colorful flowers elevates any dish or dessert to a feast for all the senses.

Many herbs produce edible flowers that captivate the essence of the herb. The flowers of herbs offer a light hint of the flavor of strong herbs and are a visual delicacy as a garnish.

Be mindful with flowers. Eat only flowers that you are sure are edible. There are as many poisonous flowers as there are edible flowers. Be certain they have been grown without pesticides. Flowers from commercial florists are beautiful but are laden with hazardous chemicals. Do not eat flowers that you have picked from the side of the road, as the exhaust and emissions from automobiles are not wise to ingest.

Flowers are the sensual, visual gifts of nature that seduce bees, bugs, birds, and bats to generously pollinate plant life. Be cognizant that every flower will bear at least one fruit or a handful of seeds. Pick with discretion and respect. The future of the plant is in the hands of your consideration.

There are many varieties of edible flowers, of which I will only delve into a few of the more familiar and available persuasion.

Borage

Borage has sweet, small trumpeting light-purple flowers with a delicate, vegetal flavor.

Broccoli

Broccoli has small, dainty white flowers with a delicate broccoli flavor.

Calendula (Calendula officinalis)

A member of the composite family, this annual prefers cool weather. It has a slightly bitter flavor. Christians called calendula "Marygold" because it bloomed during the festivals for the Virgin Mary. It is also known as a "pot marigold."

It has bright yellow to orange, thin daisylike petals. Marigolds have been called "poor man's saffron" as they are used to color culinary dishes, as saffron does, but at a fraction of the cost. They are perfect as a garnish on sweets or in savory dishes.

Medicinally known as an anti-inflammatory and antiviral, calendula, like echinacea, boosts the immune system to increase the particle-ingestion capacity of white blood cells. It also encourages collagen production to ensure healthy tissue and growth repair. Calendula is native to Asia and southern Europe. It grows twelve to eighteen inches in height.

Fresh Herbs and Flower Ice Cubes

Ice cubes infused with fresh herbs or edible flowers make an elegant addition to a glass of fresh water, lemon water, lemonade, or iced tea. Simply sprinkle an ice-cube tray with fresh herbs, fill with water, and freeze. Choice herbs and flowers to freeze include rose, lavender, mint, chamomile, sage, fennel, whole cloves, and whole allspice.

Chamomile *(Matricaria recutita)*

A member of the aster family, this annual prefers partial shade to full sun. It is mild and sweet in flavor. Native to eastern Europe, it is recognized in the pharmacopoeia in twenty-six countries. A mild sedative, it is commonly used as a calming tea. Chamomile has anti-inflammatory and antiseptic properties. With a yellow center surrounded by dainty white petals, it looks like a tiny daisy. It's a perfect garnish for sweets or salads.

Chives *(Allium schoenoprasum)*

A member of the amaryllis family, this hardy perennial prefers partial shade to full sun. Chives are hollow, grasslike stalks prized as a culinary herb with a mild oniony flavor. Chives produce light-purple, round, clustered, fluffy flowers in mid-spring. Good in salads and to garnish savory dishes, chives are native to northern Europe. They are easy to grow and reach ten to eighteen inches in height.

Daylily *(Hemerocallis)*

A member of the lily family, this perennial prefers full sun to partial shade. Each mature flower lasts for less than a day. Daylilies can be eaten as a bud or as an open flower. They have a vegetal, sweet flavor. Delicately crunchy and sweet, they are excellent in salads.

Daylilies flower in tall, clustering stalks in early spring. They are yellow-orange to tawny in color with a touch of orange, yellow, and red. The inside of the bloom is lightly speckled. Darker-colored flowers tend to be more bitter, and lighter-colored flowers tend to be sweeter. Daylilies have a fibrous root, not a bulb, and are related to lilies, but are not a true lily. The flowers have been known to lift the spirit. Traditionally, the crown and root are used medicinally.

Gardenia

Gardenia has large, white flowers that look like loose roses. They are very fragrant and mild in flavor.

Hibiscus

Hibiscus has a single layer of delicate, broad, red petals with a sweet flavor.

Honeysuckle

Honeysuckle has small, golden to white, trumpeting flowers that are very fragrant—like sweet honey.

Hyssop

Hyssop has small, clustering purple flowers with a sweet flavor like licorice and anise.

Jasmine

Jasmine has very fragrant, white to golden flowers with a sweet, perfumelike flavor.

Johnny-jump-up

These flowers are very similar to pansies. They come in a wide variety of colors, including purple, yellow, orange, and maroon. They have a mild vegetal flavor.

Lavender

Lavender has delicate lilac-purple flowers clustered on tall stalks. They are mild and sweet.

Lemon

Lemon trees produce small, white flowers. They have a delicate, sweet flavor. Be mindful that for every flower picked, there will be one less piece of fruit.

Nasturtium (Tropaeolum majus)

Native to Peru, this annual prefers full sun. It is named from the Latin words *nasus,* meaning "nose," and *torguere,* meaning "twist"—probably for its zesty, strong, spicy, peppery flavor. Good for salads and savory foods, the colorful, hearty flowers have smooth, round leaves with pale-green veins. Nasturtiums grow in six colors: cream, tangerine, deep mahogany, bright scarlet, cherry-rose, and soft salmon. This sprawling plant grows six to twelve inches tall.

Orange Blossom

Orange trees produce small, white flowers. They have a delicate, sweet flavor. Be mindful that for every flower picked, there will be one less piece of fruit.

Pansy *(Viola wittrockiana)*

A member of the violet family, this annual prefers cool weather. Pansy hybrids have been grown for more than 100 years. Dainty pansies are related to violets and Johnny-jump-ups. The French called this flower *pensée,* meaning "thinking of you." With bright hues of purple, blue, deep maroon, yellow, and red, they are beautiful on desserts. The face of the flower is two to five inches across. Pansies have a sweet, delicate flavor.

Pea

Pea shoots produce tiny white to yellow flowers with a sweet, vegetal, pea flavor.

Rose *(Rosa)*

A prickly shrub, rose prefers full sun. Roses existed 40 million years before humans walked the Earth. They are indigenous to the Northern Hemisphere, but none is native to the Southern Hemisphere. The rose family is the harbor for a generous botanical portfolio, including apples, pears, and many berries. There are more than 200 natural varieties of roses, and more than 20,000 man-made varieties. The first cultivated roses are on record from the Shen Nung dynasty in China from 2737–2697 B.C.

From white and classic red to purple, yellow, orange and every shade in between, roses have a delicate, fragrant flavor that should be used sparingly. Be sure to use only organically cultivated flowers. Commercial flowers, such as from a florist, are heavily laden with chemicals, pesticides, and preservatives. They beautifully decorate sweets or garnish a salad. Wonderful in fresh chilled tea or lemonade, roses are the essence of love.

Sage *(Salvia officinalis)*

A member of the mint family, this perennial prefers full sun to light shade. Native to Mediterranean regions, sage was named from the Latin word *salvare,* meaning "to save." Grown in monasteries in France and Switzerland, it was brought to England in the fourteenth century.

Sage is a culinary herb with gray-green, oblong, pebbly-textured leaves. Vibrant blue to violet flowers blossom in mid to late summer. It has a strong, herbal aroma and flavor, and is good with dishes flavored with tarragon, thyme, and oregano.

Signet Marigold (Tagetes tenufolia)

A member of the composite family, this annual prefers full sun. It is native to New Mexico and Argentina. Diminutive single flowers bloom bright yellow to orange. It is strongly scented and spicy like tarragon.

Squash Blossom (Curcubita pepo)

A member of the vine-fruit family, this annual prefers full sun. Squash is a generous vine. Squash flowers precede the fruit of the plant (such as zucchini, butternut, and acorn squashes). Each flower will bear a squash, so for each flower you pick, you will have one less fruit. Pick conscientiously or use picking as an opportunity to thin out an overbearing squash crop.

Each vibrant yellow to orange flower is about four inches across. Tender and mildly sweet, they be eaten as a closed or open blossom.

Sunflower

Sunflowers produce generous flowers, with bright, mildly sweet petals.

Tulip (Tulipa)

A member of the lily family, this bulb flower prefers full sun. Tulips have a beanlike flavor. They are one of the most highly prized flowers, especially in Holland.

Violet

Violets are brilliant to deep-purple flowers with a pansy-like face and a mildly sweet, vegetal flavor.

Spices

Spices are aromatic and flavorful substances from precious plants—bark, berries, buds, flowers, fruits, rhizomes (roots), seeds, or sprouts—used to enhance the flavor of food, whereas herbs are the fragrant leaves of plants. Most spices are described as "aromatic" or "pungent." Some spices, such as cinnamon and nutmeg, are aromatic without being hot; others, such as hot chilies, are pungent without much aroma. Most are a combination of the two.

Spices have long been revered as treasure. Playing a major role in economic development in many countries and civilizations for centuries, spices have been regarded as invaluable for their role in folk medicine and in modern medicine. Until well into the industrial revolution, spices were a commodity valued more than gold.

There is record of spices used as long ago as 3500 B.C. by the Egyptians to flavor food, for cosmetics, and in embalming practices. The spice trade was exclusively controlled by Arabs for 5,000 years. Spices were brought and grown through the Middle East and the Mediterranean to reach Europe. Arabs maintained control of the spice trade even throughout the powerful Greek and Roman civilizations.

After the fall of the Roman Empire in the fifth century, the Western world fell into the Dark Age, and the exotic dynamics of spices in Europe melted into the shadows.

Through the religious unrest of the Crusades, Muslims and Christians clashed over many things held precious to the hearts of all: religion and spices. Woven into the fabric of Muslim belief is the close association of spices and spirit.

Most spices are from India, Malaysia, and the East Indies. To arrive in Europe, spices had to be guarded through a long and arduous land route through Asia, Africa, and Arabia.

By the age of discovery in the 1400s, European seafarers were obsessed with finding a route to India and the Far East. Hence, the New World of the Americas was "discovered" by Europeans in pursuit of discovering a more feasible commercial route to the Far East for the spice trade. The Americas did not have the same spices sought after in the East. The New World did have the unprecedented gifts of chili peppers, vanilla, and allspice and a wealth of indigenous food and medicine never seen by the rest of the world.

Selecting Spices

Whole spices maintain their complex flavors much longer than ground spices. The subtle tastes and essential oils are present in whole spices and dissipate after being ground. Many spices are readily available in markets and store well, which is useful for spices that are not used regularly but are essential to lift the dynamics of a dish. Avoid cracked or hollow pods and be sure that spices are not faded or musty smelling.

Storing Spices

Spices are best stored in airtight glass jars and containers in a cool, dark place. Heat and moisture will compromise the flavors. Whole spices will keep for several months, even up to a year if mindfully stored. Ground spices begin to lose flavor after a few weeks or months, depending on how fresh they were upon purchase.

Freezing Spices

Storing spices in airtight containers or zip-lock bags in the freezer extends their shelf life—especially of the precious varieties that are hard to obtain or do not get used regularly.

Fresh, frozen spices, such as ginger and hot peppers, will keep in the freezer for up to six months. To use frozen ginger, grate what is needed from the frozen root and return it to the freezer.

Spices that have been frozen may be slightly limp when they have thawed, but their flavor will not be impaired.

Grinding Spices

Grinding or crushing spices releases their aroma and flavor. There are several methods, discussed below, depending on the spice. It is best to grind spices as needed, rather than in advance, to preserve the full flavor.

Mortar and Pestle

Pounding spices in a mortar and pestle is an ancient and traditional method. It is ideal for grinding small quantities.

Good seeds for a mortar and pestle include coriander, cumin, fennel, cardamom, caraway, dill seeds, mustard seeds, and fenugreek.

Pepper Mill

Typically used for grinding peppercorns, peppermills are good for larger seeds and "berries," including coriander, fenugreek, peppercorns, allspice, and cloves.

Electric Coffee Grinder

Using a coffee grinder is a quick and very effective method to pummel spices. It is particularly good for larger quantities.

Hand Grater

This is the choice method for custom amounts of larger-sized spices, such as nutmeg and fresh roots, including ginger and turmeric.

Allspice *(Pimenta dioica)*

Allspice is prepared from the seeds of a generous, broad-leaf tree from the myrtle family. Native to India and the West Indies, allspice's first recorded use was by Mayan Indians, who used it as a spice and for embalming long before the Spaniards reached the West Indies.

The fragrant aroma and taste is like an ambrosia of cloves, nutmeg, cinnamon, and black pepper. Fresh crushed leaves make an aromatic potpourri.

> *Origin:* Jamaica, South America
> *Taste:* Pungent, peppery-sweet
> *Aroma:* Fragrant, sweet, spicy
> *Traditional Cuisine:* West Indian, Indian
> *Culinary Uses:* Adds a warm, soft flavor to curries, cakes, jams, fruit pies, soups
> *Complements:* Pickling mixes

Anise *(Pimpinella anisum)*

A substitute for licorice, anise is known to ease the stomach and balance blood sugar.

> *Origin:* Middle East
> *Taste:* Similar to licorice
> *Aroma:* Slightly sweet
> *Traditional Cuisine:* European, Middle Eastern, Indian
> *Culinary Uses:* Cakes, candies, sweets, breads, soups, drinks
> *Complements:* Breath fresheners, licorice

Asafetida

A strong spice used in place of garlic and onion in the Ayruvedic tradition because it is considered to be milder and less aggravating to the system. Use it sparingly.

Origin: India, Pakistan
Taste: Pungent, oniony, garlicky
Aroma: Strong, pungent
Traditional Cuisine: Indian
Culinary Uses: Vegetables, pulses, pickles

Bay Leaf *(Laurus nobilis)*

Bay leaf is originally from Asia Minor and the Mediterranean regions. Bay leaves were fashioned into laurel crowns for emperors and heroes in Rome.

The towering fifty-foot tree has pale-yellow to green flowers. The leaves of the tree are dried and used to season soups and stews. The flavor is pungent, warm, and strong; use it sparingly.

Origin: Mediterranean, Asia Minor
Taste: Savory, warm
Aroma: Deep, sweet, woody
Traditional Cuisine: Mediterranean
Culinary Uses: Soups, stews, broths
Complements: Thyme, garlic, vegetables

Caraway *(Carum carvi)*

Caraway is one of the oldest spices known. Evidence of caraway seeds was found in preserved food remains from the Mesolithic period, more than 5,000 years ago. Caraway was also found in the tombs of ancient Egyptians to ward off evil spirits.

Caraway is a member of the parsley family and is traditionally associated with rye bread and sauerkraut. It has been chewed to sweeten the breath. A crescent-shaped, pale- to dark-brown seed, caraway has a sweet, peppery flavor with a hint of fennel.

Origin: Central Europe
Taste: Slightly warming, bitter
Aroma: Pungent
Traditional Cuisine: Eastern European, Jewish
Culinary Uses: Cabbage, breads, soups, sauerkraut, vegetables
Complements: Honey, garlic, oregano, rye

Cardamom *(Elettaria cardamomum)*

Cardamom is an herbaceous perennial bush of the ginger family. It is an ancient, favored spice that is said to have been grown in the garden of the king of Babylon in 720 B.C.

Cardamom is a dynamic spice that can complement sweet and savory food with a pungent, warm flavor with lemon overtones and the distinct hint of eucalyptus and camphor. It is good for whitening teeth and sweetening breath. It effectively exorcises garlic breath. It is favored in chai spice, curries, and garam masala. It is excellent in carrot cake and pumpkin breads.

Origin: India, Sri Lanka
Taste: Bittersweet, strong
Aroma: Sweet and pungent
Traditional Cuisine: Indian, Chinese, Thai
Culinary Uses: Chai spice, sweets, curry, garam masala
Complements: Curry

Chilies *(Capsicum annum)*

There are more than 150 varieties of chili peppers. Chilies are a nightshade plant like all peppers, tomatoes, and eggplants, native to Central and South America. Evidence of chili peppers was found in pre-Columbian Peru.

Columbus was the first European to taste the chili pepper. It was a great prize to bring back to Europe to spice bland food. Chilies were amicable for seafaring journeys with a generous shelf life of two to three years when properly dried.

Favored worldwide, their hot and spicy flavors spark taste buds and increase digestion. A little bit carries a long way.

Origin: Central America
Taste: Mild to fiery hot and spicy (Many varieties available—from mild to unbearably hot)

Aroma: Faint
Traditional Cuisine: Central and South American, Indian, Southeast Asian
Culinary Uses: Any savory dish, salsa, hot sauce, oils, pickles
Complements: Pepper, ginger, garlic

Cinnamon *(Cinnamomum zeylanicum)*

This is a familiar, warm spice with a home-baked aroma that complements most sweets. Freshly ground cinnamon from whole sticks is incredibly superior to powdered cinnamon. The aroma of the essential oils is intoxicating.

Origin: Sri Lanka
Taste: Delicate, sweet, warm
Aroma: Sweet, woody
Traditional Cuisine: Middle Eastern, European
Culinary Uses: Sweets, desserts, mulled wine and cider
Complements: Nutmeg, ginger, vanilla

Cloves *(Eugenia caryophyllus)*

Cloves were named from the Latin word *clavus,* meaning "nail." Cloves are a strong spice, long favored for culinary and medicinal uses. Cloves are the dried, unopened flower bud of the tropical evergreen tree of the myrtle family. They are used to numb the mouth and flavor cigarettes. Use sparingly to complement sweets and curries.

Origin: Indonesia
Taste: Sharp, hot, bittersweet
Aroma: Warm, sweet
Traditional Cuisine: Indian, European, American
Culinary Uses: Sweet and savory dishes, desserts, curries
Complements: Nutmeg, cinnamon, allspice, ginger, garam masala

A fragrant ornament can be made with a fresh orange and a handful of whole cloves. Pierce the orange skin with the sharp end of the clove. Cover the orange generously with cloves and hang from a string.

Cumin *(Cuminum cyminum)*

Cumin seeds have been used for more than 5,000 years and were found in the Egyptian pyramids. Cumin, like caraway, is an herbaceous perennial of the parsley family. Strong and spicy-sweet, it has a pungent-bitter background flavor. Freshly ground cumin seeds are superior to cumin powder. Cumin is excellent in guacamole.

> *Origin:* North Africa
> *Taste:* Pungent, slightly bitter
> *Aroma:* Strong, slightly sweet
> *Traditional Cuisine:* Mexican, Indian, Middle Eastern
> *Culinary Uses:* Vegetables, guacamole, pickles, salads, relishes
> *Complements:* Chili, saffron, cinnamon, coriander

Curry Leaf *(Murraya koenigii)*

Curry is an individual spice from the leaves of a subtropical tree originally from Sri Lanka. A medley of spices—including the irreplaceable curry leaf—is commonly known as curry. As the name implies, this spice yields a strong, warm, curry flavor.

> *Origin:* India, Sri Lanka
> *Taste:* Mild, like curry
> *Aroma:* Warm, spicy
> *Traditional Cuisine:* Indian, Southeast Asian
> *Culinary Uses:* An essential part of the spice mix known as curry

Fenugreek *(Trigonella foenumgraecum)*

Prized as a balancing herb in Ayruvedic medicine and used by the ancient Egyptians, fenugreek is originally from India and southern Europe. In India, fenugreek is grown for its angular seeds and to restore the soil, as it is known to be a nitrogen-fixing plant. Nitrogen-fixing plants have the ability to draw nitrogen from the air and feed it to the soil. It is like a "self-feeding" plant, because nitrogen is one of the most essential elements of fertile soil.

The fenugreek plant grows about two feet high with light-green leaves that look like clover or pea leaves. Ten to twenty seeds are harvested from each pod.

Bright to dull yellow in color with a tangy, burnt-sugar flavor, fenugreek is the aromatic part of curry spices.

Origin: Mediterranean
Taste: Astringent, bitter
Aroma: Strong
Traditional Cuisine: Indian, North African, European
Culinary Uses: Pickles, vegetables, curries
Complements: Red pepper, garlic

Ginger (*Zingiber officinale*)

An upright, tropical rhizome, or root, that grows three feet high with elegant lance-shaped, purple-tinged flowers. Ginger was referenced as early as 500 B.C. by the great philosopher Confucius. It aids digestion and increases circulation.

Origin: Southeast Asia
Taste: Spicy, slightly bitter
Aroma: Fresh, warm, sharp, lemony
Traditional Cuisine: Asian
Culinary Uses: For sweet and savory dishes, pickled, seaweed, vegetables, sweets
Complements: Garlic, curry

Mustard (*Brassica alba*)

Mustard is an ancient spice and is mentioned in the works of both Hippocrates and Pythagoras. Mustard is well favored in American cuisine as a condiment. Fresh mustard seeds are quite spicy. They make a good pickling spice.

Origin: Europe, Asia, America
Taste: Spicy, bitter, aromatic
Aroma: Subtle
Traditional Cuisine: Indian, European, American
Culinary Uses: Condiment, hot mustard sauce, pickling, salads
Complements: Garlic, fresh herbs
Varieties: White and yellow from Americas, black and brown from Europe, brown
   from India

Nutmeg and Mace *(Myristica fragrans)*

Nutmeg and mace are from a tropical evergreen tree that grows to sixty feet in height. The tree only produces nutmeg fruits after fifteen to twenty years, and then produces 1,500 to 2,000 fruits a year. The fruit is the size and color of an apricot and splits when ripe to reveal a brilliant red aril, called mace, plastered in entwined webbing around the dark shell of the nutmeg kernel.

Nutmeg is a narcotic and an exceptional spice for sweets. The nut of nutmeg is best fresh grated. Fresh is so far superior to ground. Its flavor complements cinnamon and vanilla. It is excellent in chai or egg nog–flavored drinks.

Origin: Moluccas
Taste: Sweet, aromatic
Aroma: Warm, like cinnamon
Traditional Cuisine: Southeast Asian, European
Culinary Uses: Sweets, desserts
Complements: Cinnamon, vanilla

Paprika *(Capsicum annum)*

Paprika is made from the powder of a mild pepper. It varies in spiciness depending on the heat of the pepper. It is a quintessential Hungarian spice brought by the Turks.

Origin: South and Central America, Eastern Europe
Taste: Hot, mildly sweet
Aroma: Warm, spicy
Traditional Cuisine: Hungarian, Middle Eastern
Culinary Uses: Grains, vegetables, sauces, soups
Varieties: Mild and sweet, hot, spicy

Pepper *(Piper nigrum)*

Pepper is a culinary staple and one of the most popular spices worldwide. Pepper is known as the king of spices. In the Middle Ages, dowries, rent, and taxes were commonly paid in part by pepper. It enhances the flavor of foods and adds hot undertones.

Origin: Southeast Asia
Taste: Clean, hot
Aroma: Warm, spicy, woody
Traditional Cuisine: Most countries
Culinary Uses: Infinite uses in practically any dish
Varieties: Black, brown, green, pink, red

Poppy *(Papaver somniferum)*

The poppy seed is well regarded in the Middle East as a good addition to savory and sweet foods, for medicinal purposes, and as a narcotic. The opium poppy has been prized for ages as the source of opium. High in protein and healthy oil, poppy also makes a beautiful garnish. In America, we find poppy seeds usually only on breads and bagels.

Origin: Mediterranean
Taste: Sweet, nutty
Aroma: Pleasant, nutty
Traditional Cuisine: Indian, European, Middle Eastern
Culinary Uses: Sweets, halava, grains
Varieties: Blue from Holland, cream from India

Saffron *(Crocus sativus)*

Saffron is the most expensive spice in the world and is treasured for its brilliant color and subtle flavor. Even today, the precious spice saffron, the stigma of a crocus flower, is sold by the gram. More than 200,000 stigmas must be hand harvested to yield one pound of saffron.

Origin: Asia Minor
Taste: Bitter
Aroma: Distinct
Traditional Cuisine: Indian, European
Culinary Uses: To color and flavor rice, cakes, liqueurs

Star Anise *(Illicium verum)*

Star anise is traditionally used in Japan as incense. It forms an eight-pointed star with a shiny, amber-colored seed. It is harvested from trees, which will grow and bear for more than 100 years. Like anise, it has a sweet, strong licorice flavor. It is an essential part of the spice blend known as Chinese 5 spice.

> *Origin:* China
> *Taste:* Warm, sweet, licorice
> *Aroma:* Sweet, fragrant, cinnamon-like
> *Traditional Cuisine:* Chinese, Vietnamese
> *Culinary Uses:* As part of Chinese 5 spice
> *Complements:* Cinnamon

Tamarind *(Tamarindus indica)*

A dark-brown fruit from the pod of the tropical, semi-evergreen tamarind tree. The six- to eight-inch pod has a sticky pulp, loaded with tartaric acid, which has a wonderful sweet-tart fla-

Spices and Herbs Used in Various Parts of the World

EAST			NORTH AND CENTRAL AFRICAN
ASIAN			
JAPANESE AND CHINESE	THAI AND PACIFIC RIM	INDIAN	
basil	basil	cardamom	chilies
cilantro	chilies	chilies	chives
coriander	cilantro	cinnamon	cinnamon
garlic	coriander	cloves	cloves
ginger	curry leaf	cumin	garlic
green onion	garlic	curry leaf	ginger
	ginger	fennel	mint
	mint	fenugreek	saffron
	parsley	garlic	
	tamarind	ginger	
	turmeric	mint	
		saffron	
		tamarind	
		turmeric	

vor. It is excellent in Caesar salad dressing and chutney and is traditionally used in curry. It is available in sticky blocks in ethnic stores.

Origin: Southeast Asia
Taste: Sour, fruity
Aroma: Slightly sweet
Traditional Cuisine: West Indian, Indian, Thai
Culinary Uses: Curries, chutneys, soups, condiments
Complements: Curry, spicy foods, garlic, ginger

Turmeric *(Curcuma domestica)*

A brilliant yellow-orange tropical rhizome, or root, with a similar shape to fresh ginger root, turmeric is the spice that gives curry its traditional color. It is used as a dye (and it will stain anything). In Malaysia, a paste of turmeric is made and spread on the mother's abdomen and umbilical cord for spiritual and medicinal purposes. Turmeric is quite bitter, hot, and peppery. It is valued for its blood-building properties. Although it is most widely available powdered, it is incredible as a fresh root.

WEST			
MEDITERRANEAN		**AMERICAS**	
ITALIAN	MIDDLE EASTERN AND GREEK	CONTINENTAL	MEXICAN AND SOUTH AMERICAN
basil	cilantro	basil	chilies
black pepper	dill	black pepper	chocolate
garlic	garlic	caraway	cilantro
marjoram	marjoram	cinnamon	cinnamon
oregano	oregano	garlic	coriander
parsley	parsley	oregano	cumin
rosemary	poppy	vanilla	garlic
sage	thyme		paprika
thyme			parsley

Origin: Southeast Asia
Taste: Pungent, hot, peppery
Aroma: Fresh, peppery
Traditional Cuisine: Indian, Southeast Asian
Culinary Uses: Curries, beans, grains
Complements: Mustard, garlic, ginger

Vanilla *(Vanilla planifolia)*

One of the most divine, intoxicating spices, vanilla is the stamen of a luminous, grayish-yellow-green orchid flower that grows on a vine up to eighty feet long. The long pods contain thousands of seeds. It takes up to six months to cure vanilla. Vanilla is more fragrant than it is flavorful. Intoxicating.

Origin: Central America
Taste: Sweet, divine
Aroma: Intoxicating, sweet
Traditional Cuisine: European, American
Culinary Uses: Sweets, chocolate

11

Sundries

Sweeteners

Sweetness makes the world go round. Honey and sweet fruits have been highly prized presumably since before recorded history. Sweetness is a multibillion-dollar industry, and sugar is everywhere, masked by seemingly innocent names.

Sugar is essential for life. Our brains run on glucose, a simple sugar, into which all other sugars are broken down. Our brains do not differentiate among the sources of the sugar, whether a piece of fruit, a candy bar, vegetables, honey, table sugar, starch, or whole grains. The brain simply requires the sugar. The body, on the other hand, certainly can differentiate among the sources and types of sugar. The empty calories of refined sugar burn out quickly, leeching minerals in the process.

Refined sugar upsets the body's natural balance. Refined sugar passes into the bloodstream too quickly. It also shocks the stomach, which is thrown into an acidic condition as it tries to cope with the situation. The acidic condition quickly depletes minerals, especially calcium. Stress is put on the pancreas to produce the right amount of insulin to regulate the blood sugar before the entire body goes into shock. The rush of energy from refined sugar is quickly exhausted, and havoc is left in its wake.

Our bodies are designed to process whole foods. Whole foods, like fruit and grains, have a brilliant balance of sugar and minerals. Sugar runs the brain, and minerals support the body. Mineral-rich sugars are released into the bloodstream in a regulated manner and extend the energy available from sugar for a longer period of time. Balanced sugars from whole foods do not tax the body and bloodstream, and provide a long, strong energy without the classic "sugar crashes" associated with refined sugar, which is devoid of minerals.

Date Sugar

Date sugar is made from dried, pulverized dates. It is very sweet, as dates contain plenty of naturally occurring sugars. Date sugar does not dissolve well, but it is an excellent ingredient for sweets.

Evaporated Cane Juice and Sucanat

Evaporated cane juice is literally organic sugarcane that has been juiced and dehydrated into crystallized granules. It is not heated to high temperatures and is rich in minerals and many nutrients. It is not bleached or refined in any way.

Sucanat is a trademark for crystalized dehydrated sugarcane juice. It is a wonderfully sweet and nutritious sugar. It has a golden-brown color and is as sweet as commercial sugar. Cane juice is certainly concentrated sugar and should be used in moderation.

Fruit Juice Concentrate

Concentrated fruit juice makes a great, unrefined sweetener. Fruit juice concentrate is sold as a sweetener, but organic frozen fruit juice concentrate also works well. Neither is raw.

Grain Sweeteners

Malted grain, also called malt syrup, is relatively nutritious with at least half of the nutrients found in whole grains. Malted grain syrups digest and metabolize more slowly than many sugars because they contain a good amount of complex carbohydrates. This regulates the absorption of sugar into the bloodstream and smooths out the radical rush associated with refined sugar.

These sweeteners are called "malt syrup" because maltose is the sugar that naturally occurs when the grains are sprouted to produce the syrup. Malted grain is not raw, but it contains many nutrients and minerals.

Granulated Barley Malt

This sweetener is made from sprouted, slow-cooked barley, dried until granular. It has a pale-brown color and a very mild sweetness.

Barley Malt Syrup

Barley malt syrup is a mild sweetener made from sprouted barley and water, slow-cooked into a very thick syrup. Mild and pleasant tasting, it has a golden-amber color.

Brown Rice and Brown Rice Malt Syrup

Brown rice syrup is made from brown rice that has been simply slow-cooked for a very long time into a very thick syrup. Mildly sweet, it has a pale golden-yellow color. Brown rice malt syrup is made from rice that has been sprouted before it is cooked. Both brown rice syrup and brown rice malt syrup are very gentle on the blood sugar, providing long-term energy.

Honey

Honey is a mixture of flower nectar, a sweet substance secreted by flowers, and bee enzymes. The main sugars in honey are fructose and glucose. Honey is sweeter than sugar and is absorbed directly into the bloodstream.

Honey contains all of the essential amino acids and a high concentration of essential nutrients. It is rich in carbohydrates, B-complex vitamins, and vitamins C, D, and E.

Raw honey is the only type of honey worth considering. Raw honey is rich in amylase, an enzyme that breaks down sugar. Honey that has been heated or filtered is devoid of enzymes and many of the precious nutrients. Unfiltered honey will contain small amounts of bee pollen, which is rich in nutrients, protein, all of the essential amino acids, and enzymes.

Maple Syrup

Maple syrup is a gift from the maple tree. For only three to four weeks in the spring when the nights are below freezing and the days are warm, sap flows up from the roots of the sugar maple.

The sap is distilled or (more commonly) boiled to concentrate the sugars into a syrup. The Native Americans traditionally gashed the trunk of the maple tree with a tomahawk (not harming it), and channeled the sap with wood funnels. They would allow the sap to freeze. The watery part of the sap would freeze first, and the ice would be removed, leaving pure, unrefined maple syrup. Alternatively, they would concentrate the sugar by dropping hot rocks into a container of the sap to evaporate the water.

Maple syrup is graded: Grade A, Grade B, and Grade C. Grade A maple syrup is considered to be the best, with a light and amber color, a thicker viscosity, and a clean sweet flavor. Grade B is usually less refined and darker, a bit thinner with a stronger maple flavor. Grade C is usually only available from maple syrup farms and is the least refined, quite watery with a strong

maple flavor. I prefer Grade B and Grade C (whenever I can find it), because they are less refined and have more minerals. I also enjoy the quintessential flavor of maple that the "lower"
grades embody.

Be sure to buy 100 percent pure maple syrup. Most commercial "maple syrup" that many
of us grew up with, classic with pancakes and waffles, is not pure maple syrup at all, but a mixture of corn syrup, sugar, caramel color, and artificial flavoring. This type of syrup is almost as
bad as soda pop and should be avoided.

Molasses

Molasses is the liquid that is separated from raw sugar during the process of sugar refining. Molasses is very rich in minerals. It is a thick syrup with a deep, dark-brown color and a strong
taste. Be sure to use only molasses that is a byproduct of organic sugar, as commercial sugar is
grown and processed with horrendous amounts of chemicals.

Refined Sugar

Highly refined, commercial sugar is sold on the sly under less-assuming names, like cane sugar,
natural cane sweetener, raw sugar, and turbinado sugar. If it is not organic, do not be fooled by
the guise of harmless and healthful names. It is still sugar.

Brown Sugar

Brown sugar is white sugar with molasses or caramel color added. It has been colored to appear
more wholesome. Brown sugar is just as harmful as white sugar.

Cane Sugar

The name appears more wholesome, but it is none other than white sugar.

Fructose

Fructose is a very refined sugar from corn syrup. It is not from fruit sugar as the name implies.
It wreaks havoc on blood sugar and depletes the body of minerals.

Raw Sugar

Raw sugar is not raw. It is simple coarsely ground white sugar that has not been bleached as
much as granular white sugar.

Turbinado Sugar

Turbinado sugar is sold along with health food under the guise of healthy sugar. There is nothing healthy about it. It is simply coarse white sugar that has been named after the turbine in which it is refined. This very successful marketing plan has fooled many consumers.

Xylitol and Sorbitol

Both xylitol and sorbitol are typically refined from commercial glucose and sucrose. Neither is recommended as a healthy sugar source or alternative.

Stevia

Stevia is a phenomenal herb native to South America and a member of the chrysanthemum family. Stevia does not contain any sugar but does contain glycosides, which taste very sweet to the tongue. Studies in Japan conclude that stevia *tastes* 300 times sweeter than sugar (sucrose).

Stevia does not affect blood sugar and does not cause cavities. It is an excellent alternative for anyone with blood sugar fluctuations or imbalances such as candidiasis, or anyone who cannot tolerate sugar or has a condition such as diabetes.

Stevia is strictly regulated by the FDA and is not "approved" as a sweetener. It can only be sold as a supplement. Meanwhile, excitotoxins and known carcinogens, such as aspartame, continue to be sold and mass-marketed as sugar alternatives. Stevia is the all-natural alternative to sugar and chemicals.

Stevia has been shown to actually help aid and rejuvenate the pancreas, the organ that takes the brunt of sugar misuse and abuse.

Stevia is sold as white powder or the less-refined green powder. It is also sold as a liquid, similar to an herbal tincture. The liquid may be clear or colored. In both cases, powdered stevia is simply mixed with water or alcohol to form a liquid.

Stevia has a very strong flavor. It is very sweet with a slight licorice flavor. A very small amount goes a very long way.

I have found that it is best to use stevia to boost the sweetness of a dish. For instance, fruits, maple syrup, or raw honey can be used in moderation with the addition of stevia. The flavor of the sweetener is carried by the stevia as if a lot of sweetener has been used.

Oil

Choosing a high-quality and nutritious oil is a learning process. As with most packaged food, labels are very misleading. Many of the steps of commercial processing are detrimental to the nutritional content of the oil, and are not required by law to be listed. Solvents, degumming, deodorizing, and pressing all leave room for a huge margin of compromise.

Fatty acids are the main components of fats and oils. There are about twenty fatty acids that the body needs to maintain normal function. Two of these, though, the body can't make on its own and must receive through diet—omega-3 and omega-6 fatty acids. Omega-6s are commonly available in many foods, so most people don't have to worry about meeting their requirements of this nutrient, but most don't get enough omega-3s in their diet. Omega-3s can be found in high amounts in flaxseed oil, and in moderate amounts in canola oil, walnut oil, wheat germ oil, and soybean oil.

Types of Fats in Oil

The fats found in oils can be saturated, monounsaturated, or polyunsaturated.

Saturated Fats

These are the "bad" oils. Saturated fats are usually solid at room temperature and are the ones that contribute to atherosclerosis and heart disease. Coconut, palm, and other tropical oils are high in saturated fats.

Monounsaturated Fats

Unsaturated fats used in place of saturated fats can lower your risk of heart disease. Unsaturated fats are much healthier than saturated fats. Monounsaturated fats are generally liquid at room temperature, but may solidify when cold. As these fats are the most resistant to oxidation, a process that can cause cell damage, these are considered the healthiest fats. Oils composed of monounsaturated fats include olive, peanut, avocado, and canola oils.

Polyunsaturated Fats

Polyunsaturated fats remain liquid at room temperature and in the refrigerator. Oils containing polyunsaturated fats include corn, safflower, sunflower, and cottonseed oils.

Oils to Absolutely AVOID!

· Cottonseed oil
· Fried oil
· Hydrogenated oil
· Margarine
· Shortening

Methods of Oil Extraction

There are four basic methods of extracting vegetable oils: expeller-pressing, solvent extraction, cold-pressing, and the Omegaflo® process.

Guide to Oils

OIL	TYPE	CONTENTS	COMMENTS
Almond oil	Monounsaturated	Omega-6 (26%) Omega-9 (65%) Saturated (9%)	A light oil with a slightly sweet flavor. Good for sweets and dressings.
Coconut butter	Naturally saturated	Lauric acid (43–53%) Omega-9 (9%) Saturated (89%)	Organic, unrefined, cold-pressed coconut butter is solid at room temperature. Very rich and buttery consistency and lower in calories than most fats and oils. Some unrefined coconut butter has a distinct coconut smell and flavor. Omega Nutrition has an excellent coconut butter that is clean-tasting without a strong smell. Excellent for sweets. A perfect butter replacement in any dish. Because of its naturally saturated-fat content, coconut butter is the safest and most stable oil for high temperatures.
Flax oil	Superpolyunsaturated	Omega-3 (57%) Omega-6 (34%) Omega-9 (18%) Saturated (9%)	Flax oil has a fairly strong, earthy flavor and a rich golden color. For balanced taste, it is best to mix with another, sweeter oil. It is the richest source of omega-3 of any oil and should be refrigerated at all times.
Hazelnut oil	Monounsaturated	Omega-6 (15%) Omega-9 (76%) Saturated (7%)	Hazelnut oil has a delicate aroma and flavor. Rich, deep golden-brown color. Delicious in marinades and sweets.
Hemp oil	Superpolyunsaturated	Omega-3 (20%) Omega-6 (58%) Omega-9 (11%) Saturated (9%)	Hemp oil is one of the most nutritious oils with all of the omegas, as well as GLA. It is a deep golden-green color and should be refrigerated at all times.
Olive oil	Monounsaturated	Omega-6 (8%) Omega-9 (82%) Saturated (10%)	Olive oil varies greatly in color and taste. Some varieties are golden and fruity, others are more green and rich. Always choose cold-pressed organic olive oil. A very versatile oil. Although all oils are best left raw, olive oil can tolerate temperatures up to 300°F for safer sautéing.
Pistachio oil	Monounsaturated	Omega-6 (31%) Omega-9 (54%) Saturated (12%)	Pistachio oil is highly prized as a culinary treat. Deep-green color and rich, sweet flavor. Excellent in pesto, marinades, and dressings.
Pumpkinseed oil	Polyunsaturated	Omega-6 (79%) Omega-9 (20%) Saturated (20%)	Pumpkinseed oil is a deep-green oil with a rich flavor. Good for dressings and sauces. Pumpkinseed oil can tolerate medium heat.

Guide to Oils *(continued)*

OIL	TYPE	CONTENTS	COMMENTS
Safflower oil	Polyunsaturated	Omega-6 (79%) Omega-9 (13%) Saturated (8%)	Safflower oil has a rich flavor and is very versatile. Be sure to use only unrefined, organic safflower oil. Golden in color and can tolerate medium heat.
Sesame oil	Monounsaturated	Omega-6 (41%) Omega-9 (46%) Saturated (13%)	Unrefined sesame oil has an authentic sesame taste. Sesame oil contains sesamol, a natural preservative, making it a very stable oil. Excellent for Mediterranean and Asian cuisines.
Sunflower oil	Polyunsaturated	Omega-6 (69%) Omega-9 (19%) Saturated (12%)	Sunflower oil is a golden color with the delicate flavor of sunflower seeds. Excellent in salad dressings. Be sure to use only unrefined, organic sunflower oil.

Expeller-Pressed, Unrefined, and Refined Oil

The material (nut, seed, grain, or bean) is cleaned and hulled. This is usually done mechanically, without heat. The material is then cooked at low temperatures (110°F to 180°F) for easier extraction. The material is crushed in large batches by a giant auger or screw to press out the oil. The material may be subjected to heat of 160°F to 190°F during this process. If the material does not undergo any further processing, it can be labeled "expeller-pressed" or "unrefined." However, many oils continue through further refinement.

Once the oil has been pressed, it is then degummed, which strips away the lecithin, chlorophyll, vitamin E, and minerals. It is subject to an alkaline solution to refine the oil and separate unwanted material (primarily nutrients).

Next, the oil is bleached, which removes the natural carotenes (vitamin A) and other nutrients along with it.

The oil is further deodorized by means of very high temperature steam distillation (more than 450°F). It is then often winterized, or prepared for storage, for further clarifying by cooling and filtering to render a colorless, odorless, tasteless, nutritionally void, clear oil with a long shelf life.

Oils that are labeled "partially refined" may be subject to any part or all of this detrimental process.

Solvent Extraction

Oil that is extracted by means of solvents does not have to be labeled as such. There are no laws subjugating the labeling of a "process," only the requirement of listing ingredients. Because solvents are extracted after they are exposed to the material, the solvent is not considered an "ingredient."

Extraction by means of solvents removes more oil from the material than expeller-pressing. The material is cleaned and hulled. It is then crushed into flakes by mechanical rollers.

A petrochemical solvent, most likely hexane or heptane (gasoline), is exposed to the material to extract the oil from the solid. After the extraction, the solvent is removed by being boiled off or evaporated at a temperature of about 300°F. It is currently unresolved whether any of the solvent remains. Hexane and heptane are very toxic materials, even in very small amounts.

Cold-Pressing

There is no legal definition of *cold-pressed*. It would seem that cold-pressed oils would involve a process without heat. This is untrue. There is no commercial process that maintains this type of extraction, except for small producers of olive oil.

In the 1950s, oil entrepreneurs attached the term *cold-pressed* to oils in the hope that this would appeal to health-conscious customers and would fetch a higher price. It worked, and the label stuck. In reality, these oils can be heated, degummed, bleached, and refined.

The Omegaflo® Process

The Omegaflo® process has the most integrity of any oil extraction process. It is used by Omega Nutrition to produce the best oil products on the market. It is designed to protect the precious and delicate essential fatty acids naturally found in seeds and nuts. Only organic material is used. The oils are always refrigerated from pressing to purchase.

The material is cleaned and hulled. It is cold-pressed in small batches in an oxygen-free and light-free environment. No further processing or refining is used. The oil is packed in opaque bottles and flushed and sealed with inert gas. The result leaves all nutrients intact.

Precious Components of Oil

These are the components of oil that we do not want removed in the pressing and refining process:

- *Carotenes*—Carotenes are the precursors of vitamin A. They are the red and yellow pigments in vegetation and food. They are necessary for good vision and strong immunity and help maintain mucous membranes and healthy hair, skin, nails, glands, and bones. Carotenes are passed on into cold-pressed, unrefined oils.
- *Chlorophyll*—Chlorophyll, plant's "blood," is almost molecularly identical to hemoglobin and therefore helps build our blood. Chlorophyll aids digestion and disinfects the intestinal tract. It's found in decent amounts in hemp seed oil and pumpkin seed oil.

- **Lecithin**—This substance is essential for brain function, since the brain's protective myelin sheath is made up mostly of lecithin. It is also important for healthy nerve tissue and for a healthy liver.
- **Vitamin E**—Vitamin E is the vitamin for longevity. A powerful antioxidant, it improves circulation, strengthens cell walls, and enhances cell-membrane integrity. Vitamin E regulates reproductive health and contributes to healthy skin, nails, and hair.

Vinegar

The word *vinegar* is derived from the French words *vin aigre,* meaning "sour wine." The "mother" of vinegar is a medley of bacteria, specifically *mycoderma aceti,* which is introduced to a liquid such as apple cider, wine, fruit, rice, or beer. The bacterial activity converts the liquid into a weak solution of acetic acid, which makes it sour. Some high-quality vinegar is sold "with the mother," meaning some of the original starter is included.

There are many kinds of vinegar made from many ingredients. Many varieties of vinegar are very acidic and kill healthy bacteria in the intestines. This includes distilled white vinegar and most wine vinegar. The exceptions are apple cider vinegar, umeboshi plum vinegar, and unfiltered brown rice vinegar, all of which have a balanced acidity.

Apple Cider Vinegar, Unpasteurized and Unfiltered

Apple cider vinegar is made from fermented apple cider and has a sweet-and-sour flavor. Apple cider vinegar is very high in minerals and promotes healthy digestion.

Apple cider vinegar should always be in stock in a good pantry. It can be used to balance many marinades and dressings or to complement and balance the strength of garlic, onion, and cabbage. Apple cider vinegar can replace lemon juice in most dishes for a tangy dynamic. Be sure to buy organic, raw, unfiltered apple cider vinegar.

Apple cider vinegar has been prized as a tonic for ages. It is a combination of alkaline elements and minerals and is stored as glycogen in the body for a direct source of fuel and energy.

With a mild 5 percent acidity, apple cider vinegar normalizes the body's acid-alkaline balance. Many vinegars are extremely acidic to the body and kill healthy bacteria in the intestines. Unlike most vinegar, apple cider vinegar supports a healthy digestive system and promotes balance of beneficial bacteria, ridding the guts of unwelcome overgrowth.

> Apple cider vinegar is one of the finest glass, mirror and surface cleaners. It is a natural disinfectant with a price that can't be beat.

Apple cider vinegar has antiseptic qualities with an acidic nature that is very cleansing and balancing to the digestive tract. The pectin in unfiltered apple cider vinegar promotes healthy bowels and elimination. The phosphorus prevents the buildup of putrefied bacteria in the intestines. The potassium encourages healthy cell growth and fluid balance in the cells and body.

A tonic of 1 tablespoon of apple cider vinegar in 8 ounces of water is very balancing taken first thing in the morning or a half hour before a meal.

Balsamic Vinegar

Balsamic vinegar is one of the most flavorful and prized vinegars. It is made in Italy from the white Trebbiano grape and gets a deep, rich color and pungent sweetness from aging in barrels of various woods and in graduating sizes for several years.

Unfortunately, balsamic vinegar is very acidic, and too much of it can be detrimental to healthy bacteria in our intestines. Many types of balsamic vinegar contain sulfites, an unwelcome preservative. Some balsamic vinegar contains natural sulfites that are not harmful to the body. Look for sulfate-free vinegar or vinegar with naturally occurring sulfites.

It is possible to responsibly enjoy the celebrated flavor of balsamic vinegar occasionally. Mixing and matching vinegar is a good formula. I recommend using a balanced vinegar such as apple cider vinegar as a base and a small splash of very good balsamic vinegar for splendid flavor.

Brown Rice Vinegar

Brown rice vinegar is made from fermented brown rice and is quite mild and slightly sweet and acidic. Brown rice vinegar is very tasty in Japanese preparations and can be enjoyed in moderation.

Umeboshi Plum Vinegar

Umeboshi plum vinegar is the pickling brine of umeboshi plums. It is the essence of umeboshi and is prized for balancing organic acids.

Umeboshi plum vinegar has a dynamic tangy, salty, sour flavor. An excellent "safe vinegar" with balanced acidity. It's perfect for salads, dressings, sauces, and dips.

Wine Vinegar, Red and White

Red wine vinegar and white wine vinegar are made from wine from fermented grapes. Wine vinegar has a sharp flavor. They are very acidic and reek havoc on healthy flora in the intestines. Wine vinegar should be used very sparingly or avoided completely.

Salt

Salt (sodium chloride) is a universal seasoning. It has been a valuable commodity throughout the ages for flavor and has been used as a preservative for ages. There are many kinds of salt, including sea salt, rock salt, and table salt.

Quality sun-dried sea salt is good for you; it is abundant in both essential and trace minerals. Celtic sea salt (see page 165) has more than eighty vital minerals, including magnesium, sulfur, potassium, calcium, silica, iron, manganese, and phosphorus.

Chloride—part of sodium chloride—is a component of our powerful digestive juices, hydrochloric acid. Salt is considered a digestive aid, strengthens digestion, and balances poor food combinations.

Beyond being pleasing to the palate and waking up digestive juices, salt is an essential partner in the sodium-potassium "pump" in every cell, necessary to maintain fluid balance and a healthy acid-alkaline balance in the body. Without sodium, the nervous system cannot function. However, sodium deficiency is not a concern in the American diet. The current guideline for daily salt consumption is about 3,000 to 5,000 milligrams (3 to 5 grams), less than ½ teaspoon, but average consumption is somewhere around 12,000 to 17,000 milligrams (12 to 17 grams!)—more than 3½ teaspoons of refined salt every day.

The Origin of Salt

Salt is formed out of the highly saturated solution of the sea. Salt precipitates into a solid form on smooth surfaces and crystallizes as the liquid evaporates. If the crystallization is slow and steady, the resulting crystals will be larger. If the process is hastened, the crystals will be smaller. Commercially produced salt is dried at very high temperatures and manipulated to produce uniform grains.

Rock salt and table salt are mined from dry salt beds where oceans once were. Rock salt has been leeched by rainwater for thousands of years and is usually devoid of some of the minerals found in fresh sea salt.

Natural sea salt should be gray and slightly moist as it is sun-dried or dried at low temperatures to preserve the precious minerals. Common table salt is dried at temperatures in excess of 3,000°F and has been stripped of all essential and trace minerals.

Types of Salt

Alae Salt *(Hawaiian Sea Salt)*
Alae salt is a mixture of sea salt and red Hawaiian clay. The red clay adds a supplement of natural iron and a beautiful soft-red color.

Edible Rock Salt *(Redmond Salt or RealSalt)*
Rock salt is mined from ancient sea-salt deposits in the earth, like common table salt. Unlike common table salt, this salt is not chemically purified. Good rock salt is rich in natural minerals and has a clean taste.

Fleur de Sel
Fleur de sel (meaning "flower of salt") is perhaps the finest salt available. For thousands of years, Fleur de Sel has been hand harvested from the top of shallow ponds of evaporating seawater on an island off the Atlantic coast of France. Fleur de Sel is composed of small crystals of porous, moist salt with slightly sweet, complex flavors.

Kosher Salt
Kosher salt is mined and processed the same devaluing way that table salt is. The only difference is that it is produced in a machine that makes coarser, larger grains of salt.

Sea Salt *(Sel de Mer)*
Sea salt is salt from seawater. Good sea salt is sun-dried and evaporated from seawater which preserves the precious trace minerals. Good sea salt should be moist and gray in color. It is available in coarse or fine grains.

Commercially produced sea salt is dried at high temperatures (3,000°F) and is therefore devoid of minerals. It is white and free-flowing.

Sea salt comes in several varieties:

- *Celtic sea salt*—Sun-dried sea salt harvested in Brittany using 2,000-year-old Celtic methods.
- *Lima sea salt*—Sun-dried sea salt harvested in western Europe and the Americas.
- *Maldon sea salt*—Sun-dried sea salt harvested in the Atlantic waters of England.
- *Si salt*—Sun-dried sea salt harvested in Mexico.

Table Salt *(Common Salt)*

Table salt is mined from ancient sea salt deposits in the earth. It is chemically demineralized and recrystalized as small, uniform grains. Table salt is primarily sodium chloride, although it usually contains additives such as magnesium carbonate to keep the salt from clumping.

Miso

Miso is a salty, savory, high-protein, fermented paste, rich in B vitamins and good cultures. Miso has been around for millennia. There is a record of miso's being used more than 2,500 years ago in China. The ancient Chinese called it *chiang* (pronounced *jang*). It is believed to have been brought to Japan in the seventh century by Buddhist priests.

Commonly made of soybeans, rice, or barley; salt; water; and a live culture, miso is used as a seasoning, like bouillon or soy sauce, and as a salty thickener in sauces.

Aspergillus oryzae, a live culture, is used to "start" the fermentation process, which digests the beans and grains into a savory paste with the consistency of soft peanut butter. The health-giving microorganisms of the culture predigest the miso to create an abundance of live enzymes and cultures, which feed a healthy balance of flora in the intestine.

The live cultures from miso are very alkalinizing for the body. The lactic-acid-forming bacteria, *lactobacillus* and *pediococcus,* aid digestion and assimilation.

Miso contains all eight of the essential amino acids necessary to assimilate protein. Miso is 12 to 20 percent protein, which is easily assimilated by the body, since it is a predigested protein. It is a precious source of plant-based B vitamins.

There are three traditional types of miso: barley, rice, and soybean. Generally, darker miso indicates a longer period of culturing and a stronger flavor. The lighter the miso, the mellower and sweeter the flavor.

Barley Miso *(Mugi Miso)*

Traditional Miso
Traditional barley miso is cultured for one to three years.

> *Color:* Dark brown
> *Texture:* Smooth and firm
> *Flavor:* Strong, salty

Carbohydrate: 21%
Protein: 13%
Salt: 13%

Mellow Barley Miso *(Amakuchi Mugi Miso)*

Mellow barley miso is cultured for only a few weeks to a few months.

Color: Light to dark brown
Texture: Smooth and firm
Flavor: Salty, not as sweet as mellow rice miso

Carbohydrate: 30%
Protein: 11%
Salt: 10%

Rice Miso *(Komé Miso)*

Red Miso *(Akamiso)*

Red miso is cultured for one to three years.

Color: Dark russet to reddish-brown
Texture: Soft and chunky to smooth and firm
Flavor: Rich, savory, and salty with sweet undertones

Carbohydrate: 19.1%
Protein: 13.5%
Salt: 13%

Light Yellow Miso *(Shinshu Miso*)*

Light yellow miso is cultured for less than one year.

Color: Light yellow to yellow-brown
Texture: Smooth and soft
Flavor: Mellow, salty, slightly sweet

*Named for an ancient province of northern Tokyo.

Carbohydrate: 19.6%
Protein: 13.5%
Salt: 12.5%

Mellow Red Miso *(Amakuchi Miso)*

Mellow red miso is cultured for six to twelve months.

Color: Light red to light brown
Texture: Smooth and soft
Flavor: Mellower than red

Carbohydrate: 27.9%
Protein: 12.6%
Salt: 13%

Mellow White Miso *(Shiro Koji)*

Mellow white miso is cultured for only a few months.

Color: Pale yellow to cream
Texture: Smooth and soft
Flavor: Mellow, sweet, and salty

Carbohydrate: 36%
Protein: 11.1%
Salt: 5.5%

Soybean Miso *(Mame Miso)*

Soybean miso is fundamentally different from rice miso and barley miso because it is made from a bean, not a grain. Hence, soybean miso generally requires longer aging.

Hatcho Miso

Hatcho miso is cultured for more than two years.

Color: Deep brown
Texture: Chunky, rich
Flavor: Deep, mellow sweetness, savory aroma

Carbohydrate: 12%
Protein: 21%
Salt: 10.6%

Natto Miso

Natto miso is made from soybeans, whole barley, barley malt, kombu, ginger, and sea salt. Natto miso is a hearty chutney and a delicious, balancing condiment.

Color: Cinnamon brown
Texture: Hearty, chunky
Flavor: Sweet and savory

Carbohydrate: 24%
Protein: 18%
Salt: 11.5%

Gourmet Pantry Extras

There are a few good treats that make a pantry capable of impromptu gourmet twists. A little bit of dynamic, distinguished, mature flavor goes a long way. It is best to use one or two primary flavors at a time rather than overwhelm a dish and lose the dynamic flavors.

Cacao Beans

Theobrama cacao chocolate, made from cacao beans, is known as the "food of the gods" in many languages. Cacao beans grow on the tropical evergreen cacao tree. Cacao is dried and processed to produce chocolate, cocoa powder, and cocoa butter.

Raw cacao beans can be found in specialty and ethnic markets. They are flat, dark-brown bean pods with a thin skin. Cacao is deliciously rich and bitter. Raw cacao beans can be ground and used in lieu of cocoa powder or chocolate. Fresh cacao beans must be sun-dried and peeled before using.

Capers (Capparis spinosa)

Capers are a sweet-tart flower bud of a low-growing bush with round thick leaves. The tree yields ornamental pink flowers with long tassels of purple stamens. The flowers open in the morning and are dead by midday.

Capers grow largely in Mediterranean regions where it is warm and dry. The caper buds are picked by hand and wilted in the sun. They are typically pickled with vinegar, olive oil, and a salty brine and packaged in jars. It is best to give capers a rinse before using them.

Cocoa Powder

Pure cocoa powder is made from fermented, roasted, and ground cacao beans. Cocoa powder is not considered to be "raw," but small amounts of it can be used in addition to carob to create an authentic chocolate flavor.

The word *chocolate* comes from *xocolatl,* the Aztec word meaning "bitter water." The unsweetened drink that the Aztecs made from pounded cocoa beans and spices was probably quite bitter.

Conventionally, the cacao beans are removed from their pods and fermented, dried, roasted, and cracked, separating the nibs from the shells. The nibs are ground to extract the cocoa butter, a natural vegetable fat, of which cocoa beans contain up to 54 percent, leaving a thick, dark paste called chocolate liquor.

The chocolate liquor is dried and ground into cocoa powder or further refined, adding lecithin, cocoa butter, and sweetener to make chocolate.

Nama Shoyu

Nama shoyu is a live, unpasteurized soy sauce. *Nama* means "raw" or "unpasteurized." Nama shoyu is aged several months to several years, usually in cedar kegs. It has a salty, savory, full-bodied flavor.

Nama shoyu is a staple condiment for flavor and seasoning in a living kitchen. It is excellent in marinades, dressings, and anywhere tamari or soy sauce is traditionally called for.

Nama shoyu is made from soybeans and wheat cultured with *Aspergillus oryzae,* or "koji" culture, which is also used to culture miso. Because it is unpasteurized, it is rich in naturally occurring enzymes and live beneficial organisms, such as *lactobaccilus,* for a healthy flora balance in your guts. (See the Resource Guide for a good source for nama shoyu.)

Nutritional Yeast

Nutritional yeast is a yellow, flaky yeast generally grown on molasses. It has a wonderfully "cheesy" flavor and is abundant in many nutrients, minerals, and vitamins. It is excellent to add to pâté and seed and nut cheeses to develop a cheesy flavor. Nutritional yeast is rich in B vitamins. Although it does not have naturally occurring vitamin B_{12}, it is commonly fortified with it.

Nutritional yeast has sixteen amino acids and fourteen minerals and is 52 percent protein. It is especially high in phosphorus.

Olives

Olives are a great stock for every pantry. Olives come in many colors, sizes, and flavors. Olives are a fruit that must be "cured" before they are edible. Olives picked fresh from a tree are terribly tannic and inedible. A brine, made from salt and water, is the usual bath for curing olives. Look for olives that are cured in sea salt for the best quality and nutritional choice. Avoid olives that have been treated with preservatives.

Olives were widely cultivated in Mediterranean regions and were enjoyed extensively by the Greeks and Romans. The remains of olives have been found in Egyptian tombs dating back to before 3500 B.C.

Olives grow on gnarly trees with small, silvery leaves. The trees grow very slowly and are not considered prime for choice productivity until they are fifty to seventy-five years old and will then produce fruit for centuries.

The two basic categories of olives are green olives and black olives. Green olives are younger olives and tend to be lighter and fruitier in flavor. Green olives can be found stuffed with anything from garlic to hot peppers. Black olives are ripe, more mature varieties. The older the olive, the more wrinkled the skin (just like us humans!). The flesh of riper olives tends to be softer and more flavorful.

Sun-dried olives are a savory variety of olives. Olives labeled "sun-dried" are likely to be cured and stored in well-tended conditions. Most sun-dried olives are dark, wrinkly, and very rich in flavor.

Olives will keep for a long time in the refrigerator. Opened olives can be stored in their brine for several months. If a white moldiness forms on the surface, it is an indication that the brine is oxidizing. The olives are still safe and perfectly edible to eat when well rinsed.

Pickled Ginger

Pickled ginger is a popular Japanese condiment, traditionally served with sushi. The best varieties are very simple without preservatives. Pickled ginger is a wonderful condiment that refreshes the palate between dishes.

Raw Carob Powder

Carob grows on a tropical tree in a long, leathery pod with a sweet edible pulp that is usually dried and ground into a powder. Carob is also called "locust bean" and is found in many processed foods. Carob is naturally sweet and is often used as an alternative to chocolate and cocoa. Much commercial carob is toasted, so be sure to look for "raw" carob.

Sun-Dried Tomatoes

Sun-dried tomatoes are a flavorful addition to many dishes and sauces. Sun-dried tomatoes are best purchased as dry pieces or halves and can be stored indefinitely in a cool, dry place. Look for organic sun-dried tomatoes. Some companies are very mindful of processing and preservation of nutrients and dry their tomatoes at low temperatures. However, most commercial companies process their sun-dried tomatoes at high temperatures. This destroys delicate flavor and precious nutrients and minerals. If you are uncertain about a particular product, call the company to inquire about the procedure and temperatures they use to dry the tomatoes. Be certain to use sun-dried tomatoes that do not contain the preservatives sulfur dioxide or sulfites.

Sun-dried tomatoes can be soaked in fresh water until soft and then blended for thickening sauces. They can also be cut into small pieces and added directly to a marinating dish to soak up the flavor.

Marinated sun-dried tomatoes can also be purchased in a jar. Be mindful of the ingredients as most manufacturers use inorganic oils and sneak in preservatives.

Umeboshi Plums

Umeboshi plums are a prize. They are pickled, unripe plums that have been soaked in the sunshine with brine and shiso leaves, or beefsteak leaves, for flavor and a brilliant deep-pink color.

Umeboshi plums have an unusual and wild salty-sweet-tart flavor. They are very nutritious and are valued for balancing elements. Because they embody such a dynamic range of flavors and are very good for digestion, eating an umeboshi plum with every meal is a prescription for health according to some macrobiotic traditions.

Umeboshi Plum Paste

Also called bainiku, umeboshi plum paste is puréed umeboshi plums and shiso leaves. The paste is very convenient for adding to sauces and marinades.

Available in health food stores and Asian markets, it is fairly expensive, but a little bit goes a long way and it keeps fresh for a long, long time.

Vanilla Extract

Vanilla extract is an essential component of a sweet pantry. Vanilla extract is a dark amber-brown liquid and the most common form of vanilla beans available. The vanilla bean is the stamen of a gorgeous, grayish-yellow-green orchid native to tropical America. It is a sensually fragrant, long, dark pod that contains thousands of tiny seeds. It was traditionally cultivated and processed by the Aztecs, who used it to flavor their *xocolatl,* an unsweetened chocolate drink.

Vanilla extract is made from vanilla beans that are steeped in alcohol or glycerine to extract the flavor. The mixture is then aged for up to several months.

Wasabi

Wasabi is a Japanese variety of horseradish from a root of an Asian plant. Wasabi is dried into a pale-green powder that is mixed with water to make a sharp, potent, fiery paste traditionally served with sushi and sashimi. Wasabi is uniquely hot and spicy. The heat tingles the sinuses, and too much certainly makes the eyes water. Wasabi is very cleansing for the sinuses and mucous membranes.

Wasabi is most commonly sold as a dry powder or as a paste. It can be mixed with mustard, horseradish, and gardenia. Be sure to check the ingredients, as many varieties have artificial colors and preservatives. Some specialty and Asian markets carry fresh wasabi, which can be grated like horseradish.

The Prime
Raw Foods Kitchen
Equipment and Tools

The kitchen is a temple and should be a good friend. It is where magic and alchemy interface with mouthwatering pleasure. Stocking the raw foods kitchen with basic amenities is simple when the needs of a savvy chef are known.

There are three basic categories of equipment for a smooth-running kitchen:

1. *Manual Equipment:* knives, cutting boards, and kitchen gadgets and tools.
2. *Electrical Appliances:* blenders, food processors, and juicers.
3. *Bowls, Platters, Dishes, and Plates:* mixing bowls, salad bowls, serving bowls, dishes, platters, and plates.

The basic stock for a kitchen should start simply and grow with skill and use. Culinary equipment is an investment. Good-quality equipment can last a lifetime if it is cared for. It is better to make an intelligent purchase of good-quality equipment than load the cupboards with shabby, unused goods. It is nice to have all the toys your heart desires, but it is possible to get away with minimal accessories if you know your needs.

Manual Equipment

Good Knives

Every kitchen should have at least three good knives: a large chef's knife, a small paring knife, and a quality serrated knife (with a blade like a saw).

There are many quality brands available. Shapes and handles are the elements to look for. The best-quality knives have the base of the blade running all the way through the handle for a lifetime of sturdy service.

Chef's Knife

A chef's knife is the workhorse of the kitchen. It has a large curved blade that can be used for most cutting, slicing, chopping, dicing, and mincing. Chef's knives vary slightly in size. Find one that has a comfortable handle that feels good in your hand. It should have a good feel of weight, not too flimsy, not too heavy, and not cumbersome. Treated properly, this knife can be with you for a lifetime.

Paring Knife

A paring knife is a small knife with a slightly curved blade. It is not much longer than an index finger. This little guy makes it easy to work with small ingredients, and is safer than a chef's knife for details.

Serrated Knife

Serrated knives come in all shapes and sizes. What distinguishes a serrated knife from other knives is the blade. A serrated blade is scalloped like a saw. This type of blade makes cutting certain produce much easier. Tomatoes are a classic example. A serrated knife will cut through the skin of a tomato cleanly and easily. A super-sharp straight-edged knife can do the task, but a dull knife will more than likely mush the tomato. Serrated knives are also great for slicing sushi and other soft-skinned fruits, such as plums and apricots, without mauling them.

Knife Sharpener

Quality knives are only good when they are sharp. Sharp knives are also much safer to work with, with less risk of slipping and cutting your precious fingers instead of the produce.

There are three basic types of knife sharpeners: cylinder sword sharpeners, mechanical wheel sharpeners, and sharpening stones.

Serrated knives should be sharpened with care. Serrated knives can be gently sharpened on a sharpening steel or the fine-grain side of a whetstone. They should not be sharpened on a wheel sharpener. Having serrated knives sharpened professionally is ideal when available. Many culinary stores provide this service.

Cylinder Sword Sharpener (Sharpening Steel, also called "Butcher's Steel")

This is a long, round, heavy, metal sharpener with a surface not much rougher than a fine nail file. It is held in one hand, and the knife blade is swept toward the tip of the sword at a 20- to 30-degree angle five or six times on one side and then on the other. It takes a little coordination but is very effective.

Sharpening steels are best for knives that are only mildly dull. Knives that are very dull must be sharpened on a whetstone first and fine-honed on a sharpening steel. It is best to choose a sharpening steel that is longer than the knife to be sharpened.

Mechanical Wheel Sharpener

This is a small sharpener with two sets of stacked metal wheels that are fitted with a little give so that they slightly overlap. A valley between the wheels is where the knife is sharpened. Wheel sharpeners are usually handheld. Some types rest on the counter. The blade of the knife is drawn through the valley again and again until sharp. These sharpeners are inexpensive and are very easy to use.

Sharpening Stone (Whetstone, Oilstone)

A sharpening stone is typically a rectangular stone made from carborundum (silicon carbide), which feels like a very fine pumice stone. Some whetstones must be lubricated with water or oil, and some sharpening stones can be used dry. Follow the manufacturer's instructions. The blade of the knife is drawn across the stone at a 20- to 30-degree angle away from the blade, five or six times on one side and then the other for sharpening. If the two sides of the stone have different textures, the knife should be sharpened first on the coarser side and finished on the finer-grain side. Whetstones are a good tool for knives that are very dull. Sharpening stones are inexpensive, but take a little skill to be used effectively.

Cutting Board

A good, hefty cutting board is the foundation of the kitchen. There are wooden and plastic cutting boards. There are also very thin cutting surfaces for travel and easy storage.

Wooden Cutting Board

Wooden cutting boards are the highest quality. Knives are protected by the natural give of wood. I recommend using one side of the board for fruit and the other side for vegetables, especially garlic and onion, to avoid mixing flavors (like onion and mango). If the board is not designed for both sides to be used, a separate board can be used for pungent produce or fruit.

There has been question if wood is sanitary or if it can get moldy. Wood has natural resins that are antiseptic. As long as the wooden cutting board is well washed and thoroughly dried after use, there is no problem. Avoid cutting boards that have a finish. The finish is not meant to be ingested, but over time it will be nicked and pieces could end up in your meals.

Plastic Cutting Board

Plastic cutting boards are usually less expensive than wooden cutting boards. Some folks say that plastic is more sanitary than wood, but plastic is not for eating, and after prolonged use it will inevitably end up in food. Very hard plastic cutting boards, which are designed to reduce the risk of plastic getting in food, are so hard that they dull knives quickly.

Thin Plastic Cutting Board

These are very handy and inexpensive. They are thin sheets of durable plastic that can sustain even a heavy, sharp knife. They store easily and are great for traveling or to have on hand for a party, when extra cutting boards are needed.

Dry Measuring Cups

A set of measuring cups is a standard, inexpensive basic to have in any kitchen. As culinary skills develop, measuring cups might be traded in for eyeing amounts and mixing to please a seasoned palate. A standard set of measuring cups will include a ¼-cup, ⅓-cup, ½-cup, ¾-cup, and 1-cup measurer. Stainless steel is the way to go over plastic. Plastic off-gasses and leeches into food over time and is best avoided whenever possible. Stainless steel will last for the rest of your life.

Liquid Measuring Cups

Glass or Pyrex liquid measuring cups are essential for exacting a good measure for liquids like water, juice, shoyu, and vinegar. They have a handy pinch on the rim for easy pouring. A set including 1-cup, 2-cup and 4-cup measurers is ideal. If choosing only one, a 2-cup measurer will serve best for overall use.

Measuring Spoons

A set of measuring spoons is a simple aid for measuring small amounts of herbs, spices, shoyu, vinegar, honey, maple syrup, sea salt, and so on. After some quality time in the kitchen, a "splash," "drizzle," or "pinch" may become more frequent language. Although following recipes provides a sound base from which to work, always season to your own taste.

A standard measuring spoon set will include ⅛ teaspoon, ¼ teaspoon, ½ teaspoon, 1 teaspoon, and 1 tablespoon.

Grater/Shredder

A grater or shredder is an indispensable tool. There are a variety of shapes and sizes that can be used for grating or shredding carrots, apples, ginger, beets, sweet potatoes, and any firm vegetable.

Graters with four or more sides that can stand on their own are versatile and sturdy. Each side has different-sized holes for grating various levels of fine shreds. The finer sides are good for ginger and delicate carrots, and the finest side can double as a zester for citrus.

Peeler

A sturdy peeler can get lots of action peeling carrots, cucumbers, beets, apples, pears—you name it. It is a good tool for creating long ribbons of carrot for delicate dishes and garnish. I love a peeler with a generous rubber handle that is kind to the paws and prevents a hand from cramping from a zealous grip.

Citrus Zester

A citrus zester is a handy goody for a beginner's or veteran's kitchen. It is designed to grate or peel the delectable thin outer skin of citrus, like lemon, without the bitter white pith beneath. Citrus zest is a wonderful ingredient with the quintessential flavor of citrus.

There are two types of zesters: toothed zester and file zester.

Toothed Zester

This is a small zester, not much longer than the width of your palm with a row of teeth for grating the zest. This type of zester makes beautiful citrus shavings that make a delicate garnish as well as a tasty ingredient. There is also a larger raised tooth below the other teeth that can carve larger curls of peel for good looks or flavor.

File Zester

A file zester is usually six to nine inches long with a flat face and small grates for zesting citrus skin. These zesters are brilliant. No matter how firmly the citrus is grated, only the most choice, colorful outer layer of skin is shaved very delicately. Lovely.

Garlic Press

A good garlic press makes dealing with garlic a clean pleasure. Pressed garlic has a lighter, more delicate flavor than minced garlic because it excludes the bitter center stem. All garlic presses have a flat face of holes that the garlic is squeezed through. Some presses have a face on a moving hinge for more pressure with less effort. Others have a flat face that applies direct pressure to press the garlic through the holes. A quality heavy garlic press is worth the buy, and it will last a lifetime.

Ginger Grater

This is a porcelain grater designed specifically for shredding ginger. It is an inexpensive, handy tool for ginger lovers. Ginger graters come in a variety of shapes and sizes. Some are small, flat, and rectangular, and others are small and concave. They have a flat face with rough bumps for grating. These kinds of graters make grating ginger an easy task without the risk of grating precious fingers.

Kitchen Scissors

A sturdy pair of sharp kitchen scissors is a useful tool for cutting dried fruit, sun-dried tomatoes, and nori sheets. A pair of scissors dedicated for food-only use benefits all parties involved. It will keep glue, tape, and paste from getting in your food, and food from getting in your office supplies. Everyone wins.

Saladacco (Spiralizer, Spiral Slicer)

There is a good question if a Saladacco (also called a spiralizer or spiral slicer) is a "basic" piece of kitchen equipment. It is so wonderful and handy that it has a high priority in my kitchen.

A Saladacco is a stacked plastic tool that can cut hard vegetables into threads and delicate ribbons. The top part of the machine has a flat plastic disk with teeth, which is easily turned by a handle from above. The top part fixes into the middle section, which contains a blade. The vegetable is pressed into the teeth of the disk, and the handle is turned. As it rotates, the blade produces long, uninterrupted threads of the vegetables, as delicate as angel hair pasta. Oh, this thing is great. (See the Resource Guide for ordering information.)

Rubber Spatula

Rubber spatulas are a chef's best friend. Spreading, scraping, and licking are pleasures with these guys. They are especially handy for getting all of the good out of the awkward angles of a blender or food processor. These tools will be welcomed and used again and again.

Small Wooden Spoon

A small wooden spoon, the size of a traditional metal teaspoon or tablespoon, is necessary for spooning honey and miso, to protect the delicate enzymes. Metal is very reactive and destroys the precious goodies in both raw honey and miso. I like to use wood whenever possible, as it is a gentle, respectable surface.

Bamboo Sushi Roller

A bamboo sushi roller is essential for tight, professionally rolled sushi that can be cut to perfection. Bamboo sushi mats will set you back a dollar or two and are available in health food stores and Asian markets.

Strainer

A fine strainer is a handy tool for draining soaked goods such as nuts and sun-dried tomatoes. Two strainers are better than one—one small strainer (four inches across) for details and a large strainer (six to eight inches across) for larger duties. Stainless steel is a better choice than plastic. Stainless steel is very sturdy and will last a lifetime. Plastic off-gasses and leeches into food over time.

Steamer

A basket steamer is a handy and easily stored tool for steaming vegetables. It can also double as a strainer on the sly. Some steamers sit above a fitted pot. This is a set that works very well. Additionally, there are steaming units (equipped with a timer) that sit on the countertop for those who do not want to mess with the stove.

Hand Citrus Juicer

A hand citrus juicer is a great tool for squeezing fresh lemon, orange, and lime juice. There are a few kinds of hand juicers, most of which are equally easy to use. They are usually made from glass, metal, or plastic and are not much larger than a fist or two. Most models sit on the counter with a blunt, ribbed spike. A citrus fruit, such as a lemon, lime, or orange, is cut in half and pressed, squeezed, and turned on the spike to extract the juice. The juice is caught in the bottom part of the juicer in a little moat. Some models have a strainer over the moat to catch seeds and extra pulp.

Another type of hand citrus juicer is a similar blunt spike with ribs attached to a post handle. The citrus half is held in one hand and the spike is ground into the half, squeezing it to extract the juice. It takes a little coordination and can be a spot messy.

Mortar and Pestle

A mortar and pestle is one of the most ancient pieces of culinary and medicinal equipment. It is a heavy bowl with a rounded pounding stick. Generally made from heavy stone such as marble, a mortar and pestle is used primarily for grinding fresh spices. The delicacy of freshly ground spices is worth this easy effort. A mortar and pestle is fairly inexpensive and will last a lifetime.

Spice Grater/Nutmeg Grater

This nimble tool makes grating some spices a cinch. The grade of the holes is perfect for shaving nutmeg and cinnamon sticks. The flavor and aroma of freshly ground spices are superior to spices that are already ground. It is easy to clean and hold.

Pastry Bag

Pastry bags are a perfect tool for decorative detail. A set can be purchased with a variety of "tip" attachments for different designs. The pastry bag can be used to write "Happy Birthday" and other messages or to draw on confections. If you do not have a pastry bag, a clean plastic bag with a flat corner (not a pleated corner) will work. Simply spoon in the creamy goods, snip off a small corner, and squeeze the cream through the hole.

Melon Ball Spoon (Melon Baller)

A melon baller is a spoon in the shape of a perfect half circle designed to scoop melon into balls for a pretty presentation. Melon ball spoons can be used for any melon, including cantaloupe, Crenshaw, honeydew, and watermelon. It's also great for papaya.

Serving Spatula

A good serving spatula can make or break the presentation of many desserts. I recommend a thin, flexible, trianglular server. This will serve for most pies and cakes with ease. Stainless steel is a better choice than plastic.

Glass Jars

Glass jars of all shapes and sizes are useful for soaking, sprouting, and storing. Mason jars are ideal because the ring that screws onto the jar is separate from the lid. A piece of screen can be secured by the ring, making it useful for sprouting and draining.

Some health food stores and specialty markets carry "sprout" jars that have lids and screens for this purpose. In a pinch, any widemouthed glass jar can be used with screen or mesh held by a rubber band.

Hand Towels!

A lot of towels ensures a clean process. Paper towels are an unnecessary waste of precious trees. A plethora of towels encourages surfaces to be wiped and cleaned regularly. Cleanliness is of the utmost importance. Keeping your hands dry will preserve your precious skin. Take a look at most chefs' mangled paws. Towels that are 100 percent cotton are the way to go. Avoid synthetics, especially anything with polyester, which is not very absorbable.

Canvas or Reusable Grocery Bags

Bringing a reusable bag to the market takes only a smidge of effort but returns many personal and planetary rewards. Many markets offer a 5- to 20-cent discount for every bag you use. A good, sturdy bag will protect your fresh produce from being crushed and bruised better than a paper or plastic bag. Reducing disposable waste is a growing priority in our global reality. Taking personal responsibility for conscious consumption is the next step toward the bigger picture and the protection of our children's future.

Electrical Appliances

Blender

A blender is a basic, yet essential, piece of equipment. It is a requisite for making dressings, sauces, soups, and smoothies. There are inexpensive models that are good to start with; later you may want to invest in a high-end blender. Look for a blender with variable speeds to control how fast the blade whips. Blenders cost from $30 to $200.

Food Processor

A good food processor makes fine cuisine a dream. It is a necessary tool for any new or seasoned chef. There are different sizes for different needs. A 7-cup, 9-cup, or 11-cup processor is a fair choice for regular household use.

I recommend investing in a good food processor if possible. The difference between a good food processor and a cheap, shabby one is worth the money. A good food processor has a heavy, strong motor that will not give up. (I have one that survived years in a restaurant kitchen and is still kicking.)

Different brands frequently have the same functions. They usually come with several attachments that serve different purposes. There is an S-shaped blade that sits in the bottom of the carafe used for grinding, mincing, and chopping. By the way, this is the only blade used for the recipes in this book. Most brands also have a shredding and slicing blade, both of which are flat disks with holes or crescents to create the desired design. There are several good brands on the market, but Cuisinart is my trusted brand for a great machine with a reasonable price tag, $160 to $200 (and worth every penny).

Juicer

A juicer is, of course, essential to the raw foods kitchen. Most home juicers are designed for vegetables and fruit (except citrus). Citrus juicers are best for citrus. Some juicers have other attachments that can be used to make pâté, hummus, and frozen sorbet. (See Chapter 15 for more information on juicers.)

Bowls, Platters, Dishes, and Plates

Bowls, platters, dishes, and plates in different shapes and sizes are necessary for preparing and serving beautiful cuisine. Glass and ceramic are the best choices. Start with a few pieces and add more as your needs grow. Yard sales are a good place to find inexpensive pieces (and recycling is cool).

Mixing Bowls

A good set of mixing bowls is a must-have basic. Glass or stainless steel is the best material. Avoid plastic whenever possible (for personal and global health).

A set of three to six stackable bowls is a good start and build from there. Having a second medium-large bowl is useful to have on hand. Mixing bowls can double as serving bowls for casual everyday use.

Generous Salad Bowls

A beautiful salad bowl will make preparing and serving salad a pleasure and a charm. Wooden salad bowls are an ultimate choice. Ceramic or glass bowls are also good and are usually less expensive.

Pie Plates

Glass and Pyrex pie plates are essential for well-served pies, tortes, and vegetable quiches. A 10-inch pie plate is standard. However, a variety of sizes and depths makes assembly of various dishes easy.

Torte Pans

Torte pans resemble metal pie plates, but they are made up of two pieces. A ringlike housing separates from a flat circular bottom. Torte pans can make freestanding pies, tarts, and tortes for gorgeous presentation. They are available in every size from 4 to 14 inches. They are relatively inexpensive, so having a few sizes on hand helps to suit the company to be served.

The Next Level: Gourmet Kitchen Equipment

The needs of a seasoned chef grow into new toys for the kitchen. Kitchen equipment is a long-term investment that can provide a lifetime of pleasure and health. Ceramic knives, special cutting tools, glorified blenders, and dehydrators make culinary masterpieces a reality.

Ceramic Knives

Someone who loves me very much gave me two ceramic knives as a gift—a chef's knife and a paring knife. At first sight, I knew I would love them, although it took me a few months to get comfortable with them. I was very concerned that I would break them. While ceramic knives will break if dropped on a marble floor, they are sturdy enough to handle the tough stuff. I do not use them to pound garlic or to regularly cut very dense vegetables, such as jicama, but now they are my first choice for chopping, slicing, and cutting almost anything.

The deal with ceramic knives is that they are made of a nonmetallic mineral (clay). Metal is a very reactive compound, which is why a wooden spoon should be used for spooning live miso and raw honey, as explained earlier. The claim is made that ceramic knives need to be sharpened only once every two years (when used daily). They must be sent back to the manufacturer for that task, however. My knives are still as sharp as the day I got them, so I am convinced of the claim so far. I have had some of them for ten years.

Ceramic knives do require a bit of special handling and storage. I keep them in a knife block on the counter to protect them and in a special homemade box when traveling.

Mandoline

A mandoline is a clever slicing-dicing manual machine. It cuts vegetables into thin slices and strips in a snap. A mandoline is a rectangular machine made of metal or plastic with a very sharp blade in the middle for paper-thin slicing. A set of razor-sharp teeth can be fitted to the blade to produce matchstick slices when vegetables slide by. There are various-sized teeth for wider and more delicate cuts. Mandolines vary in price and quality. They range from $40 to $250.

Double Boiler

A double boiler is a pan that fits inside of another pan. The pan beneath is filled with water, and, as the water heats, it gently warms the food in the upper pan. This way, the heat does not directly heat the food. This is a great way to safely and gently warm food without the risk of losing enzymes and nutrients to high heat. Double boilers are excellent for making soups, sauces, and marinated vegetable dishes.

Vita-Mix Vita-Prep

The Vita-Prep by Vita-Mix is a glorified blender that can whip at extremely high speeds. The Vita Mixer is the Rolls Royce of blenders. The high-powered motor can pummel just about everything. The Vita-Prep can perform any food-processing task and can be used like a blender for creams, smoothies, and sauces. It can even grind grain into flour and seeds into powder.

The Vita-Mix Home Model has one speed. The Vita-Mix Total Nutrition has variable speeds (I recommend this one). Call Evergreen Trade at 1-800-422-7980. The quality and versatility of Vita-Mix products ensure a long and useful life, but they come with fairly expensive price tags.

Coffee Mill (Spice Grinder)

A small coffee mill is a brilliant little gadget for grinding fresh spices. These appliances are relatively small and can be stored out of sight easily. A coffee mill can also be used to grind small amounts of nuts and seeds. It is especially good at grinding flaxseeds. Coffee grinders are relatively inexpensive and will last a long time if used respectfully (not overloaded), cared for, and cleaned.

It is fine to use the same mill for coffee and spices. Just clean between uses with a damp towel.

Dehydrator

A dehydrator is an essential piece of equipment for the savvy gourmet. A dehydrator is a low-temperature oven with four to nine trays that slide or stack with mesh sheets so that air can freely circulate. A dehydrator is warmed by a heating element, usually a simple coil. The better varieties of dehydrators have a fan to circulate air and a thermometer to regulate temperature.

Dehydrators are indispensable for making fresh, live crackers, chips, flat breads, cookies, veggie burgers, and savory snacks.

The Excalibur Dehydrator is my favorite tried-and-true brand and has a reasonable price of $150 to $225.

Teflex Sheets

Teflex sheets are reusable plastic sheets that sit flush on Excalibur Dehydrator trays. These sheets make peeling breads, crackers, cookies, and fruit leather from the surface of the trays a cinch. They can be washed and reused for years.

Part Three

*

Raw Foods Preparation Techniques

13

Balancing and Developing Flavors

Balancing flavors is an easy science to learn but takes a lifetime to refine. As life seems to be all about the details, great food is all about the sauces.

Our tongues can taste only a few very rudimentary flavors: sweet, salty, sour (pungent), spicy, and bitter. So much of the flavor that we taste is actually from the reaction of our sense of smell, which triggers the olfactory gland to stimulate chemical reactions in our brains that flood our senses with euphoric pleasure associated with taste.

Oil is the foundation from whence all flavors emerge. Salt is the savory essence to round out and bring forward the balance of flavors. Pungent and sour flavors cut through and counterbalance the base of the oil. Piquant and savory spices detail the balance of flavors with subtle or strong under- and overtones. Ah, and a touch of sweetness finishes the balance and sets off flavor as a complement to the salt.

Balancing these elements with the use of different ingredients is an easy approach to creating balanced flavors. Choosing components from various ethnicities is a simple way to develop a diverse variety of recipes. For instance, for an Asian infusion, use miso, sesame, umeboshi plums, and shoyu; for an Italian flare, use olive oil, garlic, sea salt, and basil. It is easy to get the hang of the technique of balancing flavors when you understand the simple science.

Oil

Oil carries flavor. In all classic sauces and dressings, good oil is the base from which delectable flavors bloom. It is essential to use high-quality oils. It is possible to make sauces and dressings without any fat at all, although the maturity—the full body—of the flavor usually leaves a lot to be desired.

Oil makes everything taste good. Choosing high-quality oil nourishes desires and cravings with satisfying integral nutrition. The oil in a dish, sauce, or dressing does not have to be refined. Nuts, seeds, avocados, coconut, nut butters, tahini, and olives are excellent whole-food oil bases to work with. High-quality oils like cold-pressed olive oil, sesame oil, walnut oil, hemp oil, and coconut butter carry the elements of flavor brilliantly.

Oils have a muted undertone of flavor, unlike bolder elements of flavor. They can be nutty, fruity, woody, or mild. Mixing and matching oils is a creative way to subtly mold the flavor of a dish or dressing. Although hemp and flax oils are some of the most well balanced and nutritious, they have a strong flavor that is not appealing for every recipe. In savory dressings and dishes, I like to use the base of a tastier oil and add in a touch of hemp oil or flax oil as a nutritional supplement. Remember that oil is a delicate and sensitive compound that should be treated with respect. Be mindful to buy a top-quality oil and store it properly. Don't skimp on the good stuff; you are worth every ounce.

Salt

Salt is an essential compound for life and makes everything taste better. Salt is an electrolyte that is responsible for the electric pulse that fuels the trillions of cells in our bodies. It is also the broadest flavor the tongue recognizes. There are many salty options to balance and season a dish or dressing, including sea salt, shoyu, miso, and seaweed.

Pungent and Sour Flavors

The acidic tang of pungent and sour flavors counterpoises the basic oil element. Pungent and sour flavors are the medium-high note that cuts through the base of oil to make way for other flavors.

Classic and nouveau pungent and sour elements include vinegar, mirin (a sweet rice wine vinegar with a smooth, delicate flavor), sake (a traditional Japanese rice wine), umeboshi plums, and wine. Some fruity pungent and sour flavors also include a sweet element such as orange or other citrus juice, tart apple, and pineapple. Ooh la la, the dynamics develop.

Piquant and Savory Spices

The spicy flavor as realized by the tongue is not limited to hot, fiery spices. Spices are the seductive winds of flavor. Sought after from the dawn of adventure, spices awaken the spirit of food and arouse the senses. Spices can be used as a subtle solo flavor or commingled for an emerging bouquet of finesse.

Fresh herbs and whole spices are the empyreal choice for superior, dynamic flavor. If some fresh spices and herbs are unavailable, dried or preground spices will do the trick.

In developing flavor, it is easier with a small amount of spices. It is always easier to add more spice if necessary, but it is not possible to take away the spice once it's been added. Too much of an overwhelming spice can be difficult to balance.

Fresh herbs have a more delicate flavor than spices. With fresh herbs, it is generally the more, the merrier. However, starting with a mellow flavor leaves room for adding additional spices or herbs for a dynamic, well-seasoned flavor.

Sweetness

Ah, the sweet balance of flavor. Sweetness is the harmonic high note of flavor. Sweetness is one of the basic fundamental flavors. A hint of sweetness simply makes the tongue taste *more* flavor. More flavor makes for a more dynamic sensual delight.

A touch of sweetness balances salty flavors and entices other flavors to emerge. In savory flavors, the sweet element is typically a subtle balance and not designed to stand out on its own.

Most ingredients used for pungent flavor, such as vinegar and citrus and fruit juices, have a delicate hint of sweetness that perfectly balances a flavor. Additionally, honey; maple syrup; sweet vegetables, such as ripe tomatoes, carrots, snap peas, and fresh corn; and fruit work wonders. Try sliced apples or pears tossed with arugula and a seasoned vinaigrette, grapes with a walnut and endive salad, plums diced into a savory salsa, or a handful of golden raisins or pomegranate seeds in a wild rice dish.

14

Chopping and Cutting Techniques

An essential element for preparing great food is a good knife and a few fundamental knife skills. A sharp knife and a deft hand can create a great variety of textures that bring out flavor and season a dish with shape and color. The bouquet of balanced flavor in a sumptuous dish is awakened by aroma and texture. A variety of texture hosts a party in your mouth.

Vegetables, herbs, and fruits that are cut well take on a new dynamic of flavor. The difference between a ripe tomato cut with a sharp serrated knife into neat slices is quite different from the same tomato smashed and mauled by a dull knife and sloppy skills. Fresh produce blooms in flavor to meet the cut. Likewise, a finely shredded carrot will be much sweeter and juicier than the same carrot that has been chopped. Different textures complement different dishes. A few techniques broaden the delectable variations of simple food to a symphony of flavor and texture.

Mincing

Mincing is a very fine-chopping technique to cut food into very small pieces. Strong flavors like garlic, ginger, hot peppers, and onions are commonly minced to integrate flavor evenly. (A chunk of raw garlic can be very overwhelming.)

A large chef's knife is the best for thorough, even mincing. The produce is typically sliced and then minced, chopping back and forth until the food is finely chopped into very small pieces.

A good technique is to hold the knife in your right hand, placing your left palm or fingers on the top of the blade, and then to rock the blade on its curve for quick, regular chopping. A food processor can quickly mince vegetables in a jiffy.

Dicing

Dicing vegetables produces larger pieces than mincing vegetables. Diced vegetables are usually an eighth- to quarter-inch cubes. Tomatoes, bell peppers, sweet onions, and cucumbers are commonly diced for salads, marinades, and chutneys.

The produce is typically sliced and then cut across the slices to make small cubes. The result is a great texture that mixes well and releases and absorbs flavor.

Slicing

Slicing is a broad term for cutting vegetables into various shapes, such as discs, strips, or wedges. Recipes that call for "sliced" vegetables usually explain the nature of the cut for the best results.

A cucumber or zucchini is generally sliced across the seeds to make discs. A carrot is usually sliced to make similar round slices. A bell pepper can be sliced lengthwise to make colorful strips or across the seeds to make pepper rings. A tomato can be sliced across the seeds to make round tomato slices or cut in half through the top and cut into wedge slices. An apple or a pear can also be cut in half and into slices or across the seeds for a larger slice.

Peeling

Firm vegetables and fruits can be easily peeled with a tool designed for peeling. Softer fruits and vegetables can be peeled with a small paring knife.

The skins of root vegetables, such as carrots, beets, and sweet potatoes, is rich in minerals and does not need to be peeled if the vegetable is scrubbed clean. However, peeling these vegetables lends a cleaner flavor and a uniform color for fine culinary presentation. Similarly, the skins of cucumbers, apples, and pears are valuable goodies that do not need to be peeled other than for specific culinary techniques and texture. It is a good idea to peel any produce that is not certified organic (or is not from your own garden), as pesticides and chemicals tend to be concentrated in the skin.

A peeler is a good tool for peeling fruits and vegetables such as carrots, cucumbers, squashes, eggplant, beets, burdock, sweet potatoes, yams, apples, and pears.

A paring knife is good for peeling fruits such as papayas, mangoes, cherimoya, sapotes, and persimmons. Some fruit is simply peeled by hand, including bananas, oranges, grapefruit, and tangerines.

Julienne Cut (Matchsticks)

Julienne is a cutting technique in which the food is cut into matchstick-sized pieces. For example, to make julienne carrots, first peel the carrot and cut in half or in three pieces. Cut one piece in half lengthwise. Lay the flat face down on the cutting board and cut slices lengthwise to make flat pieces. Stack a few flat pieces and slice them lengthwise again to make delicate matchstick-sized pieces.

Julienne vegetables like carrots and cucumbers are great for sushi rolls and add beautiful shapes, color, and texture to salads and marinated dishes. They also release and absorb flavor. Matchsticks can also be cut with a mandoline (see Chapter 12).

Shredding

Shredded vegetables add great flavor to any dish and provide juicy, delicate texture to salads and marinated dishes. Vegetables can easily be shredded with a hand grater. The finer the shred, the sweeter the flavor, especially with carrots.

Chiffonade

Chiffonade is a technique for leafy greens, such as lettuce and spinach, and fresh herbs, especially basil and sorrel. The leaves are stacked and rolled into a cigarlike shape. Then they are sliced with only a few strokes of the knife to make delicate strips. This is a quick technique that produces fine results.

Zesting

Fresh citrus zest, an ingredient for dynamic flavor, is easy to create with the right tool. There are a few types of zesters (see Chapter 12). To zest lemon or orange, simply shaved off the flavorful delicate outer skin with a zester (a grater can also be used). Be certain not to grate down to the white, inner skin of citrus, as it is quite bitter.

"Spiralizing"

Firm vegetables can be sliced into delicate ribbons with a great piece of equipment called the Saladacco (see Chapter 12). A piece of a firm vegetable, such as a carrot, beet, or winter squash, is rotated on a sharp-toothed blade to cut fine pasta-sized strips for garnish or as an ingredient in marinated dishes.

Vegetable Ribbons

Firm vegetables can be peeled to the core with a peeler to make wider ribbons. Simply peel the vegetable, such as a carrot or daikon radish, with a peeler, and keep peeling in one long strip, rotating the vegetable until there is nothing left to peel. Vegetable ribbons are great for sushi rolls or in soups.

Techniques for Specific Vegetables, Herbs, and Fruits

Garlic

Garlic has a strong flavor that works best when it is well distributed in a dish. For blended dressings, soups, sauces, and pâtes, the garlic will be thoroughly pulverized to release flavor and does not need to be chopped or minced.

When adding garlic to a dish, it should be finely minced or pressed through a garlic press (see Chapter 12). A garlic press does an excellent job of excluding the bitter heart of the garlic clove and pressing out only the choice, firm flesh.

The center "sprout" in garlic cloves can be very bitter and may be the element that causes heartburn in sensitive people. The center of a garlic clove can be removed for a sensitive palate before mincing. Simply cut the garlic clove in half and pull out the white or pale-green sprout. Then go about mincing the rest of the clove with no worries.

Ginger

Ginger has a wonderful, warming flavor that works best when it is well distributed in a dish. The ginger in blended dressings, sauces, soups, and spreads will be pulverized by the natural events of processing. To add ginger to a dish that will not be blended or processed, it is best to shred or finely mince it for an even release of flavor.

Mincing Ginger

Ginger can also be finely minced to add extra flavor to dishes. Peel the ginger and cut into fine slices along the fiber (lengthwise rather than across the fiber) for best results, then chop across the slices for even, fine mincing.

Peeling Ginger

The skin of ginger has valuable minerals and vitamins, but in older, more mature ginger roots it can be woody and fibrous. Tough skin should be peeled away before using. The best way to peel ginger is with a spoon! The edge of a spoon will easily peel the nooks and crannies of a gnarly ginger root without a mess or risk of slicing your fingers with a sharp knife in a tricky spot. Young ginger with thin, delicate skin generally does not need to be peeled for fine flavor.

Shredding Ginger

Fresh ginger can be easily shredded using a grater (watch your fingers!) to break up the fiber for good flavor. Finely shredded ginger releases its juices gracefully and evenly. Shredded ginger is great for brewing a warming tea.

Hot Peppers

Hot peppers add lively spice and kick to many dishes. There are a flurry of peppers with a range of heat—from mildly sweet to ear-burning hot. The tips of hot peppers are always more mild than the upper parts of the pepper. The seeds are where the real fire is. To keep the heat more mild, remove some or all of the seeds before chopping.

Remember that the heat and flavor of hot peppers develop with a little time, so start slow and add more to taste. Using an extra pinch of dried hot peppers is a good way to sensitively control the heat.

Onions

The flavor of onions varies significantly depending on the variety. Sweet onions, Maui onions, and Vidalia onions are the most mild. Red onions are quite a bit sweeter and more mild than yellow or white onions. Green onions are excellent raw and add a nice touch of color and texture to many dishes.

Dicing Onions

To dice onions by hand, first cut the onion into reasonably thick slices. Stack the slices and cut into strips, trying to keep the stack intact. Turn the cut slices, and cut again, across the slices for neat diced cubes.

Onions can also be diced in a food processor. Cut the onion into chunks and chop in pulses in the food processor. When dicing onions in the food processor, be careful not to chop too finely (unless that is your design).

Mincing Onions

To mince onions by hand, follow the dicing instructions and then continue to chop, rocking the knife back and forth over the onions until finely minced.

Onions can be easily minced in a food processor. Cut the onion into chunks and chop in pulses to desired size. Be careful not to blend until soggy. If the onions are chopped too finely for taste, press through a strainer to wick away excess juice.

Slicing Onions

Rings of sliced onions are a nice addition to salads and marinated dishes. To slice an onion, cut off the end and slice into the outer layer of skin. Lift this flap to easily peel away the top layer. This makes it easier to cut and reduces the chance of slipping. If the whole onion is not going to be used, it is best to remove the skin only from the part being used. The remaining skin protects the onion during storage.

Fresh Herbs

Chopping fresh herbs properly and thoroughly lends the best flavor to dishes without large awkward pieces, fibrous stems, or mushy texture.

Fresh herbs should be thoroughly dried before chopping. Remove all large stems for best results. It is not necessary to bother with small delicate stems, as they can be finely chopped without detection.

Using the chiffonade technique described on page 194 makes thoroughly chopping herbs easy.

Fresh herbs can be easily chopped in a food processor. Use at least 1 to 2 cups of loose herbs at a time for best results. Remove any large stems and chop the herbs in pulses until fine.

Apples and Pears

Cutting apples and pears into slices is a cinch. Cut the apple or pear in half lengthwise. Lay the flat face down and cut in half again from stem to bottom. With a paring knife, make a V-shaped cut to remove the core and seeds. Cut into slices as thin as desired.

Another neat way to cut apples and pears is across the seeds to make round slices. In an apple, the seeds will form a star. The core can be cut away with a circular motion of the knife in each slice.

Avocados

Removing the Seed

Cutting an avocado and removing the pit without mauling the fruit is an easy trick. Cut the avocado in half from the stem around to the bottom on both sides. Twist the halves to separate. With a chef's knife, gently push the blade into the avocado pit and twist the knife to pull out the seed. To plant the pit (it just might grow!), stick three toothpicks around the circumference of the pit so that it can stand suspended, hovering in a drinking glass. Fill the glass with enough water to submerge the bottom third of the pit. Change the water once a week as the roots grow. When the roots are three to four inches long, the pit can be planted in a flowerpot with organic potting soil.

For Neat Avocado Slices

With a sharp paring knife, slice the avocado into wedges while it is still in the skin. Make thin or thick slices as desired. Scoop the slices out with a spoon, or gently peel the skin away by hand or with a paring knife.

Citrus Fruits

Fresh lemons and oranges are excellent additions to sauces, dressings, soups, marinades, and drinks.

Fresh lemon zest makes a great appearance in many dishes or as a lovely garnish. It is a good idea to zest or grate the skin of lemons or oranges just before using the fruit to have the zest on hand. Fresh citrus zest can also be dehydrated for longer storage.

Also a slice of fresh lemon makes a nice garnish for salads or on the rim of a glass. For a wedge of lemon or orange to squeeze into a drink or over a salad, cut from stem to navel and into quarters or wedges to suit your needs.

Juicing Citrus

When using a juicer, rolling a lemon or other citrus fruit on the counter with good pressure from your palm is a good way to break up the cellulose inside to extract more juice from the flesh.

Lemons and oranges can be cut in half, across the seeds, or from stem to navel for different uses. For juicing, it is best to cut citrus fruit across the seeds. It is a good idea to cut a slice from the center of a lemon or orange before juicing for a pretty presentation on a glass of fresh juice.

Coconuts

Coconuts require a fairly serious knife to open them (like a machete). Young coconuts can be opened with a cleaver or an old, sharpened knife that you do not care about.

Young Coconuts

Young coconuts have "eyes" on one side that can be penetrated with a thin knife. Young coconuts that have been husked down are much easier to deal with than coconuts with the outside husk and skin intact. To find the eyes of a husked coconut, look on the side opposite the point. Stab at the side gently with a small knife until you hit a spot that gives a little. With a long thin knife, carve out an eye or two for a straw or to drain the coconut water.

Alternatively, young coconuts can be cracked open with a kitchen cleaver. To open the coconut, stand it on its side and give it a good whack with the cleaver near the top point. It may be necessary to rotate the coconut on its side and give it another whack. Be careful!

A safer alternative is a power drill. For real! Drill two holes in the coconut—one for a straw, and one for air to escape. It's safe, effective, and handy.

Cracking Young Coconuts

After the water has been enjoyed through a straw or drained out into a glass, the coconut should be opened for the succulent flesh inside. To crack open the coconut for meat, stand the nut on its bottom or side on a firm surface. (A towel on the floor or porch may be better than the counter.) Hold the cleaver in one hand and keep the other hand FAR away. Do not attempt to hold the nut in place. If your other hand is far away, there is absolutely no chance of hacking it with the cleaver. (I say this with veteran experience.) Hold the knife firmly, take a deep breath, aim, and give it a good whack. It may be necessary to turn the nut over and give it another whack to open it all the way. Pry open the nut and scoop out the flesh.

Cucumbers

Cucumbers are a wonderfully refreshing fruit that can be cut many ways for many pleasures. Those with tough skins are usually better peeled. Any cucumber that is not certified organic should always be peeled because pesticides and other chemicals concentrate in the skin. Cucumbers can be peeled in strips for a pretty presentation for a salad or as a garnish.

Cucumber Matchsticks

Cucumber matchsticks are a great addition to sushi rolls and add a nice texture to salads. To make cucumber matchsticks, first peel the cucumber. Cut the cucumber lengthwise. Scoop out the seeds with a spoon. Cut the cucumber in half or in three pieces. Lay the cucumber on its flat face and cut in half lengthwise. Turn the quarter piece over and continue to slice lengthwise to make matchsticks as thin or thick as you desire.

Cucumber Moons

To make cucumber moons, first peel the cucumber. Cut the cucumber in half lengthwise. Scoop out the seeds with a spoon. Lay the flat face of the cucumber down and cut into thick or thin slices as desired.

Mangoes

Mangoes are the "king of fruits" and should be handled diplomatically. Procuring neat mango slices for a pie or simply for the palate's pleasure is an easy technique that requires a little practice. After many years and many mangoes, I found the following three techniques to be the most successful at yielding the most fruit.

Cut and Peel

Stand the mango on its end with the stem facing up. The pit of the mango runs along the more narrow width of the fruit. Slice along the pit, from the stem down, sawing as close to the pit as possible without cutting into it (the pit is fibrous and woody). Repeat on the other side. Lay the flat slice with the pit on the cutting board and cut around the pit to get an extra wedge of fruit. Again, be careful not to cut into the pit. Peel the skin away from the small wedges with a paring knife or by hand if the flesh is loose.

The larger halves can be peeled whole with a paring knife or cut in half and peeled away. Experience with a knife will play a part in how neatly the skin can be peeled away. Slice the mango thinly for pies or in larger pieces for smoothies or fruit salads.

Mango Cubes on the Half Shell

Stand the mango on its end with the stem facing up. The pit of the mango runs along the more narrow width of the fruit. Slice along the pit, from the stem down, sawing as close to the pit as possible without cutting into it (the pit is fibrous and woody). Repeat on the other side.

Place each half of the mango flesh side up. With a paring knife, cut "crosshatch" slices into the flesh, making a large checkerboard pattern. Be sure not to cut into the skin. Turn the skin inside out to push out the cubes, which will still be attached to the skin. This makes a gorgeous presentation in the center of a fruit salad. Eat them right off the skin, or cut the cubes from the skin with a paring knife.

Peel First and Slice Second

For exceptional gourmet slices, this superior technique takes a little practice. It is essential to start with a nice firm mango. (Good ripe mangoes should be firm.)

Peel the mango with a paring knife. Holding the mango with a dry hand or towel, use a sharp paring knife to cut through the flesh near the stem to find the pit. Saw along the pit as closely as possible, around one side to the bottom and carefully back to the top. The whole side of the mango should come off in one gorgeous piece. Repeat with the same technique on the other side. This should leave little to no flesh on the pit and two intact sides of mango. Slice thinly, keeping the flesh as intact as possible. The sliced side can then be spread or fanned out for a beautiful layer in a pie or torte.

Papayas

Skinning and seeding a papaya for neat slices is a simple task when done in the right order. A good papaya should be firm, but give to the light pressure of your fingers. Papayas should not be stored in the fridge, unless on the verge of going bad, or to store a piece of papaya that has been cut.

Papaya Fan Slices and Spears

The best way to deal with a papaya is to cut off the very top where the stem meets the fruit. Peel the papaya with a paring knife. Cut the papaya in half lengthwise. Scoop out the seeds with a spoon. (Papaya seeds are very spicy like black pepper and add an exotic element to salad dressings. The seeds are also known as a strong antiparasitic for the intestines.)

Slice the papaya lengthwise into spears or thin slices. The thin slices can be spread or fanned out for a sweet, brilliant layer in a pie or torte.

Papayas for Smoothies and Papaya Balls

Cut off the top of the papaya at the stem. Cut in half lengthwise and scoop out the seeds with a spoon. Scoop the flesh out with a spoon for a smoothie or into neat balls with a melon baller (see Chapter 12).

Pineapples

Cutting a pineapple well makes a great difference in yielding the most fruit without losing a lot of the flesh with the skin. The core of a pineapple is quite fibrous. This is where the enzyme bromelain is most concentrated. The core is not the most choice for eating, but it is excellent for juicing.

To remove the spiky decorative top, it is not necessary to cut it off. Simply grab the top with one hand and the pineapple with the other hand and twist the top right off.

Cut off the bottom and top of the pineapple so that it can sit flush on the counter or cutting board. Cut off the skin in strips from the top to the bottom. Pineapples have "eyes" where the sections of skin meet. These eyes can be scooped out individually or cut out in a strip on an angle.

Once the pineapple is skinned, there are several ways to cut pineapple flesh.

1. Stand the skinned pineapple on its flat bottom. Cut the pineapple in half from top to bottom. Cut the halves in quarters from top to bottom. Set each quarter on its long flat side and cut away the core. Save the core for juicing.
2. Stand the skinned pineapple on its flat bottom. Cut the pineapple along the core from top to bottom. This first cut will yield a nice slab of pineapple that can be cut into slices or cubes. Turn the remaining pineapple and cut along the core from top to bottom. Continue until only the core is left. Save the core for juicing.
3. Cut the skinned pineapple across the fruit into round slices. Lay each slice down and cut the core with a circular motion of the knife.

Tomatoes

There are many ways to cut tomatoes for different needs. Using a sharp serrated knife is the first step to all-around success. The "sawing" edge of a serrated knife poses little difficulty to the thin but tricky skin of a tomato. The second step is to cut out the stem neatly for clean flavor and for tender texture throughout.

Dicing Tomatoes

To dice a tomato, first cut out the stem. Cut the tomato into fairly thin slices. Stack a few slices at a time, and cut into strips, trying to keep the stack together. Turn the stack and cut across the slices for a neat diced cut.

Removing the Seeds

The seeds of a tomato are watery and succulent, though not ideal for every recipe. Tomato sauces are much thicker and richer when the seeds are excluded. Tomatoes without seeds are much easier to slice and dice for all of your culinary needs. The seeds can be set aside for other recipes to blend into soups and light dressings or for juicing.

To remove the seeds of a tomato, first cut out the top. Then, cut the tomato in half from stem to bottom. With a paring knife, carve a smile-shaped cut in the seeds to loosen any flesh from the seeds. Scoop out the seeds with a spoon.

Juicing

Fresh vegetable and fruit juice is clean fuel for energy and pure nutrition. The vitamins and minerals of fruits and vegetables are suspended in the colloidal solution of their juices. Drinking fresh juice provides the body with instant energy and bioavailable nutrients. Fresh juice will be absorbed and assimilated in as little as 15 minutes on an empty stomach. The digestive tract does not have to deal with fiber for digestion and can feed the body the nectar of energy straightaway.

Fresh juice is a terrific way to start the day or makes a great afternoon booster. It is best to drink juice on an empty stomach to appreciate and absorb the full value of the stellar nutrition that fresh juice has to offer. Fruit juices tend to be more cleansing and sugary; vegetable juices are more strengthening and building. Fruit juice and vegetable juice should be consumed separately for optimum assimilation and digestion.

Go Organic!

Choosing organic juices and organic produce for juicing is a smart and important option to exercise whenever possible. Certified organic agricultural practice is required to feed and rest the soil, which in return yields more vitamins, minerals, and other nutrients in food than in commercially grown produce. Organic produce is free from chemicals, waxes, pesticides, and fungicides. (See Chapter 2 for more information.) Modern, commercial farming methods permit an alarming amount of chemicals and pesticides for common use. Chemicals and pesticides are likely to concentrate in the skin and juices of fruits and vegetables. A fresh juice made from commercial produce will certainly have a wealth of enzymes and nutrients, but will also be concentrated with commercial chemicals. Choose organic produce for home juicing (for personal and planetary health) and seek out juice bars that use certified organic goodies. You are worth every precious effort.

Fresh Juice versus Bottled Juice

There is a significant difference between fresh juice and bottled juice. Fresh juice is alive with enzymes, vitamins, minerals, and other nutrients: the very essence of life. Bottled juice has been pasteurized (heated) to maintain a long shelf life. Bottled juice is devoid of live enzymes with diminishing nutrients and minerals. Many markets offer fresh juices that are bottled and sold in the refrigerated section for convenience. These bottled "fresh" juices are a reasonable compromise and a good fix, especially on the go. The best choice above all is a fresh organic juice made in your kitchen or a fresh organic juice made to order from a juice bar.

Juicing at Home

Home juicers have revolutionized making fresh vegetable and fruit juice in the home kitchen— not much mess, not much fuss for high-quality, fresh juice. Juicing in your own kitchen ensures the best certified organic produce, a sanitary environment, and your own personal formula for a delicious fresh elixir. (See the recipes in Part Four for many delicious and healing combinations.)

Certain juicers, such as the older Green Power juicer or the new Green Star juicer, both made by the Green Power Company, are designed to minimize the oxidation and breakdown of the vital nutrients in juice. It is possible to make a few servings of fresh juice in the morning to last throughout the day or even for two days. Of course, the fresher the juice, the more nutritious and tasty it is.

Fresh juice is a vital base for fresh blended soups and sauces. For instance, blending fresh carrot juice with avocado, fresh parsley, cilantro, and a little nama shoyu makes a delicious, savory, smooth soup.

Use Prime Vegetable Odds and Ends for Juicing

Juicing choice vegetable odds and ends is a great way to recycle the prime scraps of produce. The tops of carrots and beets and the bottoms of celery can be scrubbed and used for juicing. Tougher outer leaves and bottom stems of romaine and other lettuce are prime juicing material, as are the stems of spinach, kale, and chard. Large cores of organic apples are a sweet addition as well as any remnants of chopped vegetables like bell pepper, cucumber, tomato, or stems of herbs like parsley and cilantro.

There is no shame or waste in using vital vegetable odds and ends for juicing. As long as the vegetable pieces are cleaned and free from bruises and damage, they are perfect juicing material. Be sure to choose only prime extra pieces for juicing. Keeping a container in the fridge to store these odds and ends for juicing is a neat way to handle the goods. The ends of vegetables from preparing dinner can be part of the next morning's juice.

Juicers

There are many kinds of juicers on the market, with a wide range of price tags. There are five types of vegetable and fruit juicers available: (1) masticating juicers, (2) triturating juicers, (3) centrifugal juicers, (4) juice presses, and (5) electric citrus juicers. The descriptions below not only discuss how each type of juicer operates but also provide specific brand names that are recommended as the best home-juicing products.

1. Masticating Juicers: Champion, Oscar, and Samson

The Champion, Oscar, and Samson juicers are masticating juicers that grind produce much the way our mouths do and press the juice through a screen to be collected. These juicer products are affordable, versatile pieces of equipment. The Champion Company packs a well-stocked warranty for a high-powered piece of equipment that performs a myriad of tasks.

These juicers have two "plates." One "plate" has screens to press juice through, and the other is a "blank plate" made of solid plastic for homogenizing.

The "blank plate" enables the juicers to homogenize, or grind whatever is pushed through it. It can grind produce, nuts, beans, grains, and frozen fruit without pressing the juice out to create smooth pastes like almond butter, hummus, and frozen fruit sorbet.

The Champion, Oscar, and Samson juicers provide excellent capabilities for a reasonable price tag ($225–$300).

2. Triturating Juicers: Green Power, Green Star, and Angel

The Green Power and Green Star juicers (see page 205) and the Angel juicer are triturating juicers that can do everything the Champion can do with a higher level of quality. The Green Power and Angel juicers are about the same size and shape.

A triturating juicer has two cylindrical twin gears that turn toward each other, chewing, grinding, and pressing the juice from the fiber. This is done at a low speed to ensure that nothing will ever be heated. It is very effective and extracts almost every drop of juice available from produce.

The juice produced from this method is of the highest quality. It is as good as a juice from a juice press and is known to maintain freshness and nutrients for longer periods of time. Because of the shape of the gears, it can manage all kinds of produce, even very fibrous greens, without getting tied up.

These machines can also grind and homogenize produce, nuts, beans, grains, and frozen fruit without pressing out the juice the way a Champion does. It is the best machine for frozen ice creams because it does not heat up the way a Champion will and produces even, firm, perfect results. These machines are the best home juicers on the market. They are more expensive than Champion juicers (Green Power $400–$600; Angel $1,200–$1,500) and are an investment worth every penny. All things considered (with prodigious juicing experience), the Green Power juicer is the ultimate choice for home juicing.

3. Centrifugal Juicers: Juiceman and Acme

Centrifugal juicers, or basket juicers, such as the Juiceman juicer or the Acme juicer, shred produce and use centrifugal force, or outward-spinning momentum, to extract the juice from the fiber. These machines are relatively inexpensive, but are limited to only juicing. They cannot grind or homogenize. Juice extracted in this manner is known to oxidize fairly quickly.

4. Juice Presses: Norwalk

Juice presses like the Norwalk juicer involve two steps to juice. First, the produce is shredded into pulp. Second, the ground produce is wrapped in a porous cloth and hydraulically pressed to extract the juice from the fiber. The juice press is very efficient and designed for maximum preservation and minimum oxidation of the juice. The grinding mechanism can also be used to homogenize produce, nuts, beans, grains, and frozen fruit.

The juice press will heat up. The mechanism that grinds the produce is subject to friction that heats up the juicer after a few minutes. Therefore, it is not the best for frozen fruit ice cream because the ice cream melts before you get a chance to eat it. These machines are very expensive (at least $1,500), and juicing and cleaning are quite laborious.

5. Electric Citrus Juicers

An electric citrus juicer makes juicing lots of lemons, oranges, or grapefruits a snap. Electric citrus juicers are reasonably small and easy to store and decently inexpensive ($35–$150). They are very useful and helpful for any fresh citrus juice lover. An electric citrus juicer may not be the first mechanical kitchen tool to buy, but it certainly lends a helping hand.

16

Sprouting: Amplified Nutrition in a Simplified Form

1. Sprouts Are a Miracle Food.

Sprouts can be grown any time of the year, without soil, maturing in three to five days even without sunshine and rival almost any food in nutritional value. Sprouts will grow year-round in any climate with very little effort to provide vital, organic, locally grown produce (as local as your own kitchen!).

2. Sprouts Are One of the Most Nutritious Foods of All Time.

Sprouts are abundant in all essential amino acids (the building blocks of protein), vitamins, minerals, chlorophyll, and enzymes. Sprouts are perhaps the most vital of all fresh foods. Any seed, nut, grain, or bean can be germinated and sprouted for a tremendous boost in vitamins, minerals, and enzymes. The process of germination breaks the complex nutritional matrix of a seed (nut, grain, or bean) into simpler compounds. The nutrition is digested into a simpler form and made more bioavailable for the body to use.

Seeds, nuts, grains, and beans can grow two to ten times their size in only three to five days. Nutritional content increases many times over. In many cases, three- to five-day sprouts have more nutrition than the plant will have at any other time in its life, in some cases by more than 600 percent.

3. Soaking and Sprouting Makes Seeds, Nuts, Beans, and Grains More Digestible.

Soaked and sprouted seeds and nuts are more digestible than their dry counterparts. To begin with, this is simply because they are plump with water, which helps for easier digestion. Second, the metabolic change in sprouting seeds, nuts, grains, and beans wakes up a flood of enzymes. For auxiliary support, soaking and sprouting wick away the enzyme inhibitors and tannins found in the skins of seeds and nuts, which act to pragmatically slow down digestion.

The process of germination (sprouting) simplifies the dense nutritional complex of a seed (nut, bean, or grain) and makes it more available and easier to digest. Complex carbohydrates and starch are broken down into simple sugars. Protein is broken down into amino acids. Fat is broken down into free fatty acids.

Sprouts are practically predigested. The metabolic process of sprouting provides an animated wealth of enzymes. Any food eaten with fresh green sprouts will be easier to digest.

More nutrition and energy made available for less work and stress yield vital health and generous dividends. Good deal.

What Are Sprouts?

Sprouts are seeds, nuts, beans, or grains that have been geminated with water. This initiates the growth process. Sprouting transforms seeds from a dry, dormant storehouse of nutrition into a wealth of bioavailable vitamins, minerals, and protein that is rich in enzymes for easy digestion.

Sprouts are fresh, vital, infantile plants. They are incredibly rich in vitamins and minerals. Sprouts are a simple food and are very easy to digest for optimum assimilation of nutrients.

Sprouts are becoming more popular and more available. For instance, alfalfa sprouts are commonly found in salads and on sandwiches. Crunchy bean sprouts are another widely available sprout often found in Chinese foods. Wheatgrass is grown from sprouted wheat "berries" that have been planted in soil to grow into young grass.

Sprouts are nutritional powerhouses. Any means of incorporating and munching sprouts on a regular basis is a champion of choices.

Sprouting Increases Nutrition

Sprouting actually increases the nutritional value of foods. A seed contains more concentrated nutrition than the plant on which it grew. As a plant matures, energy is collected and focused into producing a seed for reproduction. The seed is the storehouse of essential energy. When the seed is germinated, the potential energy is awakened and the complex concentration of energy is broken down into a simpler, more available state, which is easier to digest.

Imagine that in each almond exists the potential for an almond tree, or that in each tiny alfalfa seed exists the potential future of a plant that grows roots up to 100 feet deep into the earth. The potential energy of these foods is unleashed by the process of growing, which begins with sprouting.

A profound metabolic change happens in the germinating process, which pours energy into cellular growth. The nutritional energy of the food is repatterned. The seed begins to transform its stored energy into the active, growing energy of a plant.

For example, sprouting a grain, such as wheat, breaks down the complex carbohydrates into simple sugars. In a more simple form, less energy is required for digestion. The simplified structure is accompanied by an increase in certain vitamins and minerals because the seed is designed to "feed" itself until roots grow to feed from soil. Our example of wheat shows that a three-day wheat sprout has 300 percent more vitamin E than the dried seed. The gluten and protein are made more digestible so that the body can absorb more of the nutrients. The result is more nutrition and energy for less work. More yield for less effort? A dream come true. Everyone can relate to that.

A Host of Enzymes

Sprouts are a veritable fortune of enzymes. As the complex nutrition of a dry seed is unlocked during germination, a complete metabolic change occurs that wakes up the cells of the seed, and they begin to grow. The metabolic activity of these cells requires a team of enzymes to work as catalysts for the change. Sprouted seeds (nuts, beans, and grains) are teeming with enzymes and life!

Simply put, sprouts are loaded with enzymes! The simplified nutritional matrix of sprouts coupled with copious amounts of enzymes equals easy and agreeable digestion of this superfood. It can be said that sprouts have more enzymes than are necessary to digest themselves and lend other food excess enzymes for easy digestion. This is true with liberal amounts of green sprouts, such as alfalfa, clover, and sunflower sprouts. This is true only with small amounts of sprouted grains and beans, however, as they are still quite complex and starchy.

Wick Away Enzyme Inhibitors!

Those nasty enzyme inhibitors found in and under the skin of many seeds and nuts are effortlessly wicked away by soaking and sprouting. Enzyme inhibitors, such as tannic acid, are unwelcome compounds that slow down digestion. These compounds are broken down and washed away during soaking. Evidence of this can be seen in the amber-brown water that is drained away after soaking seeds and nuts for six to twelve hours.

Free from these inhibiting compounds and plump with fresh water, seeds and nuts are more easy and efficient to digest. Freedom is more fun.

Sprouting Is Easy

Any *viable* seed, nut, grain, or bean will sprout. Be sure the grain and seed is not too old and that it has not been treated with any heat or chemical processes. Most certified organic sundries are good choices for quality results.

Sprouting is the basic process of germination. Sprouting seeds hydroponically (without soil) quickens this natural process. Just as in natural conditions, a dry seed that has been patiently waiting through the dormant season is awakened by water from the spring thaw. The swelling seed is watered by the spring rains and is naturally drained by the expanding soil. The seed is peaking with potential energy before the roots begin to grow to seek nutrients in the soil to feed the growing plant.

With precise conditions in the kitchen, we focus the germinating process into a few short days. In the kitchen, we harvest our sprouts before the roots begin to develop, when the energy and nutrition are still concentrated in the body of the seed. For beans and grains, a good standard of measure is that when the tail of the sprout is as long as the bean or grain itself, the sprout is at the peak of nutrition. In smaller seeds, the peak of nutrition is when the two dwarf leaves of the sprout begin to open and most of the tiny hulls fall away.

Tools for Sprouting

Sprouting requires only a few simple household tools. Most sprouts can be grown in a jar, which makes the technique, maintenance, and cleanup very easy.

As sprouting becomes part of your culinary routine, it might be worth it to install a simple rack near your kitchen sink or in the laundry room that can be used to contain all of this vital activity.

Equipment for Sprouting
   ½-gallon glass jar with a wide mouth
   1 piece of screen or mesh
   1 rubber band (to secure the screen or mesh)
   Fresh water
   Seed, nut, bean, or grain of choice

How to Sprout Hydroponically (without Soil)

1. Soak

To begin, the seeds are soaked in water for 6 to 12 hours. ("Medium-soak" nuts should be soaked 2 to 6 hours, and "short-soak" nuts should be soaked only 1 to 2 hours. See the chart on pages 230–231.)

It is important to use fresh, clean water, as the seeds will absorb this soaking water and double or triple in size. Treated water or tap water should be avoided.

I prefer to use a generous glass jar for soaking. Cover the jar with screen or mesh secured with a rubber band for a good standard technique to keep winged creatures and bugs away and to make the next step a cinch.

2. Drain and Rinse

After the seeds are soaked, the water should be drained off. The seeds should be rinsed and drained again. The jar should be left inverted on a 45-degree angle (covered by screen or mesh) so that any excess water will eventually drain away.

Some seeds are ready for harvest at this point, including almonds, filberts, pumpkin seeds, and sunflower seeds.

3. Rinse and Drain Daily Until Harvest

As the seeds are sprouting, they should be rinsed two to three times a day with fresh water until ready for harvest (two to five days). Small seeds, such as alfalfa and clover, are ready when the hulls begin to break away from the two tiny leaves that unfold. Grains and beans are ready when the tail of the sprout is as long as the grain or bean.

Seeds for Hydroponic Sprouting
Small Seeds

Small sprouting seeds all look relatively the same. They range from amber yellow to pale to dark brown and are not much larger than the head of a pin. After only a few days of sprouting, these seeds grow to be ten to twenty times their original size and incredibly wealthy in vitamins and minerals. These sprouts are a great addition to salads, wraps, or as a dainty garnish for any dish.

Alfalfa Seeds

Alfalfa sprouts are one of the most popular varieties of sprouts widely available. They are small and delicate, only a few inches long. The flavor is mildly leguminous.

This tiny seed will mature into a plant with a taproot that can grow up to 100 feet into the earth. The tremendous life force of the plant is concentrated in the young sprout, which is one of the most nutritious of all foods. The seeds are amber yellow in color.

Broccoli Seeds

Broccoli sprouts have enjoyed a recent revival and are known for their exceptional levels of antioxidants and phytonutrients, which help to prevent cancers. Broccoli sprouts are small and tender like alfalfa sprouts, but fetch a pretty penny packaged in the store. The flavor is mild with the essence of broccoli. The seeds are pale to dark brown in color.

Clover Seeds

Clover sprouts are becoming as widely available as alfalfa sprouts these days, and rightly so. They have a dynamite nutritional portfolio of amino acids, minerals, and vitamins and a hearty fiber that stays perky and fresh for days. They are mild in flavor and crunchier in texture than most of the small-seed sprouts. The seeds are a mix of amber yellow and pale brown in color.

Fenugreek Seeds

Fenugreek is renowned as a digestive aid with a balancing spicy and bitter flavor. Fenugreek is a dark-yellow seed, typically larger than alfalfa or clover seeds. These sprouts are best used sparingly as the flavor is quite strong.

Mustard Seeds

Sprouted mustard seeds are a vital, juicy delicacy and packed with antioxidants. Mustard is certainly spicy and is known to get the digestive juices flowing. Brown mustard seeds tend to be mellower in flavor than yellow. Mustard sprouts are perfect as a garnish or mixed with other spicy sprouts like radish and onion.

Onion Seeds

Onion sprouts are a delicacy. With a delightful, tasteful hint like a diffused green onion, onion sprouts are a great garnish for soup or mixed with other spicy sprouts like radish and mustard. Onion seeds for sprouting can be difficult to find alone, but are often available as part of a spicy sprout mix. The seeds are pale brown in color.

Radish Seeds

Radish sprouts are a spicy tender sprout that adds a great kick to a salad or as a garnish. Their natural zesty spice acts as a great digestive aid. Full of vitamins and minerals, radish is known as an excellent source of organic sulfur, which makes beautiful skin, hair, and nails. The seeds are reddish brown in color.

Large Seeds

The larger seeds classified in this group are removed from their shells. They become deliciously plump, light, and freshly crunchy when soaked. With the ability to sprout wee tails, these seeds are unlikely to grow into a full plant without their protective shells.

After soaking these seeds for 4 to 8 hours, this classification of seeds can be drained and rinsed and are ready to use (just like that!). They can also continue to be rinsed and drained two or three times a day for a few days and their tails will grow!

Be sure to use only raw seeds. Toasted or roasted seeds will not sprout.

Pumpkin Seeds

Pumpkin seeds are the dark-green seeds from a pumpkin squash. They are abundant in healthy omega oils, fiber, and protein. Soaked and sprouted pumpkin seeds are plump, crunchy, and easy to digest. They make a delicious, nutritious base for a creamy salad dressing and are great marinated in shoyu for a snack or tossed into a wild rice dish.

Sesame Seeds

Sesame seeds are exceptionally high in calcium; they have more than 1,100 mg of calcium per 100 grams. Soaked and sprouted sesame seeds are very digestible. Blending soaked sesame seeds with a little oil and/or water into a creamy paste makes a great "sprouted" tahini.

Sesame seeds are available with or without the hull. Hulled sesame seeds are typically lighter or white and less bitter, but they contain less calcium, as much of it is housed in the hull. Soaking hulled sesame seeds will aid digestion and boost nutritional values, though they will not grow a tail.

Sunflower Seeds

Sunflower seeds are very high in healthy, polyunsaturated fat, protein, and fiber. They have a delicious nutty flavor that is light and crunchy when soaked and sprouted. Organic, raw sunflower seeds are very inexpensive and widely available. They are excellent tossed into a crisp salad with romaine lettuce or added to a marinated seaweed salad.

Nuts for Soaking and Sprouting
Long-Soak Nuts (6–12 Hours)

The nuts classified in this group are more dense and thus require longer soaking time to get crisply saturated and plump. These nuts also have a measurable amount of enzyme-inhibiting compounds in the skins, which are wicked away during the longer soaking time.

Almonds

Almonds are one of the few alkaline nuts, made even more so by soaking and sprouting. Almonds are very high in protein, vitamins (especially vitamin E), and minerals.

Light, crunchy, and delicately sweet, soaked almonds that have been well drained keep fresh in the fridge for a week easily. They can be ground into a delectable, "sprouted" almond butter or blended with water and strained to make a smooth, delicious fresh almond milk.

Hazelnuts (Filberts)

Hazelnuts have a distinguished flavor that can complement both savory and sweet foods. Rich in calcium and potassium, soaked and sprouted hazelnuts are light, crunchy, and full of flavor. The bitter flavor in the skin is usually relieved by soaking the nuts (versus roasting, which is a traditional technique).

Pistachios (Unroasted)

Pistachio nuts have a distinctively nutty and sweet flavor. Pistachio nuts that have been removed from the shell are a time-saving treat. Soaked pistachios are lighter and more delicate in flavor than dried nuts. They make an exquisite addition to a long-grain wild rice dish.

Medium-Soak Nuts (2–6 Hours)

The nuts classified in this group are softer and quite oily. These nuts are adequately saturated with water to become fresh crunch in only a few hours. From experience, the balance of oils is maintained after soaking a shorter time, and the enzyme inhibitors are sufficiently wicked away from the skins of these nuts.

Brazil Nuts

Soaked Brazil nuts are quite a bit lighter than dry Brazil nuts as they are plump with more water and less oil. Brazil nuts are very high in selenium, a powerful antioxidant for cellular protection and rejuvenation. They lend an exotic flair to dishes.

Pecans

Pecans are an exquisite nut from the hickory family, which is native to the Americas. The rich buttery kernel gets lovely, plump, and crunchy when soaked. Pecans are a choice flavor for desserts and one of the best nuts to grind into a pie crust. Soaked pecans are lighter and offer a lovely fresh crunch.

Walnuts

Walnuts are a great source of vitamins, minerals, and healthy fats. Soaked walnuts are deliciously light and more digestible. Chopped soaked walnuts are a perfect complement to a spinach and bosc pear salad with a raspberry vinaigrette.

Short-Soak Nuts (1–2 Hours)

Short-soak nuts only need to be soaked for 1 to 2 hours. These nuts do not have skins and are therefore devoid of the enzyme inhibitors typically found in the skins of seeds and nuts. They are very rich in precious oils, which transpire when soaked for too long.

Cashews

Cashews are very creamy and rich in vitamins, minerals, protein, and oil. Soaked cashews blend into an incredible cream, which is absolutely divine as a whipped frosting for sweet treats.

Macadamia Nuts

Macadamia nuts are very rich in oil and elegant flavor. They are considerably more digestible and lighter when soaked. They make a tasty base for macadamia nut ricotta "cheese."

Pine Nuts

Pine nuts are delicious and expensive due to the labor-intensive process of hand harvesting. A little goes a long way with pine nuts, as they are very rich in oil and flavor. When soaked, pine nuts get plump and lighter. They are excellent chopped or ground with a touch of nutritional yeast and salt for a very authentic Parmesan flavor.

Grains for Hydroponic Sprouting

Grains are one of the most important staple foods all over the world. Grains are rich in carbohydrates, protein, fiber, and precious vitamins and minerals.

Sprouting grains reduces the glutinous content, which results in easier digestion. The sprouting process has shown to improve the nutrition of the "germ," where all of the precious oils, such as vitamin E, are contained.

Sprouted grain is best eaten in moderation with a generous balance of fresh vegetables and sprouts like alfalfa or sunflower sprouts or, alternatively, with lots of fresh fruit. A nice combination is a breakfast cereal of sprouted grain, fresh fruit, and cinnamon, sweetened to taste with a touch of raw honey or maple syrup. Try adding dried fruit like raisins or dried figs cut into pieces. Sprouted grains are also great as a staple for making low-temperature flat breads.

These grains can be grown into grasses (like wheatgrass) for a nutritionally superior superfood.

Barley

Barley is one of the oldest cultivated cereal grains. It is very high in vitamins and minerals and can also be grown into a nutritionally superior grass (see "Cereal Grasses" on page 224). Sprouted barley is a great base for a low-temperature flat bread. Fresh sprouted barley is best used sparingly with generous amounts of fresh vegetables and herbs.

Kamut (Einkorn Wheat)

Kamut is one of the oldest varieties of durum wheat. It has much less gluten than modern wheat and more vitamins, minerals, and protein. It is a delicious alternative to wheat and a great grain for savory, low-temperature flat breads.

Rye

Rye is hearty grain with a sweet-and-sour flavor. Complemented by caraway seed, rye is a great grain for flat breads. Rye can also be grown into grass.

Spelt (Einkorn Wheat)

Spelt is one of the oldest wheatlike grains. It has a delicious flavor like wheat, but is more digestible because it has considerably less gluten. Spelt is rich in vitamins, minerals, and protein. Like kamut, it is a great alternative to wheat for breads.

Wheat

Wheat is one of the most common grains in America. It is probably best avoided unless grown into a grass for juicing. Wheat is very high in gluten, causing and aggravating allergies and food sensitivities. It is also not as high in minerals and nutrients as other grains.

Seed-Grains for Hydroponic Sprouting

The "grains" classified here are technically and botanically seeds. They are sprouted like grains, with the diverse nutritional portfolio of seeds. They are exceptionally high in protein. These "grains" have precious balanced ratios of amino acids, including lysine and methionine. These two amino acids are not usually present in grains, which prevent most grains from being "complete proteins."

The "grains" classified here all tend to be alkaline, a precious commodity in the family of staple foods.

Amaranth

Amaranth is one of the smallest and most nutritious superfoods native to South America. It is technically not a grain, but a starchy seed. Amaranth is rich in calcium and amino acids. It is made up of 15 to 19 percent protein.

Sprouted amaranth is best used in combination with other grains and seeds since it can be strong and bitter in flavor.

Buckwheat

Buckwheat is an alkaline grain with mildly mucilagenic properties. Buckwheat found intact with a hull can be grown into a green sprout planted in soil (see "Sprouts Grown in Soil" on page 222).

Buckwheat contains an exceptional compound called rutin, known for healing capillaries, reducing blood pressure, stimulating circulation, and neutralizing the effects of radiation. Buckwheat also makes great crunchy flat breads and incredible granola when dehydrated with fruits and nuts.

Millet

Millet is one of the few alkaline grains. Like amaranth and quinoa, it is not actually a grain, but a power-packed starchy seed native to South America. It is very rich in protein and very digestible. Millet is known for its antifungal properties and is great for *Candida* overgrowth and sugar imbalances. It is great tossed with fresh corn and tomatoes for a summer salad.

Quinoa

Quinoa has the highest protein content of any grain. Like amaranth and millet, quinoa is technically a starchy seed. Quinoa is another of the preciously alkaline grains.

Quinoa sprouts very quickly, after only a day or two, and is a great base for tabbouleh.

Wild Rice

Wild rice, or long-grain rice, is neither a grain nor a rice, but the fruiting seed of a tall, aquatic grass indigenous to the Great Lakes of North America. It is one of the oldest foods still in common use as a great and tasty source of protein, iron, and B vitamins.

Sprouted wild rice is a scrumptious and satisfying staple for marinated dishes with a myriad of variations using seasonal vegetables, herbs, and spices.

Legumes and Beans for Hydroponic Sprouting

Beans and legumes have quite a complex of protein and starch. Sprouting breaks down the nutrients into a simpler form for easier digestion and assimilation.

All beans can sprout, but some taste better than others. Beans double to quadruple in size when sprouting, so make sure to allow enough room in the sprouting jar.

Sprouted beans will be ready in two to five days, depending on the bean and the environment. A good standard of measure for harvest time is when the tail of the sprout is as long as the bean itself.

Sprouted beans have a very distinct flavor and can be a little hard to digest because of their starch. Chopping the beans and rinsing them through a strainer until the starch is rinsed out and the water runs clear or by gently steaming them can improve both of these elements.

The complexity of the starch is fairly relentless to the palate. To improve the flavor and digestibility, I have experimented with a few tricks with great success. These are a few good techniques to reduce the starch of sprouted beans for good flavor and easier digestion.

1. Rinse off excess starch by chopping and rinsing the sprouted beans: totally raw
2. Blanch or steam sprouted beans: lightly cooked
3. Rinse off excess starch *and* blanch or steam: integrated

Rinse Off Excess Starch

Starch is the complicated character in beans. Sprouting beans, by soaking and rinsing the beans until a sprouting tail grows, wakes up the dormant nutrition and begins to break down the complex starch. This means less work for more results. Be sure to use beans that have been sprouted until the tail of the sprouted bean is as long as the bean itself, indicating that the nutrition is generally peaking.

Although sprouted beans have a simpler arrangement of starch than cooked beans, they can still be difficult for some people to digest. Large starchy beans, such as garbanzo beans, can be tricky to digest even when sprouted. The excess starch in sprouted beans can be further reduced by chopping sprouted beans and rinsing them with fresh water. "Rinsing" the starch out of a sprouted bean is an extra step that will be applauded and assimilated by your gut. Follow these steps for chopping sprouted beans:

1. In a food processor, chop the sprouted beans in pulses until the beans are broken but not pummeled smooth.
2. In a strainer or colander, rinse the broken, sprouted beans with fresh water. Stir and rinse the beans until the water runs clear.
3. Voilà! Use the beans for various recipes, especially spreads and breads.

Blanch or Steam Sprouted Beans

Sprouted beans can be blanched or steamed for easy digestion. Blanching (quickly heating) and steaming soften the texture, mellow the flavor, and break down the indigestible starch and cellulose in sprouted beans. Weakened digestive systems greatly benefit from this approach. The texture and flavor of steamed sprouted beans are very palatable and smoother, much like a cooked bean.

Although the bulk of the nutrition is made much more digestible, some of the enzymes and nutrients are compromised by this process because of the heat. Sprouted beans have a much higher nutritional portfolio than dry or cooked beans. Even reducing these nutritional levels a touch by blanching or steaming sprouted beans yields superior results. (See Chapter 19 for more information.)

Rinse Off Excess Starch *and* Blanch or Steam

These two techniques—rinsing the starch and blanching or steaming—can be used together with superb results. Chopping the beans and rinsing away the excess starch reduce the time necessary for blanching or steaming. A flash of heat will do the trick. For one, the beans are in smaller pieces and require less heat and time to penetrate the cellulose. Second, much of the starch has already shoved off, and most of the work is done.

To integrate rinsing the starch and steaming or blanching, do the following:

1. Chop sprouted beans in the food processor until they are broken but not completely pummeled.
2. Put the chopped beans in a strainer or colander and generously rinse with fresh water until the rinse water runs clear. Carry on!
3. Blanch or steam the cleaned beans. (See Chapter 19 for more information.)

Sprouts Grown in Soil
Green Soil Sprouts

Green soil sprouts are seeds that are sprouted in their protective shell and planted in soil and grown into baby plants, a few inches tall. These are delicious fresh and crunchy delicacies.

Growing Beans into Long and Crunchy Bean Sprouts

Under the right conditions of pressure, beans can be grown into delicate, long, crunchy bean sprouts hydroponically (without soil). With a good fit, the right weight, and water, you are on your way. Mung beans and adzuki beans are the best and most tasty.

Equipment for Sprouting Beans
> 2 pieces of screen or mesh
> 1 plate
> 1 drainable container
> 1 colander and a bowl that fits inside of it
> OR
> 2 terra-cotta pots that fit inside each other with holes in the bottom (usually used
>   for potted plants)
> 1 weight (a stone or sealed jar filled with water that fits inside the bowl or pot)
> Soaked beans

Step 1: Soak

Soak ½ cup of beans in 2 cups of fresh water for 6 to 12 hours.

Step 2: Drain and Rinse

Drain off the water from soaking. Rinse and drain again.

Step 3: Put Under Pressure

(a) Put the drainable container (colander or one clay pot) on a plate and line the bottom of it with a piece of screen or mesh to contain the soaked beans.

(b) Put the soaked beans on top of the screen in the drainable container (colander or the first pot).

(c) Put another layer of screen or mesh over the beans.

continued

(d) Place the bowl or second pot on the beans and put a weight in it, such as a stone or a jar with a sealed lid filled with water.

Step 4: Water Daily

Take off the weight and the bowl or pot to rinse the sprouts two to three times a day, trying to disturb the beans as little as possible. Allow the water to drain out before returning the weight to the beans and putting the whole get-up back on the plate to catch any excess water.

Buckwheat Lettuce

Buckwheat lettuce (grown from buckwheat in the shell) is a delicate sprout that must be grown in the soil. It has a very thin, juicy, fragile stalk and small, broad, flat, tender green leaves that open to push away the dark triangular hull. The flavor is very mild and delicate. Buckwheat lettuce is a delectable addition to any green salad.

Pea Shoots

Pea shoots are perky, fibrous sprouts with delicate green leaves. They have a mild flavor like green peas. They are gorgeous in sushi cones and as a garnish for anything, especially soup.

Sunflower Sprouts

Baby sunflowers! Sunflower sprouts (grown from sunflower seeds in the shell) have a delightful fresh crunch and a delicately nutty flavor. They have an iridescent crisp stem and two perky, juicy leaves that unfold to drop the protective outer shell of the sunflower seed. These sprouts are a nutritional delicacy for every salad.

Cereal Grasses

Grass, in young stages of growth, is one of the most nutritious foods on the planet. Young grass is one of the most ultimate whole foods with all of the essential amino acids and a wealth of vitamins and minerals. Grass is like synthesized liquid sunshine. It has an incredibly high amount of chlorophyll (the equivalent of plant's blood), which is almost molecularly identical to the hemoglobin in our blood. It is one of the best purifying and blood-building tonics for blood.

Cereal grasses (as well as algae, such as spirulina and chlorella) are some of the few foods on the planet that contain the nucleic acids RNA and DNA. RNA and DNA are like the genetic map to growing new cells. With grass, we get the map (nucleic acids) and the building blocks (amino acids). All we have to do is drink and assimilate.

Studies have shown that cereal grasses and chlorophyll have been instrumental in neutralizing the effects of radiation on the body. Cereal grasses contain precious nucleic acids (RNA and DNA), which are essential for healthy cellular regeneration. This may be very important, especially when cells are damaged by radiation, which can destroy the cell's RNA and DNA. Just a snappy cellular reminder—compliments of your fresh shot of wheatgrass.

Barley Grass

Barley grass is very similar to wheatgrass, but tastes a bit more bitter. Barley is a more ancient and hearty grain than wheat with a more diverse mineral portfolio. The flavor is not as sweet and appealing as wheatgrass, which is why it is not found commercially. It is easy to find barley grass as a dried powder in supplement form.

To grow barley grass, it is essential to find whole "sprouting barley." I like to mix the seeds with wheat seeds to grow barley-wheatgrass for a sweet and bitter flavor.

Rye Grass

Rye grass is also more bitter and tart than wheatgrass. It is hard to find viable seeds, but if they can be found, these seeds are a great choice to mix in with wheat seeds when growing wheatgrass.

Spelt and Kamut Grasses

Spelt and kamut grasses are a great alternative to wheatgrass. This is because they are ancient grains that have not been hybridized. These grasses are sweet and mildly bitter. It can be difficult to find viable seeds that will sprout well.

Wheatgrass

Wheatgrass is by far the most common and popular of edible grasses. It is strangely sweet in a shuddering kind of way. I find it best in juices with parsley and served with a squeeze of lemon. It is an outstanding source of essential amino acids, enzymes, and vitamins. A shot a day and your blood will say "hooray!"

How to Grow Green Soil Sprouts and Cereal Grasses

1. SOAK

   In a glass jar with a wide mouth, soak 2 cups of seeds in 5 cups of fresh water for 6–12 hours. Cover the jar with screen or mesh and secure with a rubber band.

2. DRAIN AND RINSE

   After 6–12 hours, drain off the water. Rinse and drain again.

3. INVERT THE JAR

   Invert the screen-covered jar and place at a 45-degree angle to allow all excess water to drain away. The jar should remain inverted until it is time to rinse and drain again.

4. RINSE AND DRAIN

   Rinse and drain two to three times per day until the tails of the sprouting seeds are as long as the seeds themselves.

5. PREPARE SOIL AND TRAY

   Put 1½ inches of organic potting soil in a shallow 18-inch square or rectangular garden tray (available from nurseries).

6. SPREAD SEEDS, WATER, AND COVER

   Spread the sprouted seeds evenly over the soil. Water the tray well. Cover the freshly spread seeds with a generous piece of screen and another tray or a piece of dark plastic (like a trash bag). Indirect or filtered sunlight is best. Avoid direct sunlight. Secure the covering as necessary.

7. WATCH AND WATER

   Water the tray daily or every other day as necessary. Do not overwater or allow to dry out. Allow to grow for three to five days.

8. REMOVE PLASTIC COVER OR TRAY

   Remove the plastic cover or tray when the grasses or sprouts are reaching up to the screen covering. It is best to leave the protective screen covering gently spread out on top of the growing tray. Allow to grow one to two more days, exposed to indirect or filtered sunlight until ripe and ready for harvest.

9. HARVEST

Harvesting Green Soil Sprouts:

Soil sprouts are ready for harvest when the first two leaves are unfolding and the shells are beginning to fall off. Each seed will grow at a slightly different rate. It is best to harvest when most of the sprouts are ready, even if there are still some on the young side. Younger sprouts are more tasty and nutritious than older ones.

A sharp knife works best to saw down sections of sprouts for harvest. Sharp scissors will work, but be careful to avoid squeezing and mauling the sprouts. Work attentively to avoid clumps of dirt and small roots.

To clean and hull the sprouts, simply put the freshly harvested sprouts in a wide bowl and fill with fresh water. Gently shake and dunk the sprouts with your hand, allowing the hulls to float to the surface. Repeat as necessary. The shells are not particularly tasty as they are a bit rough and fibrous, but they will not harm you if you are unable to remove every single one.

To dry the sprouts, use a salad spinner or gently blot with a dry towel.

To store the sprouts, be mindful that they are dried well. Store them in a plastic bag, along with a dry paper towel, in the refrigerator for best results. (The paper-towel-in-a-plastic-bag trick helps to keep all greens and lettuce fresh in the fridge. Compliments of my mom.)

Harvesting Grasses:

Grasses are ready for harvest when they are about 3½ to 4½ inches tall and the grass has split its first "joint" near the soil at the base of the blade. A "joint" is where the grass has grown from one single blade into a stem where two blades will grow. It is best tasting and most nutritious to harvest when there is only one joint.

A sharp knife works best to mow down sections of grass. It is best to harvest the grass only when it is ready for juicing to maintain ultimate and vital nutrition. Sharp scissors will work, but try not to squeeze and traumatize the grass with rough paws.

It is not usually necessary to wash the grass. If you must, simply rinse the grass with fresh water and dry in a salad spinner.

If you must store harvested grasses, store them in a plastic bag along with a dry paper towel in the refrigerator. Use as soon as possible for optimal benefits.

10. COMPOST THE SOIL

After the soil sprouts or cereal grasses have been harvested, the soil can be composted and used again. Just turn the tray over and start a pile of "used" soil on the edge of your yard. Break up the mat of roots with a shovel, trowel (a small forked garden tool), or your hands.

Another technique for composting is to use a bin or a large lidded container to store the soil. Be sure to use a lid, so rainwater does not collect in the bin. (I use a 33-gallon bin.) Likewise, break up the mat of roots with your hands or a trowel. Continue to add soil as your sprouting trays expire, turning the soil regularly until the container is two-thirds full. The soil will be ready to use in only a few weeks. Eventually, with the right timing for this system, it is unnecessary to purchase additional potting soil. The soil will continue to be enriched by the decomposing roots. This system can even be used for city sprouting, although it requires ample storage space.

Clay-Grown Sprouts

The seeds classified here must be sprouted flat on clay due to their sticky and gummy nature. This is a different sprouting method that does not require rinsing and draining. It uses a 1-foot-diameter porous clay plate (like the shallow terra-cotta planters used for gardening and house-plants) to spread the soaked seeds. The clay absorbs water and gives it back as necessary, allowing the right conditions to grow delicate green sprouts. I use terra-cotta saucers that potted plants often sit in.

Chia Seeds

Chia seeds are the little known powerhouses of healthy omega oils, protein, and fiber. They are most well known for their television debut as "Chia Pets." They grow tender and dainty sprouts with a sweet and mild flavor.

Flaxseeds

Flax is one of the most well-balanced oils and the best source of the EFA (essential fatty acid) called omega-3, necessary for beautiful skin and hair. Flaxseeds can grow into delicate and delicious morsels of tender sprouts.

Watercress Seeds

Watercress is a spicy bunch! Watercress is a wild plant that grows in water streams and is cultivated for its distinguished spicy zest. As young sprouts, watercress is much more mild and delectable.

How to Sprout Using the Clay Method

1. Soak
   Soak ¼ cup of seeds in ¾ cup of fresh water until the water has been absorbed.

2. Spread and Set
   Use two clay dishes (one smaller than the other). Dunk the smaller dish in water and spread the moistened seeds evenly in the dish. (This layer should not be too thick or the seeds will suffocate.) Fill the larger dish with ½ inch of fresh water. Set the smaller dish in the water in the larger dish. Cover the dishes with a piece of screen or mesh for protection.

3. Keep Fresh and Watered
   Maintain the water levels of the larger dish as necessary (in dry climates, the water will evaporate more quickly). Do not directly water the seeds. The water will absorb through the clay dish so the seeds can drink. Indirect or filtered sunlight is best (keep out of direct sunlight). Delicate sprouts will appear and grow in a few days.

Hydroponically Grown Sprouts

SEED	DRY MEASURE (PER HALF-GALLON JAR)	SOAK TIME (IN FRESH WATER)	RINSES PER DAY (WITH FRESH WATER)	SPROUT TIME
SMALL SEEDS				
Alfalfa	2–4 tbsp	6–8 hours	2–4	4–6 days
Broccoli	2–4 tbsp	6–8 hours	2–4	4–6 days
Clover	2–4 tbsp	6–8 hours	2–4	4–6 days
Radish	2–4 tbsp	6–8 hours	2–4	4–6 days
BEANS				
Adzuki beans	1 cup	8–12 hours	2–4	3–4 days
Garbanzo beans	1 cup	8–12 hours	2–4	3–4 days
Lentils	1 cup	8–12 hours	2–4	3–4 days
Mung beans	1 cup	8–12 hours	2–4	3–4 days
GRAINS				
Millet	1½ cups	8–10 hours	2–3	1–2 days
Oats	1½ cups	8–10 hours	2–3	1–2 days
Quinoa	1½ cups	8–10 hours	2–3	1–2 days
Wild rice	1½ cups	8–10 hours	2–3	3–7 days
SEEDS AND NUTS				
Almonds	2 cups	6–12 hours	2–3	1–2 days
Peanuts	2 cups	6–12 hours	2–3	1–2 days
Pumpkin seeds	2 cups	6–12 hours	2–3	1–2 days
Sunflower seeds (hulled)	2 cups	6–12 hours	2–3	1–2 days

Soil-Grown Sprouts and Grasses

SEED	DRY MEASURE	SOAK TIME (IN FRESH WATER)	SPROUT TIME (IN A JAR)	DAYS TO MATURITY (IN SOIL)
Barley	1½–2 cups	6–12 hours	1–3 days	5–10 days
Buckwheat	1½–2 cups	6–12 hours	1–3 days	5–10 days
Rye	1½–2 cups	6–12 hours	1–3 days	5–10 days
Spelt	1½–2 cups	6–12 hours	1–3 days	5–10 days
Sunflowers (hulled)	1½–2 cups	6–12 hours	1–3 days	5–10 days
Sunflowers (unhulled)	1½–2 cups	6–12 hours	1–3 days	5–10 days
Wheat	1½–2 cups	6–12 hours	1–3 days	5–10 days

Clay Method

SEED	DRY MEASURE	SOAK TIME	SPROUT TIME TO MATURITY
Chia	1 cup	1 hour	3–5 days
Flax	1 cup	1 hour	3–5 days
Poppy	1½ cups	6–8 hours	3–5 days
Psyllium	1 cup	30 minutes	3–5 days
Sesame	1½ cups	6–8 hours	3–5 days

17

Culturing and Fermenting

Culturing and fermenting foods are ancient traditions in many cultures around the world. Fermented foods have "live" cultures and are teeming with friendly bacteria to support the balanced population of healthy flora in our intestinal tract.

Colonies of friendly flora in the intestines are principally responsible for digestion and assimilation of nutrients. Maintaining healthy intestinal ecology is essential for vital health, good digestion, a healthy metabolism, and a hearty immune system. It is the dynamic work of friendly bacteria that "digest" nutrients and food so that they are able to pass through the intestinal wall to be picked up by the blood and escorted throughout the body.

The warm, moist environment of the intestines is ideal for breeding bacteria. Maintaining a healthy internal balance is essential for propagating friendly bacteria and keeping unhealthy bacteria under control.

Eating fermented and cultured food is a brilliantly tasty way to maintain a healthy majority of friendly bacteria to support robust digestion and a hearty metabolism for systemic health.

Probiotics and Lactic Acid

Cultured and fermented food is naturally abundant in *probiotics*, a tribe of friendly bacteria. *L. acidophilus* and *L. bifidus* are common strains of probiotics of the *Lactobacillus* family and can be purchased as a dietary supplement. These probiotics are naturally found in fermented foods like miso, kimchi, sauerkraut, rejuvelac (a fizzy beverage), and seed and nut cheeses (as well as unpasteurized dairy yogurt).

Fermented food is also rich in lactic acid. Lactic acid balances the pH of the intestines, resulting in good digestion, better absorption of nutrients, and a healthy metabolism. Lactic acid acts as a disinfectant, killing unhealthy invading microbes while simultaneously helping to restore healthy microbes as the principal population.

Dr. Johannes Kuhl, a notable German researcher and scientist, documented the many health benefits of fermented food. He concludes that natural lactic acid and fermentive enzymes have a beneficial effect on metabolism and a curative effect on disease. His further studies support the idea that fermented food is "predigested" and can be tolerated and metabolized by even those with very weakened digestive systems, especially elderly folks and those suffering from gastrointestinal weakness. Lactic acid in the fermentation of vegetables (like kimchi and sauerkraut) is a magical process of alchemy. Microbes that are abundant in plants, called lactobaccillus, are capable of producing lactic acid in the fermentation of carbohydrates.

Predigested Nutrition

The nutrients in fermented and cultured foods are very bioavailable, meaning our bodies can easily assimilate and absorb them. The process of fermentation "digests" nutrients by breaking them down into a simpler state. This "digestion" is the work usually required by our own digestive systems. Therefore, our bodies do not have to do the work. Hooray! Nutrients that have been broken down are very easy to absorb. The food arrives escorted by a throng of friendly bacteria with the hard work already done. More nutrition for less work. A brilliant formula for champion health.

Daily Culture

We are first introduced to beneficial bacteria in the form of *Lactobacillus bifidus (L. bifidus)* in breast milk during the first 48 hours of mother's lactation. This culture is implanted for our lifetime and is subject to an increase and decrease in population due to food choices, medication, and environmental conditions.

There is a wide variety of cultured and fermented foods that can find a welcome place in anyone's diet (hey, wine is a live, fermented food). Simple condiments like unpasteurized apple cider vinegar and nama shoyu, an unpasteurized soy sauce, are cultured and fermented and full of healthy microorganisms. Miso, a salty paste made from fermented beans or grains, is high in protein and popular as a broth for soup and as a savory ingredient in Asian sauces,

Symbiosis and Dysbiosis

Symbiosis is a cooperative relationship between two or more organisms that is usually beneficial to each. Such is the relationship between friendly, beneficial bacteria. A little effort to populate the intestines with congenial flora is rewarded with speedy, effective digestion and maximum absorption of nutrients, including the manufacture of essential vitamins and healthy elimination.

It is the activity of the healthy microorganisms that is responsible for nutrient digestion and assimilation of food. Bacteria in the intestines actually "digest" food by breaking down nutrients to be small enough and capable of passing through the intestinal wall into the bloodstream, where they can be escorted to local needs. Brilliant. Feed the flora and you get fed.

Vitamins are synthesized in the intestinal tract with the help of friendly bacteria. They actually help *make* nutrients. Studies suggest that this is especially true for B-complex vitamins. It is perfect that vitamins are manufactured exactly where they will be absorbed. The dynamic work of colonies of bacteria in our guts makes the production of vitamins possible.

A favorable population of healthy intestinal bacteria makes for happy and healthy elimination. Food that has been properly digested easily passes out of the system. Colonies of friendly flora and plenty of fiber in the diet from fresh fruits and vegetables support regular, robust habits. Good digestion makes for good riddance. Healthy elimination should be a regular, comfortable occurrence. No mess, no fuss. Alternatively, a shortage of good bacteria leads to dysbiosis, or imbalance, and messes with the naturally genial riddance of waste from the body. Imbalanced intestines can cause cramping, bloating, and runny stools or constipation. No fun.

The intestines are subject to a variety of conditions that kill off good bacteria and feed the unwelcome, festering bacteria. Refined foods like bread and pasta, processed sugar, alcohol, and antibiotic medication wreck the precious balance of healthy bacteria and develop a susceptible environment for unhealthy breeding.

Good fortune and cellular regeneration have granted our bodies the buoyancy of resilience. Even an abused system can return to health. The body naturally seeks balance. An occasional indulgence is tolerable. A merciful nutritionist will suggest: Choose vices wisely and become familiar with a bevy of antidotes. A few coping tools to restore some organization to the system make the margins of healthy living and eating more attractive and sustainable for the long run.

I firmly believe that what you do eat is more important than what you don't eat. Eradicating all unhealthy and processed food is a tough way to clean up the diet. Alternatively, adding luscious and delicious provisions is a pleasure and more fun to concentrate on. If a savory miso soup or a seasonal farmers' market seed cheese will help annul the effects of eating processed food, the world is a better place.

Sustaining a symbiotic balance in the guts takes only a little effort and maintenance. Cultured and fermented foods are an easy, delicious way to provide an abundance of live cultures and natural probiotics to feed and populate the guts with good flora on a regular basis. Simple and easy in, simple and easy out.

dressings, and marinades. Amasake is a sweet shake made from cultured rice that can be purchased in many markets. Tempeh, a great alternative to tofu (which is very processed), is a fermented and very digestible high-protein food. Be sure to look for the word *unpasteurized, live,* or *raw* on the label to ensure that the healthy cultures have not perished in processing.

Sauerkraut and kimchi are fermented vegetable dishes rich in lactic acid, teeming with live cultures, and can be purchased in the market or made in your own kitchen. Making cheese and whey from seeds and nuts is one of my favorite techniques. Seed and nut cheese is abundant in "predigested" protein and has a wonderful flavor and texture. The action of fermentation breaks down the complex protein into more simple compounds for easy absorption. Rejuvelac is a fermented beverage made from sprouted grain. It is rich in healthy microorganisms and lactic acid.

Including live fermented and cultured food on a regular basis is a responsible proactive design for balance and systemic health. See Part Four for a smattering of delicious culinary prescriptions.

Seeds and Nut Cheese

Cheese made from seeds and nuts is one of the finest sources of predigested protein and ferments. Any seed or nut can be used to produce a delicious cheese when tended correctly under the right conditions. Seed and nut cheese is deliciously nutritious and abundant in enzymes and friendly bacteria.

Seed and nut cheese is fermented with live cultures, so the remarkable complex protein of the seed or nut is digested and rendered into a much more simple state. The simplified protein is much more bioavailable and easy to absorb. More nutrition for less work plus live, friendly bacteria is an optimum formula for health.

Fermented food creates a very alkaline environment in the intestines and feeds the population of healthy flora. This is a model environment for the production of the body's own vitamins. Live cultures from fermented food provide a delectable array of precious B-complex vitamins, including vitamin B_{12}, riboflavin (B_2), niacin (B_3), folic acid, and biotin.

Fermenting Makes Seeds and Nuts Light and Digestible

Cultured and fermented cheese is the most digestible way to eat seeds and nuts. It is a step beyond sprouting for digestibility. Seed cheese is a delicious, whole-foods, probiotic medicine. It is an agreeable base for a variety of recipes that can be seasoned to please many tastes. Macadamia Nut Ricotta (page 315) is exceptional for a Sun-Fired Tomato Lasagna Terrine (page 375). Spring Lemon and Dill Sesame Cheese (page 317), served with Pea Mole and Fresh Figs on Jicama (page 309), is superb. Cashew Cream Cheese (page 315) authentically complements spicy salsa and guacamole.

Your Choice of Seeds and Nuts

Any seed or nut can be used alone or in combination to make cheese. Certain seeds and nuts complement different flavors and recipes. Sunflower seeds and almonds have a mild flavor and are reasonably inexpensive for a basic cheese. Cashews are another great standard and can be made gorgeously smooth. Pine nuts and macadamia nuts are delectably lavish for the choice epicure. The process of making cheese from seeds and nuts is quite similar to dairy cheese and yogurt. Producing seed and nut cheese takes less than twenty-four hours. It keeps fresh for days when stored properly. See Part Four for seed and nut cheese recipes.

Kimchi and Sauerkraut

Kimchi and sauerkraut are made from fermenting vegetables. This is an ancient technique employed throughout the world for preservation of summer's bounty and for the healthy benefits of live cultures. Fermented vegetables are a great digestive aid and balance the pH of the intestinal tract.

Lactic acid in fermented vegetables is very alkalinizing and balancing for the system. It acts cooperatively as a disinfectant to diminish unhealthy bacteria and perilous microbes while simultaneously supporting the population of beneficial microorganisms.

Kimchi, also called "Chinese sauerkraut," was first mentioned more than 3,000 years ago in China's oldest poetry book. Sauerkraut is a tradition of German and Eastern European cuisine and is an indispensable provision for health and longevity. Kimchi is characterized by being spicy and hot with fiery peppers and garlic. Sauerkraut is generally mellower in flavor and color.

Kimchi and sauerkraut are made from shredded vegetables, usually cabbage, seasoned with salt and spices. The vegetables are fermented in a clean, controlled environment, under the weight of a stone. The result is a delicious dish with zing that's overflowing with friendly bacteria and enzymes. These high-fiber cultured vegetables are among the richest sources of lactobacillus.

Salt used with fermented vegetables prevents spoilage and selectively encourages the growth of beneficial microorganisms. Salt also promotes enzymatic activity and develops a tasty flavor. Sodium chloride causes the pectin (a water-soluble fiber) in the vegetables to harden, resulting in a great crispy and crunchy texture.

Weighting down the vegetables with a stone speeds the effect of the fermentation and salting and draws out the juices. The weight also prevents contact with oxygen, which can spoil the vegetables and introduce unwelcome bacteria.

Fermented vegetables support our bodies ability to manufacture vitamins. Lactic acid supports a balanced environment in the intestines that aids in the synthesis of the B vitamins. Eating cultured vegetables cultivates optimal conditions for assimilating all vitamins, especially the precious B-complex vitamins.

Most good markets will have a selection of unpasteurized sauerkraut, "veggie-kraut," and kimchi in the refrigerated section. Some stores, especially natural food co-ops, carry locally made varieties. Be certain to look for the word *live* or *unpasteurized* to ensure that the cultures have not been killed in processing. Viable varieties will be found only in the refrigerated section to retard spoilage. Varieties found in a jar on the shelf have been pasteurized for preservation.

Make Your Own Kimchi and Sauerkraut

Producing tasty fermented vegetables in your own kitchen is quite easy. Keeping clean and orderly conditions is important for cultivating good, healthy fermentation. Most kimchi and sauerkraut is fermented for several days, so sanitary, precise conditions must be maintained to discourage the growth of mold and unwelcomed bacteria.

The basic technique for employing successfully fermented vegetables requires:

1. clean, quality produce
2. a starter, like miso

3. a good vessel for fermenting
4. a hearty weight to get all of the juices flowing and to protect the process from oxygen

A huge variety of produce, herbs, and spices can be used to make a motley assortment of fermented recipes. Cabbage is a traditional and common base vegetable. Cabbage has some naturally occurring *L. acidophilus* and readily welcomes the fermenting process. It is a generous vegetable with hearty fiber that stays nice and crunchy after being fermented. It is rich in vitamin C and has a good touch of vitamin E. Cabbage is quite inexpensive and widely available in a good selection.

Procure a Good Vessel

There are three approaches to contain fermenting vegetables.

1. A traditional crock

A large, heavy, earthen crock with a water-seal lid is the best container. Crocks can hold from 1 to 5 gallons of vegetables and have flat, molded weights that fit perfectly in the vessel. The weight is devised to keep a constant pressure on the vegetables to get all of the juices going for even fermentation.

Typically, there is a moat that runs around the top of the crock that is designed to be filled with water. The edge of the lid fits into that moat and forms an airtight seal. The edge of the lid has several dents cut into it so that, as the fermenting vegetables expand and off-gas, the air can escape but none can enter. Brilliant. This design ensures a safe, clean environment that no airborne bacteria can invade.

2. Two bowls that fit together plus a weight

Two bowls that fit together can be used with a weight to approximate the accommodations of a traditional crock. Glass is the best choice. Metal is a reactive compound, and plastic is best to avoid if possible. The prepared vegetables are put in one bowl. It is best to put a piece of mesh or several layers of cheesecloth on top of the vegetable for protection from airborne invasion and to minimize exposure to air. The other bowl is placed on top of the vegetables, and a weight is placed in the bowl (like the weights in the crock) for even fermentation. A sealed jar filled with water or coins works well as a weight. A sizable stone also does the trick.

It is necessary to clean the vegetables very well when preparing and using freshly washed bowls. With this method, there is still some exposure to air, which naturally harbors airborne bacteria. Be clean, and it will be worth the while.

3. A sealing glass jar

Prepare the vegetables and pack them into a very clean glass jar that is sealed tightly. As the vegetables ferment, they will off-gas and create pressure inside the jar. There is no additional weight used in this method, as the pressure does the trick.

This is a great approach for making small batches of vegetables and trying out new recipes.

Procedures

Step 1: Keep everything clean

Remember that the world of bacteria is a wily one. It is a fine line between cultivating good, healthy bacteria and festering, malignant bacteria. Keeping everything clean and sanitary is the best way to ensure a good harvest. You are worth the effort.

Step 2: Prepare the vegetables

Wash the vegetables well. (See recipes for good formulas.) Chop, grate, and shred to desired design using clean tools and a clean cutting board. It is good to get some variety in texture. It is recommended to shred some of the vegetables in addition to other chopping preferences. The finer the produce is cut, the more quickly and thoroughly it will ferment.

A starter is added. Miso is best to jump-start the vegetables with active, live cultures. Add 1 tablespoon for every quart of vegetables to get activity launched in the right direction. After 1 successful bath of fermented vegetables is harvested, a scoop can be saved to mix in with the next batch as a starter.

Salt is added to prevent spoilage and to promote healthy, enzymatic activity. The salt also works with the pectin of the vegetables to maintain a great crunchy texture. The miso starter has a decent amount of salt. When using a previous bath of fermented vegetables as a starter, add an additional teaspoon of salt for every quart of vegetables.

A traditional technique with cabbage is to remove the whole, outer leaves of the head to put on top of the rest of the vegetables. The outer four to six leaves are sufficient. This will help for a good, even pressure of the weights. The result will also produce a whole, fermented, and seasoned leaf excellent for stuffing or wrapping an Autumn Roll.

Step 3: Wash the vessel

Just before putting the vegetables in the chosen vessel (crock, bowls, or jar): WASH the container thoroughly with hot water. I am in the habit of adding some hydrogen peroxide to the last hot rinsing water. This ensures the extermination of any lingering funk.

Step 4: Press and weight the vegetables

Crock Method: Put the prepared vegetables in the crock and pack them down. Arrange the cabbage leaves evenly on top of the rest of the vegetables. Place the weights on the cabbage leaves. Fill the water-sealed moat on the lip of the crock with water and fit the lid in the moat.

Two-Bowl Method: Put the vegetables in the first bowl and pack them down. Arrange the cabbage leaves evenly on top of the rest of the vegetables. Cover the cabbage leaves and vegetables with the piece of screen or several layers of cheesecloth. Place the second bowl on top of the screen or cheesecloth. Put the weight in the second bowl.

Jar Method: Pack as much of the prepared vegetables as possible in the jar. When it is full, try stuffing just a little more in. Screw the lid back on the jar as tightly as possible.

Step 5: Allow to ferment 2 to 7 days undisturbed

The vegetables should sit, undisturbed, for 2 to 7 days, for increasing tanginess. It is best in a dry place (not a basement or closet!). An out-of-the-way countertop works well. The established place does not have to be especially warm but should not be too cool.

The crock and jar method can be employed for the longer duration of the run. They both provide a sealed, sanitary environment for safe fermentation. The two-bowl method is exposed to air and best recommended to harvest after 2 to 3 days.

Step 6: Harvest

After 2 to 7 days, it is time for harvest. The crock will be burping, the bowls will be off-gassing, and the jars will be pressure-sealed.

Crock Method and Two-Bowl Method: When unveiling the vegetables, get ready! The aroma might be overpowering. The top leaves of cabbage sometimes become discolored and funky. If they look questionable, just toss them out. It is not worth eating food that might be ridden with bacteria.

If cabbage leaves were not used, the top layer of the vegetables may be discolored and need to be scraped off.

Scoop the cultured vegetables out of the vessels to store. Glass jars are the best for lasting freshness. Store in the refrigerator. Separate a generous scoop to be set aside as a starter for the next batch.

Jar Method: To test the jars, unscrew one. It should be pressure-sealed and pop when opened. To arrest the fermentation, put the jars in the refrigerator—simple as that.

Rejuvelac

Rejuvelac is a fermented drink made from sprouted grain and is rich in healthy microorganisms and lactic acid. Any grain can be used to make rejuvelac. Wheat has been a traditional favorite, although I prefer more nutritional grains such as quinoa or millet.

With a mild, tangy-sour flavor, rejuvelac can be taken on a daily basis as a tonic to promote a healthy population of friendly bacteria in the system. Rejuvelac is very rich in *L. acidophilus*, *L. bifidus*, and lactic acid. It is a potent, vital, and inexpensive alternative to store-bought probiotic supplements.

Rejuvelac is a great natural "starter" for seed and nut cheeses. It is also an excellent addition for tangy soups and salad dressings instead of water. The flavor is generally mild enough to be dismissed among savory flavors.

Rejuvelac is made with sprouted grain and water. A handful of sprouted grain is added to a generous jar of water and fermented for twenty-four to forty-eight hours. The fermented water is harvested as rejuvelac and strained from the grain. Adding lemon juice is recommended for flavor and as a preservative to keep the rejuvelac fresh longer.

The amount of time for fermentation depends on the environment and the desired strength of the rejuvelac. Rejuvelac brews faster in warm, moist weather. It should be sour tasting, but not foul. It is a delicate brew. If, by any means, it tastes like it has turned the wrong direction, discard the rejuvelac and start again. Fermenting requires such deliberate circumstances to encourage the growth of "good" bacteria without any overgrowth of unwelcome "bad" bacteria. It is not worth it to risk drinking rejuvelac that might have grown out of control.

18

Dehydrated and Sun-Fired Food from a Low-Temperature Bakery

Sun-drying food is one of the oldest methods of preservation. These ancient ways were once developed as an essential preservation technique to store foods. Fruits, nuts, seeds, and grains have been dried for storage for millennia. The Essene people are recorded to have made sun-dried bread from sprouted grain in the deserts near the Red Sea more than 2,000 years ago. Many cultures today still preserve the bounty of summer harvest by sun-drying foods for the dormant season when ripe harvest is a commodity.

These vintage techniques were employed out of resourceful necessity to preserve foods. By default, these techniques also preserve precious nutrients, enzymes, and delicate flavors. Today, sun-drying, dehydrating, and low-temperature baking are used to preserve food more for taste, texture, and convenience than as a means for survival.

Most of us enjoy the benefits of dehydrated food on a regular basis, whether they are sought out or eaten by happenstance. Dried fruits eaten alone or in breakfast cereal make regular visits to many a person's sweet tooth. Raisins are one of the sweetest and most popular dried fruits, especially with children, made simply from dried grapes. Fruit leathers, also called fruit roll-ups, are a high-integrity snack food that can be made in your own kitchen. Dried herbs, such as oregano and cayenne pepper, are dehydrated foods that are regular seasoning staples in most kitchens. There are some packaged "instant" miso soups that have been dried at low temperatures to keep all of the goodies provided by miso, such as live cultures, intact.

In recent years, dehyradrated "raw" products are finding market appeal on the shelves of natural food stores. Several companies are producing crunchy crackers made from flaxseeds and sprouted grains. There are also several varieties of high-energy "power bars" produced specifically at low temperatures to preserve nutrients, minerals, and enzymes.

Most of the concepts and recipes in this book are dynamically more interesting and tantalizing than the average dried-fruit trail mix.

Slow-baking and dehydrating food at low temperatures are responsible ways to enjoy the familiar textures and tastes of flat breads, sweets, crackers, and chips. Using low temperatures over a longer period of time infuses flavors into power-packed nutrition.

The techniques to make flat breads and crackers take more time in the "oven" than traditional techniques, but the results are savory and delicious and unparalleled in nutrition.

What Is Dehydrated Food?

Dehydrating is high-integrity, low-temperature "baking." Dehydrated food has been "cooked" or dried at a temperature set low enough to preserve delicate enzymes and precious nutrients. Low-temperature baking employs the same elements as traditional baking. A steady, warm temperature of dry air is employed in an enclosed environment. The result transforms dough made from sprouted grains and seeds into breads, crackers, crisps, and sweets.

Dehydrated foods can be made from fruits, vegetables, herbs, grains, beans, and seeds. Techniques can be as simple and familiar as dried fruit and fruit roll-ups and as gourmet and savory as Falafel Flats (page 457), Chili Lime Corn Chips (page 452), Portobello Patties (page 390), and Almond Biscotti (page 430).

The Benefits of Low-Temperature Dehydration

The primary design for dehydrating food at low temperatures is to achieve a tasty texture while preserving nutrients and enzymes.

Vitamins and minerals are destroyed by heat. Enzymes, the essential catalysts for metabolic actions including digestion, are also heat-sensitive and begin to be rapidly destroyed at temperatures above 110°F. Drying and "slow-cooking" food at low temperatures ensure premium preservation of nutrients and enzymes.

Delicate flavors are also protected from being jostled out by the chemical change of cooking. Slow-cooking and dehydration maintain the subtle overtones of fresh herbs and spices. Flavors have time to infuse and meld.

Breathing Deeply for Breakfast

During the first few years of exploring a raw foods diet, I was a chef at a premier retreat center on Maui. I used to bake fresh fruit muffins every morning using the best organic vegan ingredients. At the time, I did not eat any refined or cooked food, including these fabulous-smelling muffins. Although I did not want to actually *eat* the muffins, every morning I would drool over their sweet aroma as they baked. It was mild torture. One especially gorgeous Hawaiian morning, I had an epiphany while putting the muffins on a rack to cool. In that moment, I realized that most of the precious goods in these famous muffins were being baked right out of them. I smelled their essence and nutritional spirit drift out of them from the oven. I was suddenly relieved that savoring their sweet aroma was indulgence enough. After that, my mornings were more peaceful. I could live vicariously through the sweet, fresh-baked aroma. Breathing deeply for breakfast is a great way to start the day.

Parameters and Temperatures
How Low Is Low Enough?

What temperature safely preserves the good stuff? How many enzymes are actually being saved? Is dehydrated food really "live/raw" food?

There are few absolutes in life, other than death and taxes perhaps (though some even find a way to avoid taxes). Therefore, a valiant effort to protect the precious nutrients and enzymes in food is not absolute, but it is largely effective. To some extent, food starts leaking nutrition immediately after it is picked. There are certain elements that are out of our control in the modern world, but choosing the freshest food possible and setting low temperatures are within the realm of reasonable and rewarding control.

Nutrients and enzymes are delicate and tricky, but will stick around if handled sensitively. Here is a rational standard that can be reasonably applied: If our bodies' tissues can survive a certain temperature (like testing something with a finger), so can everything that makes the tissues work, such as nutrients and enzymes.

The internal temperature of our bodies is 98.6°F. That is a nice warm temperature and an environment favored for nutrient survival and absorption. Our internal tissues and organs can survive a temperature of 106°F, but not much higher. Above 106°F, the brain begins to fizzle.

A Jacuzzi or hot tub is tolerable and delicious at 110°F. By 112°F, a hot tub is pushing the limits of comfort. It is possible to survive submersion in 116°F water, but not for long. So, somewhere in that realm is a safe margin.

A sauna, which is kind of like a mammoth dehydrator, reaches temperatures of 150°F to 180°F. This window of temperature can be tolerated only for about 20 to 30 minutes before panoramic hallucinations set in. Layers of skin protect the internal organs from heating up. Likewise, in oven baking, a "crust" forms to protect the internal temperature from overheating and drying out. Bread or cake baked at 350°F for one hour will have an internal temperature of 225°F to 250°F. No enzymes can survive that, although it can be reasonably estimated that half of the nutrients and minerals will. Further inquiries into the values of the basic ingredients, like processed flour or sugar and cooked oil, will reveal that baked goods have waning, marginal nutrition. Apropos, the quality of ingredients has a significant impact on the nutritional foundation. For instance, bread made from sprouted grain has significantly more nutrition and digestibility than bread made from milled flour.

Traditional baking calls for relatively high temperatures for a shorter period of time. Dehydrating employs lower temperatures for a longer period of time. Temperatures in the low 100s are tolerable for humans and nutrients, through and through, for a much longer period of time, which is what your flat breads, crackers, croquettes, and cookies will require.

Are Enzymes Actually Saved by Using Low Temperatures?

Enzymes can survive moderate heat and cold. Based on discussion and debate with Dr. Gabriel Cousens, M.D., a prudent estimation can be made that, similar to freezing fresh food, half of the enzymes can survive lengthy dehydration. This may have more to do with oxidation and exposure to air than with heat.

In addition to conserving heat-sensitive enzymes at low temperatures, the quality and state of the ingredients used with these techniques and recipes ensure high-quality results. For instance, sprouting grains and soaking seeds increase nutritional levels and enzymatic activity. Even if some of the enzymes are sacrificed to achieve a tasty texture for flat bread, crackers, or cookies, the end result will have far superior nutrition and digestibility than conventionally baked foods.

Are Dehydrated Foods Really "Live" or "Raw" Foods?

This is not a question that is worth spinning much of a tizzy over. Dehydrated foods have been subject to some niche debate because there is processing involved and heat employed in their making. It is fair to say that dehydrated foods *are* live and raw as long as the ambient temperature used is within the safe range for enzymes and nutrients: below 110°F.

Grains, seeds, and nuts that have been dried at sensitive temperatures will remain vital and viable. My personal experience with this involved cleaning the bottom of a dehydrator and shaking the crumbs from flax crackers that had whole flaxseeds in them outside onto a flower bed. A few days later, under ideal warm and moist conditions, I noticed that the flaxseeds in the flower bed were sprouting on their own and had baby leaves emerging. Does it get more vital than that?

What Is a Dehydrator?

Dehydrated foods are best made in a "dehydrator," a simple oven specifically designed to employ low, steady temperatures. (Dehydrators are widely available for $60–$225.) Similar low-temperature baking techniques can be done in a conventional oven set at the lowest temperature with the door slightly ajar as necessary to regulate the temperature.

The best dehydrators have a fan to circulate the air to maintain an ambient temperature. A fan that circulates air generally reduces the time necessary to thoroughly dry food. A fan also makes quite a difference in the quality of a final product, providing even, dependable results. Dehydrators that are only equipped with heating elements, like a coil, and no fan require much more attention. With just a heating element, it is usually necessary to rotate the goodies in the dehydrator by hand in order to achieve regular results.

A temperature gauge is helpful and important to keep temperatures within safe margins to preserve delicate enzymes and precious vitamins and minerals. An accepted temperature standard recommends dehydrating food below 110°F for a minimum impact on enzymes and nutrients and to return maximum flavor.

Store-Bought Products

Govinda's Crackers

The company Govinda's produces several high-quality sprouted and dehydrated products. Their products include a Pizza Pizzazz, Purple Power Hemp Bar, and Raw Power Tropical Ambrosia. All of these snacks are made from sprouted grains and germinated seeds and nuts. Govinda's uses temperatures that are within the safe range to preserve nutrients and minerals.

Manna Bread (Essene Bread)

Manna bread (Essene bread) is moist, sweet bread made from sprouted grains. You can find it in the refrigerated section of health food markets. It is the least processed "bread" available, made from whole, organic sprouted grains cooked at low temperatures with varieties that include seeds, nuts, and dried fruit.

This bread is very satisfying and moist. The sprouted grains are naturally sweet because the complex carbohydrates are broken down into simpler sugars during the "cooking" process. The convenience of buying a packaged product cannot be beat.

The word *manna* means "life" in Hawaiian; therefore, the suggestion is that manna bread is full of life. Likewise, "Essene" bread refers to the ancient process of sprouted, sun-dried bread making as recorded by the Essene people thousands of years ago in the regions near the Dead Sea. Although this bread is made from sprouted grains at low temperatures, it is exposed to heat above 250°F.

Homemade Products

Cookies (6–20 Hours in Dehydrator at 108°F)

Everybody loves a cookie. Cookie dough can be made using ground nuts and dried fruit, or grains such as buckwheat and oats. The dough can be spiced to sweet perfection. Low temperatures call for a longer time in the dehydrator.

Cookies can be monitored and removed from the oven when they have a chewy texture for a treat like Oatmeal Raisin Cookies (page 433) or when they have a crunchy texture for a treat like Almond Biscotti (page 430). Served with freshly spiced chai, "slow-baked" cookies are a heavenly treat.

Crackers and Crisps (8–12 Hours)

Crackers and crisps are made by spreading seed, nut, or grain dough very thin for the purpose of drying the dough into a crunchy crisp. It is necessary to spread the dough onto a nonstick surface so that the cracker can be peeled away without undo breaking.

Flaxseeds are a great base for making crackers and crisps. When flaxseed is soaked, it becomes mucilagenic and holds together well when spread thinly. Flax has a mild flavor and takes seasoning well. Adding herbs, garlic, olives, sea vegetables, spices, sun-dried tomatoes, vegetables, seeds, and nuts affords an endless option of variations. The result is a thin, crispy cracker that satisfies most cravings for crunchy foods.

Flat Breads (10–24 Hours)

Flat breads are unleavened loaves made from sprouted grains. Making a flat bread helps to maintain a thorough consistency of the loaf at low temperatures. It is difficult to make a thick, unleavened "loaf" of sprouted bread at low temperatures with a good consistency. Sprouted grain is quite dense and can sour easily, especially in a warm temperature. (The dense, sprouted manna bread available in health food stores is cooked at temperatures above 250°F.)

Flat breads store very well for long-term storage when dried thoroughly. They are very versatile and can be used as a crust for pizza, as a crispy tortilla, or cut into pieces like a cracker.

Fruit Strips and Fruit Leather (8–12 Hours)

Fruit strips and fruit leather are some of the simplest dehydrated snacks to make. This is a great way to make use of fruit that has been bruised or just past its prime of perfection. These fruity snacks are a great treat for kids (and adults) and are a convenient food for traveling.

Blending fruit with a little juice or water only as necessary for a smooth mix makes fruit strips and fruit leathers. Spices such as cinnamon and ginger can be added. The blended fruit is poured and spread thinly onto a nonstick sheet to be dehydrated. It is essential to use a nonstick surface for this technique so that the fruit leather can be easily peeled away.

Sea Snacks (12–20 Hours)

Sea snacks are a treat worth relishing. They are made with nori sheets and a savory filling. They can be pressed into a variety of shapes and dried to a crunchy crisp.

Grind nuts, seeds, vegetables, and herbs together to make a smooth pâté. Any recipe for pâté can be used to fill the sea snacks (see Part Four). Nori sheets, pressed sheets of seaweed traditionally used in sushi rolls, are cut into small squares and rectangles to be filled with the pâté. Let your imagination and creativity run with this one: A dollop of pâté can be put in a small square of nori sheet and folded in half to make a triangle. The pâté can be formed into miniature rolls, shaped like pretzel rods. Small pouches can be fashioned to make little dumplings. If you can shape it, it is worth a try. The stuffed snacks are then dehydrated to a crunchy crisp.

Making sea snacks is time intensive, but the results are scrumptious. When I make sea snacks, I create a whole slew of them to be rationed out so that they last for a while. Sometimes I round up a bunch of kids to do the menial work of shaping and rolling (they love it).

Sea snacks that are thoroughly dried will keep fresh for several weeks sealed in a plastic bag in the refrigerator or freezer. So your condensed efforts can be savored over some time. Yum, yum.

Seeds and Nuts, Dried and Seasoned (8–15 Hours)

Seeds and nuts can be soaked in fresh water and dehydrated again for a crunchy, enzymatically active snack or as an ingredient reserved for other recipes, especially pie crusts. Soaked and dehydrated seeds and nuts are significantly more digestible than their original dry counterparts.

In soaking seeds and nuts, the germination process wakes up the dormant nutrients and en-zymes. After arousing the nutrition, dehydrating the seeds and nuts at low temperatures arrests the stimulation of development to preserve the nutrients in a heightened state. These crunchy and fresh-tasting seeds and nuts are a great stash to have on hand.

Once seeds and nuts have been soaked in fresh water, they can be marinated in shoyu (soy sauce) and spices like ginger and chili peppers before being dehydrated into seasoned, delec-table morsels. This technique is a great live alternative to roasted and seasoned seed and nut snacks.

See Part Four for plenty of great recipe ideas.

19

Blanching and Steaming

lanching and steaming are techniques that involve short-term heating with steam or hot water to help break down the indigestible cellulose of some vegetables and complex starches of sprouted beans and grains. Be advised that these techniques are not technically considered "raw food" or "living food," but are a gentle compromise that will improve the flavor and digestibility of certain foods, like "tough" vegetables and sprouted grains and beans.

Steaming is a method of cooking that uses steam vapors from hot water to cook and tenderize vegetables or sprouted beans and grains. The vegetables are briefly suspended in a steaming basket over boiling water. The steam from the boiling water is hot enough to break down tough fiber and indigestible cellulose to make some vegetables much easier to digest. With steaming, it is easy to control how much the produce is cooked, because it is not directly on a flame or burner. It is possible to steam vegetables so that they are still crunchy and vital, retaining most of the precious enzymes and nutrients.

Steaming sprouted beans and grains is helpful to break down the complex starch for a sensitive digestive system and improve the flavor for a sensitive palate.

Blanching is a quick-cooking technique in which food is submerged in hot water for a moment. Blanched almonds are a familiar example: almonds are dunked in hot water to loosen the skins for easy peeling.

Sprouted beans and grains can be briefly blanched to break down the complex starches for easier digestion. Blanching uses such a quick hit of heat that most of the nutrients remain intact.

Certain vegetables, namely those from the *Brassica* genus, such as broccoli, cabbage, cauliflower, and kale, have a large amount of cellulose and a tricky matrix of nutrients that make digesting these vegetables in a raw state difficult for many people (especially those with weakened and sensitive digestive systems). Cellulose, a very complex carbohydrate, is an indigestible fiber. The fiber in these (and many) foods is essential for a healthy intestinal tract, because it sweeps the intestines and encourages robust peristaltic action of the colon. When the attention of the intestines is focused primarily on digesting the cellulose, the nutrients are not as well absorbed or assimilated. Steaming these vegetables is a simple solution to break down the tough cellulose so digesting and absorbing the nutrients is easier and more efficient.

Eating fresh, raw vegetables is the general formula for premium nutrition. However, if certain vegetables cannot be easily digested, the result is diminishing nutritional returns. Lightly steaming certain vegetables makes them more tender and tasty with minimal harm done to the precious enzymes, vitamin, minerals, and nutrients.

Everybody has their own individual formula. What will work best for you is a continuous inquiry. For many, steaming vegetables is a good choice for good taste and optimum health.

Sprouted beans and grains provide a wealth of nutrition for a fresh balanced diet. Beans and grains are an ancient worldwide formula for a balance of complete protein and nourishing carbohydrates. Sprouting beans and grains (versus traditional long-term cooking) makes nutritious sense because it enhances these foods for optimal health. (See Chapter 16 for more information about sprouting.) Sprouting beans and grains unlocks, simplifies, and increases the dynamic nutrition for superlative bioavailability. The complex proteins are broken down into amino acids, the complex starches are broken down into simpler sugars, and the fats are broken down into free fatty acids. In these simpler forms, the nutrition is more available and easier to digest.

However, sprouted beans and grains are still quite starchy. Some (possibly many) people have difficulty absorbing and assimilating all of the potential nutrition in sprouted beans and grains. Blanching or steaming sprouted beans and grains can improve digestibility and balance flavor and texture. Sprouted beans can be chopped and then rinsed to reduce excess starch. Alternatively, or in addition, sprouted beans can be steamed or blanched to further break down the starch and unlock nutritional potential. Similarly, sprouted grains can be steamed or blanched to make them more tender, delicious, and digestible.

Both steaming and blanching are quick-cooking methods that can be exercised with minimal impact on enzymes and nutrients. Although all nutrients, vitamins, and minerals are sensitive to heat, a brief exposure to heat causes minor harm. It is important to remember that the nutritional levels of sprouted beans and grains are higher than their dried or fully cooked counterparts. Breaking down complex starch by blanching or steaming makes the overall portfolio of nutrition more available. If the nutrients of sprouted beans and grains are marginally reduced by blanching or steaming, the net gain is still further in the positive.

Again, it is important to find a formula that works for you. Each of us has a smattering of unique variables that contributes to personal success and validity. For some, steaming and blanching are unnecessary processes to render food sublime. For others, they are the keys that unlock optimum health.

How to Steam

The steaming described here uses steam from boiling water to tenderize vegetables or sprouted beans and grains. A steaming basket that fits in a pot or a steaming pan that fits right on top of a pot is the only tool needed (besides the pot). There are also steaming units that sit on the countertop with a basin of water that boils and passes the steam up through stacked layers to steam vegetables. Only about an inch or two of water is necessary to produce enough water vapor for light or thorough steaming.

The steaming discussed here is on the light side, just enough to break down some of the tough cellulose of vegetables and the complex starch of sprouted beans and grains. It is not necessary to get the water boiling before adding the steaming basket or steaming pan full of veggies or sprouted grains or beans. However, it is easier to control the elements when the water is good and boiling before suspending the goods over the steam.

Four Ways to Heat-Treat Sprouted Beans or Grains for Easier Digestion

All of these techniques achieve similar results using a different approach. Some traditions recognize the effectiveness of preparing food to accommodate individual constitutions and strength of digestive fire. Low temperatures used for longer periods tend to be more nurturing and less disturbing. This results in a gentle, soothing quality and softer texture. A quick, high heat will be more warming and heating to help with sluggish digestion. Use your intuition and inclinations to best suit your evolving needs and the change of the seasons.

Prerequisite for beans and grains: Use beans or grains that have been sprouted until the tail of the sprout is as long as the bean or grain itself, indicating that the nutrition is at its peak.

Chopping and rinsing off the excess starch of sprouted beans will reduce the time necessary for heat-treating, since whole sprouted beans are larger and more dense and chopped beans are smaller and have more exposed surface area.

1. *Steaming:* Fill a pot with one inch of water. Bring to a boil. Put sprouted beans or grains in a steamer and place it in the pot. Lower heat and cover. Steam just until softened, 1 to 4 minutes.
2. *Nituhe (Japanese long method):* In a pot, cover sprouted beans or grains with fresh water and set on the lowest heat. To maintain the highest level of enzymes, a finger

should be able to comfortably tolerate the water at all times. Allow to soak at this temperature for 30 minutes or until the beans soften. Drain and use.

3. *Temperance:* In a pot, cover sprouted beans or grains with fresh water and set on a medium-low flame until the water simmers. Reduce to low heat and cover with a lid for 5 minutes, or until the beans or grains are just starting to soften. Turn the heat off and allow to stand for 10 minutes. Drain and use.

4. *Blanching:* In a pot, bring 3 cups of fresh water to a boil. Add sprouted beans or grains, cover with a lid, and reduce heat to medium-low until water simmers again. Turn the heat off and allow to stand in the hot water for 5 to 10 minutes. Drain and use.

Times may vary. The appropriate time for blanching and steaming will depend on the type of bean. For smaller beans (lentil, mung, and adzuki), less time is necessary; for larger beans (garbanzo and white and red beans), more time is necessary. Try, experiment, and be merry.

The following foods can be steamed for easier digestion:

- Tough vegetables
- Vegetables in the *Brassica* genus, including broccoli, cabbage, and kale
- Sprouted beans, including adzuki, garbanzo, lentil, and mung
- Sprouted grains, including amaranth, millet, quinoa, rye, spelt, and wheat

Garnishing
and Presentation

The presentation of beautiful food is a feast for the senses. Colors and textures feed the aesthetic palate. Crowning a dish with a sprig of fresh herbs, a sprinkle of seeds or chopped nuts, the confetti of edible flower petals, or simply a slice of fresh lemon or orange is a thoughtful, loving touch.

Edible flowers can be purchased in many markets and at farmers' markets. Edible flowers are easy to grow at home in a flowerpot or window box and bring beautiful color to every house or apartment. Similarly, fresh herbs are easy indoor or outdoor plants that reward a green thumb with fresh flavor.

Having a variety of serving dishes, bowls, and plates is an easy step to presenting gorgeous food. Wooden and clay bowls and simple colored dishes and plates contrast and complement different textures and colors. Little dipping bowls are perfect for side sauces, chutney, or wedges of fresh lemon.

Serving food with care is a loving and spiritual infusion of good energy. Anyone who eats food that is prepared and served with care will taste the difference.

Elements for Garnishing

"These are a few of my favorite things . . ."

There are quite a few easy garnishing tricks to create a beautiful plate. A moment of attention to detail and thoughtful presentation guarantees success. Highlighting a dish with an accent of fresh lemon, a sprig of fresh herbs, or a sprinkle of seeds brings the elements to the next level for everyone to enjoy. Sprinkle, garnish, and be merry.

Citrus

Citrus fruits, such as lemons, limes, and oranges, complement many flavors and dishes and are readily available all year. Garnishing a plate with a wedge or slice of lemon is a classy touch. All it takes is one easy slice of a knife.

Wedges
A wedge of lemon or lime is a nice offering on the side of a plate for a fresh squeeze at the table. A wedge of orange makes a sweet palate-cleaning treat for the end of a course.

To cut clean lemon, lime, or orange slices, cut the fruit in half from stem to navel. Cut the half into two or four pieces depending on the size of the fruit and the size of the desired wedge. Serve on the side of each plate, separately in little dishes, or arranged on a serving plate for everyone to enjoy.

Slices and Twists
A slice of lemon, lime, or orange on the side of a plate, the top of a dish, or on the rim of a glass is a classy touch. To get a clean round slice, cut a thin slice across the seeds in the center of the fruit. This is where the fruit is most full and round.

To make a twisted slice, first cut a thin slice across the seeds in the center of the fruit. Lay the slice flat on the cutting board. Make one cut from the center of the slice out through the skin. The slice can be scissored by the cut to look twisted to stand on its own.

A lemon, lime, or orange can be decoratively zested to make a variegated edge of a slice. Use a handheld zester with a row of round teeth at the top for the best results. Zest the skin in strips from the top to the bottom of the fruit for pretty, striped slices.

Lemon Zest
Decorative lemon zest is a delicate garnish with a lift of refreshing flavor. Choose wisely when garnishing dishes with lemon zest, as the flavor will accent the meal. Lemon zest is especially good for soups, spreads, dips, and desserts.

The best zest for garnishes is made with a small, handheld zester with a row of round teeth at the top. This zester makes delicate, curly peels of lemon, orange, or lime for pretty presentation.

Other Fruits

Sliced fruit makes a sweet garnish. Complement the flavors of a dish and provide a sweet treat to cleanse the palate between courses or at the end of a meal. With regard to food combining for optimal digestion, it is best to serve only a few slices of less sweet fruit. Sliced apple or pear or a wedge of orange are nice choices. A few pomegranate seeds or a small bunch of grapes is tasteful. Try a piece of enzyme-rich pineapple or papaya. Steer away from very sweet and starchy fruits like bananas, dates, persimmons, and mangoes for optimum digestion.

Vegetable Ribbons and Threads

Delicate ribbons and threads of vegetables make lovely garnishes for any soup, salad, sushi roll, or entrée. There are two ways to make vegetable ribbons and threads, depending on what tools are at hand.

Peeled Ribbons

Any firm vegetables can be "peeled" into pretty ribbons with a vegetable peeler. Longer vegetables, such as carrots, cucumber, zucchini, parsnips, daikon radish, and butternut squash, are the best for longer ribbons. To peel ribbons, first peel the skin of the vegetables. Then continue to peel the vegetable in long strips to the core. The results are lovely, delicate ribbons that are great to bundle on the side or top of a dish or plate for garnish. These ribbons are also good to roll in sushi rolls for a decorative texture.

Threads

Firm vegetables can be sliced into delicate "angel hair" threads with a Saladacco (see Chapter 12). Firm vegetables, such as carrots, beets, butternut squash, daikon radish, and even sweet potatoes and yams, can be cut into spiral threads easily with this handy machine. The vegetable is rotated over a sharp blade with small teeth for a simple garnish for a gorgeous presentation.

Tomato "Flowers"

A tomato "flower" is a lovely garnish that resembles a blooming rose. It's a perfect garnish for the center of a vegetable torte or a bowl of pâté, hummus, or dip.

To make tomato "flowers," you will need a small, sharp paring knife. Larger tomatoes are the easiest to skin.

1. Hold the tomato in one hand and the knife in the other. Peel away the skin of the tomato in a strip ½ inch to 1 inch wide around the middle part of the fruit. Try to peel a thin strip of skin without much flesh. Try not to break the strip if possible so that you end up with one long piece of skin. On larger tomatoes, two strips of skin can be peeled. If it does break, do not worry. It can be pieced together.

2. Lay the skinned strip facedown on the cutting board (with the smooth skin facing up). Make two to four evenly spaced incisions along one edge of the strip. The incisions should cut through only a quarter of the way through the strip. Be careful not to cut more than halfway through the strip. Roll the skin, inside out, from one end to the other. The result will be a pretty, inside-out bundle that resembles a rose. The incisions will help the flower "blossom" and fan out a bit. If the strip should split or break when peeling, roll the strip inside out into a small bundle and continue rolling the bundle with the broken piece. A toothpick can help to hold the flower together if necessary.

Edible Flowers

Edible flowers are an aesthetic delight. Flowers bring a loving touch to the table. There is a wide variety of edible flowers that suit all types of dishes, including calendulas, marigolds, roses, gardenias, impatiens, pansies, violets, and nasturtium flowers. Use the petals to create a colorful confetti or use the entire flower. A sprinkle of petals or a full blossom is a tasteful touch that delights all the senses.

Other Flowers and Plants

Adorning a plate with other flowers or decorative cuttings makes a lovely presentation. Be sure to tell fellow dining friends that the garnish is not edible or set it aside before serving the meal. Any pretty flower in bloom is a nice touch. Be creative and forage for what is at hand—for example, a bundle of acorns complements an autumn meal.

Try adorning the table with pretty bunches of leaves or stalks of flowers. Natural decorations bring a festive air and the essence of creative fun to celebrations.

Sprinkling Seeds and Nuts

Sprinkling seeds or chopped nuts on salads, soups, or sauces for contrast is a great finishing touch. Try black and white sesame seeds, chopped almonds or walnuts, pine nuts, pumpkin seeds, or delicate poppy seeds. For soups, sauces, sushi rolls, and vegetable dishes, the thoughtful pinch of garnish makes a loving addition.

Try to match the flavors and contrast the texture for tasteful results. A little bit goes a long way, so sprinkle lightly.

Fresh Herbs

Freshly chopped herbs or a decorative sprig of herbs make a great garnish. Save a few choice leaves or the decorative top of herbs when preparing a recipe to garnish the dish before serving.

Basil flowers, from the top of the plant, are a lovely addition. Try a sprig of feathery dill for soups or spreads. Curly parsley is a pretty decoration and a good breath freshener for the end of a meal. A sprig of mint in a beverage or on a dessert is a treat. Mix, match, crown, and contrast. Find delight in the details.

Part Four

*

The Recipes

21

Beverages

PEPPERMINT LICORICE TEA
MAKES 2 QUARTS.

*Licorice is a naturally sweet, earthy root that complements
the clean flavor of peppermint. Lovely.*

6 tablespoons dried peppermint leaves
3 tablespoons licorice root
8 cups fresh water

Combine ingredients in a 2-quart glass jar or pitcher and brew for an hour or two in the sun
or 2 to 3 hours on the counter or in indirect sun. Strain and serve over ice, or store in the
refrigerator.

Warming Tea and Brews

MACADAMIA NUT CHOCOLATE MOCHA
MAKES 2–4 SERVINGS.

*A lush chocolaty mocha with creamy
macadamia nuts and sultry vanilla.*

4 cups macadamia nut milk
   *½ cup raw macadamia nuts (raw
     almonds may be substituted if raw
     macadamia nuts are unavailable)*
   4 cups filtered water
2–4 tablespoons raw honey or
   maple syrup
Several drops of liquid stevia (optional)
1 tablespoon vanilla extract
1–2 tablespoons raw carob powder,
   or to taste

1–2 tablespoons cocoa powder,
   or to taste
1–2 tablespoons instant grain
   coffee (optional)
1 tablespoon cinnamon, ideally
   fresh ground
1 teaspoon nutmeg, ideally
   fresh ground
½ teaspoon sun-dried sea salt

To make nut milk: Blend macadamia nuts and water at high speed until very smooth. Pour mixture through a strainer. Save macadamia nut pulp for other uses.

Blend macadamia nut milk, honey or maple syrup, stevia (if desired), vanilla, carob, cocoa, grain coffee (if desired), cinnamon, nutmeg, and sea salt until smooth, adding more honey, maple, or stevia to sweeten to taste. Gently warm in a saucepan over low heat for 3 to 5 minutes. Your finger should comfortably be able to tolerate the heat of the water. Do not boil!

Serve in warmed mugs with a fresh cinnamon stick.

REAL GINGER BREW
MAKES 4 CUPS.

*Fresh ginger root is an exceptional therapy for aiding digestion
and stimulating circulation. This drink is warming and soothing
solo or sweetened with a spoon of honey. When cooled, this
tea is a lively ingredient for a papaya smoothie.*

¼ cup grated ginger
4 cups fresh water
Raw honey to taste (optional)

Mix ginger with water in a small saucepan and bring to a gentle simmer. Reduce the heat. Allow to simmer for 3 to 5 minutes. Strain into a teapot or cups. Sweeten with honey to taste if desired.

Traditional Chai Spice Tea

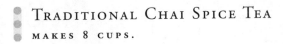

MAKES 8 CUPS.

*In this caffeine-free drink, traditional chai spices are brewed
for a spiritual experience. Sweeten and lighten to taste.*

8 cups filtered water
3 3-inch cinnamon sticks, broken
   into pieces
1 whole nutmeg, cut into small pieces
5 whole cloves
4 whole black peppercorns, bruised
   with the flat side of a knife, or
   1 teaspoon ground black pepper
6 cardamom pods, bruised with the
   flat side of a knife

1 2-inch piece fresh ginger root, grated
2 whole star anise
½ teaspoon sun-dried sea salt
Raw honey, maple syrup, and/or
   liquid stevia to sweeten to taste
Almond milk (see recipe on page 266)
   to taste (packaged almond, soy, or
   rice milk can be used instead)
2 tablespoons green tea, maté leaf, or
   rooibos leaf (optional)

Bring all spices to a gentle simmer in water and reduce to a low heat. Allow to simmer covered for 20 to 40 minutes until very aromatic. Pour liquid through a strainer. Save spices to use again. They can be used several more times, reducing the amount of water by 1 cup each time to maintain the potency of the tea. Sweeten to taste with raw honey, maple syrup, and/or liquid stevia. Add almond milk for desired taste. Warm over a low heat for 1–3 minutes or as necessary. Add green tea, maté, or rooibos as desired. Store unused portion in a glass jar in the refrigerator.

Smoothies

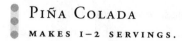 PIÑA COLADA
MAKES 1–2 SERVINGS.

*Simple, quintessential piña colada, made
exceptional by fresh ingredients.*

> 1 cup young coconut meat
> 1 cup frozen pineapple
> 2 cups coconut water or fresh
>   orange juice

Blend all ingredients at high speed until smooth.

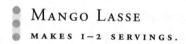 MANGO LASSE
MAKES 1–2 SERVINGS.

*Mango lasse is a sweet Indian delight traditionally
made with yogurt. The cashews make this a
creamy treat for breakfast or dessert.*

> ¼ cup whole raw cashews
> 1 cup fresh coconut water, or fresh
>   water as necessary to blend
> 1 ripe mango, pitted
> 1 teaspoon non-alcohol vanilla extract

> 1 teaspoon cinnamon
> 1 teaspoon cardamom
> 1 cup orange juice, frozen in an ice
>   cube tray

Blend cashews and coconut water or fresh water at high speed until smooth. Add mango,
vanilla, cinnamon, and cardamom and blend until smooth. Add frozen orange juice and blend
until slushy.

Serve immediately.

PEACHY KEEN SMOOTHIE

MAKES 1–2 SERVINGS.

*Peaches and cream are the perfect complements. Fresh almond milk
is sweet and alkaline to help make this a creamy delight.*

2 cups fresh almond milk (see
    page 266)
4 peaches, pits removed, peeled and
    frozen
1 teaspoon non-alcohol vanilla extract
1 tablespoon raw honey, or 2 soft
    dates, pitted

Blend almond milk with frozen peaches, vanilla, and raw honey or dates at high speed until
smooth.

Milks

Any nut or seed can be used to make milk. Nut milks are nutritious drinks, naturally packed
with vitamins, minerals, and protein. They are excellent alternatives to dairy milk or packaged
and processed soy and rice milks and can be used in cereal, tea, and anywhere "milk" is needed.

The basic technique is to blend nuts or seeds with water and strain off the excess pulp leaving a creamy, delicious beverage or a great base for soup. The variations on this theme are
many. Using more nuts or less water will yield thicker milk. Using fewer nuts or more water
will make lighter milk. Plain nut milk can be flavored with a sweetener like vanilla, carob, or
cocoa. Coconut water used instead of filtered water is divine. Spices are a sumptuous addition.
Fresh or dried fruit can be added. And certainly, frothy milkshakes can be whipped up.

The pulp left over from making milk can be used again to make a lighter milk, or the
amount of water can be reduced to maintain the same richness. It is a very efficient and affordable alternative to dairy milk and processed, packaged soy and rice milk.

Nut milk keeps fresh in a sealed glass jar in the refrigerator for several days. Any extra nut
milk can be frozen into ice cube trays for smoothies and milkshakes.

The Real Deal About Cow's Milk

Cow's milk isn't as good for you as you probably think!

1. Modern commercial dairy farming involves the heavy use of growth hormones and antibiotics, in order to produce more, supposedly healthier milk. The problem is that these hormones and antibiotics get into the milk the cows produce, and when we ingest them, they have far-reaching effects on our health, including possible endocrine and reproductive problems and the development of "super" strains of bacteria that are resistant to the constant low doses of antibiotics they are subjected to.

2. More than 60 percent of the human population is either lactose-intolerant (meaning their bodies do not produce the enzyme to digest the main sugar in milk, lactose) or allergic to milk. If more than half of us can't drink milk, it can't be as necessary to good health as many think it is.

3. Dairy products cause excess mucus production in the body. Excess mucus production can ultimately affect our digestive and immune systems.

4. Dairy milk really isn't as nutritionally packed as we are led to believe. We are all told that we need milk in order to get sufficient amounts of calcium, vitamin A, and vitamin D. But truth be told, milk is not a very rich source of these vitamins naturally; it's generally fortified with them. And most green vegetables have more calcium than milk! Eat your veggies and you'll be just fine.

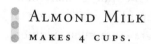

ALMOND MILK
MAKES 4 CUPS.

*A naturally sweet, versatile, alkaline, fresh milk
that's great for every need.*

1 cup soaked raw almonds (soaked
    4–8 hours)

4 cups filtered water
Pinch sun-dried sea salt

In a blender at medium, then high speed, blend ingredients until smooth. Pour through a strainer to separate remaining pulp. Save the pulp to use again for a lighter milk.

VANILLA WHOLE MILK

MAKES 4 CUPS.

A sweet and delicious fresh milk with the elegant essence of vanilla.

1 cup soaked raw almonds (soaked
   4–8 hours)
4 cups filtered water
Pinch sun-dried sea salt
1 tablespoon non-alcohol vanilla
   extract

½ vanilla bean (optional)
3 tablespoons raw honey or maple
   syrup, or 3 soft dates, pitted

In a blender at medium, then high speed, blend soaked almonds, water, and sea salt until smooth. Pour through a strainer into a pitcher to separate pulp. Pour liquid back into the blender and blend in vanilla extract and bean (if using) and sweetener until smooth.

CREAMY CANTALOUPE MILK

MAKES 4 CUPS.

A delicious breakfast drink for a summer morning.

Seeds of 1 cantaloupe
3 cups water
1 cup cantaloupe flesh
Pinch cinnamon

In a blender at medium, then high speed, blend cantaloupe seeds and water until smooth. Pour through a strainer into a pitcher to separate pulp. Pour liquid back into the blender and blend in cantaloupe and cinnamon until smooth.

Herb and Flower Ice Cubes

Fresh herbs, like mint and edible flowers, suspended in frozen ice cubes make classy additions to fresh juice, coconut water, sun tea, or a gorgeous glass of fresh water. As the ice melts, the drink is infused with delicate flavors and the lovely touch of gourmet magic.

MINTED ICE

MAKES 1–2 TRAYS OF ICE CUBES.

Great in lemonade, iced tea, or simply fresh water.

> 1 bunch mint
> Fresh water

Remove the mint leaves from the large stems. The pretty, delicate tops of the sprigs can be left whole for a nice visual. Fill each compartment of the ice cube tray with several leaves (3 to 5), and fill the tray with fresh water. Freeze until solid and ready to use.

CONFETTI ICE

MAKES 1–2 TRAYS OF ICE CUBES.

Pot marigolds come in shades of yellow, pale to brilliant
orange, and deep crimson with beautiful small petals
that look like confetti in ice.

> 4–6 pot marigold or calendula flowers
> Fresh water

Remove the petals from the flowers and sprinkle in each compartment of an ice cube tray. Fill with fresh water, and freeze until solid and ready to use.

continued

RASPBERRY LEMON ICE
MAKES 1 TO 2 TRAYS OF ICE CUBES.

*Beautiful in lemonade, orange juice,
and sparkling or fresh water.*

2 dozen raspberries
1 lemon, thinly sliced and cut into small wedges

Slice the lemon thinly with a sharp knife. Cut each slice into eight wedges. Place a raspberry or two and a piece of lemon or two in each compartment of an ice cube tray. Fill with fresh water, and freeze until solid and ready to use.

STRAWBERRY AND CREAM MILKSHAKE
MAKES 1–2 SERVINGS.

*Strawberries and cream in a milky shake is a dream. The beet
brings a brilliant flush to this frothy blend.*

¼ cup whole raw cashews or raw
  macadamia nuts (raw cashew pieces
  can be used)
4 soft dates, or 2½ tablespoons raw
  honey or maple syrup
1 tablespoon vanilla extract

1 teaspoon beet powder or
  1 tablespoon shredded beet
1½ cups fresh coconut water or apple
  juice
1½ cups frozen strawberries

In a blender at medium, then high speed, blend nuts, dates (or honey or maple syrup), vanilla, beet, and coconut water or apple juice until super-smooth. Break apart frozen strawberries and blend in until smooth.

Farmacy Fresh Juices

Fresh juice is quite delicate and should be consumed immediately after it is extracted. The process of juicing exposes the nutrients in the fresh juice to oxygen, which begins to break these precious goodies down. Certain juicers are designed to minimize oxidation and preserve the life of the juice, but the golden rule remains: the fresher, the better.

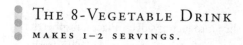

The 8-Vegetable Drink
MAKES 1–2 SERVINGS.

Eight vegetables in a delicious and flavorful juice make a true V-8. Excellent for an afternoon boost.

4 carrots
3 celery stalks
2 kale leaves
2 tomatoes

1 cucumber, unpeeled
1 small beet
½ cup loose parsley, stems included
1 clove garlic

Juice all vegetables. Drink immediately.

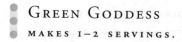

Green Goddess
MAKES 1–2 SERVINGS.

A delight of fresh, juicy greens and the sweetness of perky apples in a gorgeous, pale green tonic.

2 cucumbers
3 celery stalks
4 outer leaves of romaine lettuce
2 green apples, seeds included
1 lemon, peeled

Juice all ingredients and serve with a slice of lemon.

Bottled Juice

Bottled juice has very little value in the face of fresh pressed juice. Bottled juice on the shelves of the market has been pasteurized in packaging to preserve freshness and establish a long shelf life. Pasteurization heats the juice or, at the least, the bottle, and destroys precious nutrients that are heat- and light-sensitive. Organic bottled juice is a good stand-in for smoothies, though fresh juice is unsurpassable in its nutritional integrity.

"Fresh" bottled juice is available in the refrigerated sections of many markets. These are juices that have been pressed or squeezed and bottled fresh for the day. In some areas, there are "fresh" bottled juices produced in larger batches and sold for several days before expiring.

"Fresh" bottled juices are convenient and certainly more nutritious than pasteurized bottled juices. Far and away, though, fresh-made juice is a fountain of vital, fresh nutrition and life.

WHEATGRASS AND CITRUS TWIST
MAKES I SERVING.

The lemon really balances the strong,
sweet flavor of wheatgrass to boot.

 1 ounce fresh wheatgrass juice
 ½ lemon, peeled

Squeeze lemon juice into the wheatgrass and swirl or stir. Drink immediately.

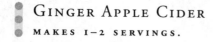

GINGER APPLE CIDER
MAKES 1–2 SERVINGS.

*Perfect for an autumn afternoon or as
a refreshment for a soccer game.*

6 red apples (Fuji, Red Delicious,
   Braeburn, etc.)
1 2-inch piece fresh ginger
1 lemon, peeled

Pinch cinnamon
Pinch nutmeg
Pinch sea salt

If the apples are organic, do not remove the seeds. Cut into slices that will fit through the juicer. Cut lemon into quarters and remove any seeds.

Juice apples, ginger, and lemon together. Combine, and stir in cinnamon, nutmeg, and sea salt.

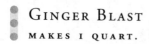

GINGER BLAST
MAKES 1 QUART.

*A feisty ginger ade using whole lemons, fortified with all of the
nutrients of bee pollen. Add a pinch of cayenne for an extra kick.*

1 lemon, outer skin removed
2 tablespoons shredded or finely
   minced ginger
1½ tablespoons bee pollen
¼ cup raw honey
Several drops of liquid stevia
   (optional for extra sweetness)

½ teaspoon sun-dried sea salt
2 tablespoons aloe vera, peeled
   (optional)
Pinch cayenne pepper (optional)
2 cups orange juice
2 cups fresh water

Cut peeled lemon into quarters and remove the seeds. In a blender, blend all ingredients at medium, then high speed until smooth and frothy.

Soups

"Of soup and love, the first is best."

—SPANISH PROVERB

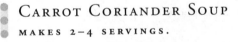 CARROT CORIANDER SOUP

MAKES 2–4 SERVINGS.

This is one of my favorite simple soups. Fresh carrot juice and creamy avocado are a luscious match.

2 cups fresh carrot juice

2 teaspoons minced fresh ginger (add more for a little more warmth)

1 medium avocado, pit removed, and cut into large chunks

½ cup fresh loose cilantro

¼ cup fresh loose parsley

2 teaspoons coriander seed (whole coriander seed freshly ground is best)

1 tablespoon organic extra-virgin olive oil (optional)

2 tablespoons nama shoyu

Pinch sun-dried sea salt, or to taste

2 green onions, outer skin removed, and finely sliced

Fresh crushed coriander seed or white and black sesame seeds

Blend carrot juice, ginger, and avocado at medium-high speed until smooth. Remove cilantro and parsley leaves from the main stems. Add in de-stemmed herbs, coriander seeds, oil, and nama shoyu. Pulse at medium speed until well mixed but with small pieces of herbs still visible. Season with a pinch of sea salt, if necessary, to taste. Sprinkle green onions on top. Serve chilled. Garnish with crushed coriander seed or white and black sesame seeds as available.

CREAMY MISO SOUP
MAKES 2–4 SERVINGS.

This soup also makes a great dipping sauce for sushi rolls.

2 Roma tomatoes or 1 large tomato, cut into halves and seeded

1 medium avocado, pit removed, and cut into chunks

2 cups coconut water; or 1 cup fresh-squeezed orange juice + 1 cup water

1 lemon, juiced

2 tablespoons white miso

2 tablespoons red miso

(If only one type of miso is available, use 4 tablespoons white miso or 3 tablespoons red miso.)

1 tablespoon minced ginger

1 clove garlic

½ cup fresh water, or as necessary to thin

3 tablespoons chopped parsley

¼ cup finely chopped green onion, outer skin removed

4 teaspoons hulled hemp seeds or sesame seeds

2 teaspoons orange zest (optional)

In a blender or food processor, blend tomato, avocado, either the coconut water or the orange juice and water, lemon juice, miso, ginger, and garlic until smooth. Add ½ cup or more fresh water as necessary to thin the soup to desired consistency. I like it to be thick. Add chopped parsley and pulse until mixed in. Sprinkle with chopped green onion and hemp seeds or sesame seeds and, if desired, orange zest.

Serve at room temperature or gently warmed.

Sweet Corn Bisque with Spicy and Sweet Pepper Relish

MAKES 2–4 SERVINGS.

A sweet creamy soup made from fresh corn, smooth almond milk, and just the right spices. Try with or without the complement of a spicy relish.

Bisque

4 ears fresh corn
2 cups thick almond milk (see page 266)
¼ cup chopped cilantro
1 clove garlic
2 teaspoons fresh ground coriander seeds
1 teaspoon fresh ground cumin seed
Sun-dried sea salt to taste

Relish

1 dry chipotle pepper
1 red bell pepper
½ cup cilantro leaves
5 mild green olives, pitted
1 tablespoon organic extra-virgin olive oil
Sun-dried sea salt to taste
Fresh ground black pepper to taste

To make the bisque: Saw fresh corn kernels from the cob. Blend corn, almond milk, cilantro, garlic, and coriander and cumin seeds until smooth. Season with sea salt to taste and set aside.

To make the relish: Cut the top off the dry chipotle pepper. Slice the pepper in quarters. Remove the seeds for a milder relish. Soak the pepper in water until soft enough to mince. Chop the chipotle pepper, red bell pepper, cilantro, and olives very finely. Mix together and season with olive oil. Add sea salt and fresh black pepper to taste. Allow to stand to develop flavor.

COOL CUCUMBER AND DILL SUMMER SOUP WITH CHIPOTLE CHUTNEY

MAKES 2–4 SERVINGS.

This is a refreshing summer soup with cool cucumber and the clean flavors of lemon and dill. Serve with or without the spicy chutney.

Soup

3 cucumbers, peeled and seeds
   scooped out
4 tablespoons pine nuts
2 tablespoons raw tahini
   (sesame paste)
½ cup lemon juice
1 tablespoon lemon zest
1 tablespoon raw honey
½ cup water
¼ cup chopped fresh dill, or
   1½ tablespoons dried dill
2 tablespoons chopped parsley
1 teaspoon sun-dried sea salt,
   or to taste

Chutney

½ cup diced tomato, seeds removed
1 tablespoon chopped chipotle
   peppers
1 tablespoon chopped parsley
2 teaspoons minced ginger
1 teaspoon organic extra-virgin
   olive oil
1 tablespoon raw honey
Pinch sun-dried sea salt

Garnish

lemon zest

To make the soup: In a food processor or blender, blend cucumbers, pine nuts, tahini, lemon juice, zest, and honey until smooth. Add water a bit at a time as necessary to thin. Add dill and parsley and pulse to mix in. Add sea salt to taste. If using dried dill, you may add an additional 2 teaspoons to season to taste. Chill soup.

To make the chutney: In a small bowl, combine tomato, chipotle peppers, parsley, and ginger. Add olive oil, honey, and sea salt. Allow to stand to develop flavor for at least 15 minutes. The chutney can be prepared ahead of time and will keep fresh for days in the fridge.

To serve: Serve soup in a broad shallow bowl. Dollop chipotle chutney on top of each serving. Garnish with lemon zest.

Gazpacho Pesto Best

MAKES 4–6 SERVINGS.

Sun-dried tomatoes and pesto are a superb complement to a traditional favorite.

½ cup sun-dried tomatoes

1 cup fresh orange juice (approximately 1 to 2 oranges squeezed)

2 tablespoons apple cider vinegar

1 teaspoon sun-dried sea salt

1–2 cloves garlic

1 small sweet onion, chopped (approximately ½ cup)

¼ cup pine nuts

¼ cup walnuts

4 Roma tomatoes or 2 medium tomatoes, seeded and diced (approximately 2 cups)

1 medium cucumber, peeled, seeds scooped out, and diced (1 cup)

½ cup chopped tender celery, from the center of the bunch

1 cup chopped fresh basil

¼ cup chopped parsley

1 teaspoon oregano (best fresh)

2 tablespoons organic extra-virgin olive oil (optional)

1–2 teaspoons sun-dried sea salt, or to taste

Fresh ground black pepper to taste

Cover sun-dried tomatoes with orange juice, apple cider vinegar, and sea salt for 5 to 15 minutes, or until very soft. This can be done ahead of time and kept on hand in the fridge. (If you are using sun-dried tomatoes from a jar and they are already marinated, do not soak the tomatoes: simply drain them, mix with the preceding ingredients, and proceed to the next step.) In a food processor or blender, blend softened sun-dried tomatoes and soaking mixture until fairly smooth. Add garlic, chopped onion, pine nuts, and walnuts, and pulse until fairly smooth. Add in the tomatoes, cucumber, celery, basil, parsley, and oregano. Pulse until mixed but not smooth. Drizzle in olive oil, if desired, and season with sea salt and black pepper to taste. Allow to stand to develop flavors (30 minutes to overnight).

Serve chilled in a broad shallow bowl.

Red Bell Pepper Cascadilla Soup
MAKES 2–4 SERVINGS.

*Cascadilla is akin to a south-of-the-border gazpacho.
Fresh coconut water can be replaced with fresh orange
juice for a sweet, tangy flavor. All the right herbs
make this soup heavenly every time.*

1 red bell pepper, seeds and stem
    removed, cut into quarters
    (approximately 1½ cups)
1 cup fresh coconut water or fresh
    orange juice
2 tablespoons white miso
1 clove garlic
2 tablespoons lime juice (lemon
    juice or apple cider vinegar
    may be substituted)
2 medium tomatoes, seeded and
    diced
1 medium cucumber, peeled, seeded,
    and diced

2–4 tablespoons organic, cold-pressed
    sesame oil or olive oil (optional)
2 green onions, chopped to the top
¼ cup chopped parsley
¼ cup chopped cilantro
1 tablespoon chopped dill
2 teaspoons freshly ground
    coriander seeds
2 teaspoons freshly ground
    cumin seeds
2 teaspoons fresh ground black
    pepper
Pinch cayenne pepper
Sun-dried sea salt to taste

In a food processor or blender, blend bell pepper, coconut water or orange juice, miso, garlic, and lime juice until smooth. Add tomatoes, cucumber, oil (if desired), green onions, chopped herbs, ground coriander and cumin, and black and cayenne peppers. Season with sea salt to taste. Pulse until well mixed but not smooth.

    Serve chilled.

SORREL AND BABY SPINACH BISQUE
MAKES 2–4 SERVINGS.

*Fresh macadamia nut or cashew milk creates the creamy luscious
texture of this bisque. Sorrel is a leafy green, similar to spinach
but with a divine, uplifting lemony zing. White miso gently
thickens and adds to a sweet mature flavor.*

2 cups macadamia nut or cashew milk
  *½ cup raw macadamia nuts or
    whole raw cashews*
  5 cups water
2 cups loose baby spinach (Mature
  spinach can be used, though it is
  not as tender. Be sure to remove all
  tough stems.)
1 cup loose sorrel, leaf removed
  from main stem (If sorrel is
  unavailable, substitute 1 cup
  spinach + 1 tablespoon lemon
  juice + 1 tablespoon lemon zest)

3 tablespoons white miso
1 tablespoon chopped chives
1 green onion, chopped to the top
1 clove garlic, minced
2 tablespoons lemon juice
Fresh ground black pepper to taste
Sun-dried sea salt to taste

Garnish
2 tablespoons chopped pine nuts

To prepare the nut milk: Soak macadamia nuts or cashews in 3 cups of fresh water for 30 minutes. Drain. Blend nuts with 2 cups of fresh water at high speed until smooth. Strain through mesh strainer. Save pulp for other use.

To make the bisque: In a food processor or blender, blend nut milk, spinach, sorrel, miso, chives, green onion, garlic, and lemon juice until smooth. Season with pepper and salt to taste.
  Serve chilled. Garnish with chopped pine nuts.

Thai Tom Yum Coconut Soup
MAKES 2–4 SERVINGS.

Thai coconut soup is heaven at its best.
Fresh coconut makes this soup divine.

2 cups young coconut meat
2 cups young coconut water
2 tablespoons peeled and chopped
   fresh ginger
1 clove garlic
1 Thai chili pepper (a small *hot*
   pepper), adjust amount to tailor
   flavor. *Go slow! You can always add*
   more. (Any hot pepper can be
   substituted.)

3 tablespoons chopped basil
3 tablespoons chopped parsley
3 tablespoons chopped cilantro
1 tablespoon ground lemongrass
2 teaspoons oregano
2 tablespoons organic extra-virgin
   olive oil, or 1 tablespoon cold-
   pressed coconut butter (optional)
2 tablespoons nama shoyu
Sun-dried sea salt to taste

In a food processor or blender, blend coconut meat and water with ginger, garlic, and chili pepper until smooth. Add more coconut water as necessary if a thinner consistency is desired. Add
chopped herbs, olive oil or coconut butter, and nama shoyu, and gently blend. Season with sea
salt to taste.

Curried Coconut Soup
MAKES 4–6 SERVINGS.

A delicious integration of flavors spiced with curry and fresh coconut.
Tomatoes and mushrooms give delectable body to this creamy soup.

2 cups young coconut meat
2 cups fresh young coconut water, or
   more for desired consistency
1 cup fresh orange juice
½ cup avocado (about ½ medium
   avocado)

1 clove garlic
1 tablespoon minced ginger
3 soft dates, pitted
2 tablespoons curry blend
2 tablespoons nama shoyu
Pinch cayenne pepper

1 teaspoon sun-dried sea salt, or more
   to taste
½ cup chopped cilantro
2 tablespoons chopped basil

1½ cups diced tomatoes
1½ cups sliced shiitake or crimini
   mushrooms

In a blender, blend coconut meat, coconut water, orange juice, avocado, garlic, ginger, dates, curry blend, and nama shoyu until smooth. Season with cayenne and sea salt to taste. Mix in, by hand, cilantro, basil, tomatoes, and mushrooms. Allow to stand for 30 minutes to allow tomatoes and mushrooms to absorb flavor.

Warming Soups

A wonderful secret of raw foods preparation is to serve soup in a warmed bowl. It allows the flavors to bloom a little bit more and keeps the soup warm without having to heat it to unhealthful temperatures upon serving.

To warm soup bowls, place the empty bowls in the oven on the "warm" setting, or as low as the oven is able to be set for 5 to 10 minutes. Use a towel or oven mitts to remove the soup bowls from the oven to be sure to protect your precious fingers.

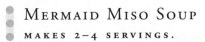

MERMAID MISO SOUP
MAKES 2–4 SERVINGS.

A lovely miso soup chock full of vegetables and herbs. Perfect any time. (It is important not to boil miso, as the precious enzymes and cultures will be killed by heat over 110°F.)

4 cups filtered water
2 cloves garlic, minced
2 tablespoons minced ginger
1½ tablespoons dried lemongrass (If
   lemongrass is unavailable, use
    1 teaspoon lemon zest.)
5 tablespoons white miso
¼ cup dry arame

2 tablespoons dry wakame, broken
   into small pieces
2 tablespoons large agar flakes
   (optional if unavailable)
1 carrot, peeled with a peeler to the
   core into delicate ribbons
1 zucchini, peeled with a peeler to the
   core into delicate ribbons

2 tablespoons nama shoyu

1½ tablespoons cold-pressed sesame
  oil (optional) (Adding oil will make
  the soup richer.)

2 teaspoons maple syrup, brown rice
  syrup, or raw honey (optional)

4 green onions, finely chopped to
  the top

2 tablespoons chopped cilantro

2 tablespoons sesame seeds or hulled
  hemp seeds

Combine water, garlic, ginger, and lemongrass in a medium saucepan and bring to just below a simmer. Turn off heat. Allow to cool for a moment. Add miso and stir until dissolved. Add arame, wakame, and, if desired, agar.

Add carrot and zucchini ribbons, nama shoyu, sesame oil, and sweetener, if desired, and stir. Add onions, cilantro, and seeds. Warm over a low flame if necessary. Your finger should comfortably be able to test the heat of the soup. This is an excellent soup to make a double recipe for. It keeps well in the fridge for several days, and the flavors marry and mature.

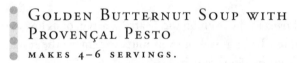

GOLDEN BUTTERNUT SOUP WITH PROVENÇAL PESTO
MAKES 4–6 SERVINGS.

Try this soup without the pesto for a quick spot of golden nutrition.

Soup

3 cups filtered water

2 cloves garlic, chopped

1 medium sweet onion, chopped
  (approximately 1 cup)

2 teaspoons sun-dried sea salt

4 cups cubed butternut squash

2 tablespoons organic extra-virgin
  olive oil (optional)

2 tablespoons raw honey or
  maple syrup

Pesto

⅓ cup walnuts

2 tablespoons pine nuts

1 clove garlic

1 cup fresh parsley leaves

½ cup fresh basil leaves

2 tablespoons herbes de Provence (or
  2 teaspoons fennel seeds
  + 2 teaspoons marjoram or
  thyme + 1 teaspoon rosemary
  + ½ teaspoon lavender)

2–4 tablespoons organic extra-virgin
  olive oil

½ teaspoon sun-dried sea salt

½ teaspoon fresh ground
  black pepper

To make the soup: In a soup pot, bring water just to a simmer with garlic, onion, and sea salt. Turn flame to low. Add cubed squash. Allow to stand over a low flame just until a fork can pierce the squash (5–7 minutes). Cover pot and turn off heat. Transfer the softened soup ingredients from the pot into the food processor. Add olive oil and honey or maple syrup and blend until smooth. It may be necessary to transfer back to the soup pot to warm again over a low flame.

To make the pesto: In a food processor, chop walnuts, pine nuts, garlic, parsley, basil, and herbes de Provence until well ground. It may be necessary to scrape the walls of the food processor with a rubber spatula to achieve a uniform consistency. Drizzle in the olive oil while processing. (The pesto should maintain a bit of texture, but be able to pour off a spoon.) Season with sea salt and black pepper to taste. Ladle soup into bowls, spoon 2 tablespoons of pesto on top, and delicately swirl it through the soup.

ALMOST CLAM CHOWDER
MAKES 4–6 SERVINGS.

This hearty soup is reminiscent of clam chowder. A simple broth is
a perfect base for flavor to bloom from.

3 cups filtered water
3 medium cloves garlic, minced
4 green onions
2 tablespoons chopped fresh ginger
3 celery stalks, chopped
1 bay leaf
½ cup sun-dried tomatoes
2 zucchini, diced
¼ cup dulse flakes
2 tablespoons raw tahini

2 tablespoons cold-pressed coconut
  butter or organic extra-virgin
  olive oil
2 tablespoons maple syrup or raw
  honey (optional)
2–3 tablespoons white miso
4 tablespoons nutritional yeast
Sun-dried sea salt, if necessary, to taste
Pinch cayenne pepper to taste
  (optional for some heat)
Fresh black pepper to taste

In a soup pot, bring water just to a simmer over a medium flame. Turn heat to medium-low. Add garlic, green onions, ginger, celery, and bay leaf. Allow to simmer and soften for a few minutes. *Do not let boil—enzymes are delicate.* Add sun-dried tomatoes, zucchini, and dulse. Cover pot and allow to stand and soften over a *very* low flame for 5 to 10 minutes. Stir in tahini, coconut butter or olive oil, maple syrup or honey, miso, and nutritional yeast. Season with sea salt, cayenne pepper, and black pepper to taste. Remove the bay leaf before serving.

Serve warm. Flavors develop as it sits. This chowder stores well.

GINGER-CURRIED PUMPKIN SOUP
MAKES 4–6 SERVINGS.

*A touch of spices and curry complements this creamy pumpkin
soup. It provides just the right warmth for a cool autumn evening.*

3 cups water
1 small pumpkin, seeds removed and
   cut into small cubes (about 4 cups)
   (Butternut squash can be
   substituted if pumpkin is
   unavailable.)
1 cup chopped sweet onion
3 cloves garlic, minced
4 tablespoons peeled and minced
   ginger
1 fresh chili pepper, chopped
1 apple, peeled, cored, and diced

2 tablespoons raw honey or
   maple syrup
2–4 tablespoons organic extra-virgin
   olive oil or cold-pressed coconut
   butter
2 tablespoons nama shoyu
1 teaspoon turmeric powder
1 teaspoon cinnamon
1 tablespoon ground coriander seeds
1 teaspoon ground cumin seed
1 teaspoon fresh ground black pepper
Sun-dried sea salt to taste

Pour the water into a soup pot. Place a basket steamer in the soup pot and bring water to a boil. Steam pumpkin with a cover on top of the pot until a fork can pierce it easily (5–12 minutes). The smaller the cubes, the less time is necessary to steam. Turn off heat. Transfer the steamer from the pot to the sink, leaving the hot water in the pot. Add onion, garlic, ginger, chili pepper, and apple to the hot water in the pot and cover with a lid.

In the sink, run the steamed pumpkin under cold water until it is cool enough to handle comfortably. Peel the skin from the cubes of pumpkin and place cubes in a blender or food processor. Add in hot water and its contents. Add honey or maple syrup, oil or coconut butter, nama shoyu, turmeric, cinnamon, coriander, cumin, and black pepper. Process. Season with sea salt to taste. The soup can be gently warmed again over low heat.

This soup keeps well in a jar in the refrigerator.

WARM CORN CHOWDER
MAKES 2–4 SERVINGS.

Fresh almond milk and fresh corn make the perfect base for flavor to blossom from in this warming chowder.

4 ears fresh corn
2 cups thick Almond Milk (page 266)
1 clove garlic, minced
2 green onions, chopped to the top
¼ cup chopped cilantro
½ teaspoon ground cumin seed
Sun-dried sea salt to taste

Saw fresh corn kernels from the cobs. In a blender or food processor, pulse corn, almond milk, garlic, green onions, cilantro, and cumin seed until mixed but not smooth. Season with sea salt to taste. Warm gently over low heat.

MINESTRONE HARVEST SOUP
MAKES 4–6 SERVINGS.

The essence of vegetable soup is embodied in this minestrone soup. All of the right herbs and spices complement a hearty, warming bowl of flavor and texture.

2 cups filtered water
1 bay leaf
1 small sweet onion, chopped
3 cloves garlic, minced
4 celery stalks, including leaves
½ cup scissor-cut pieces sun-dried
  tomatoes
1½ cups sprouted garbanzo beans
2 cups diced tomatoes, seeds removed
1 cup diced zucchini

¼ cup ground sesame seeds
½ cup chopped parsley leaves
½ cup chopped basil leaves
1 tablespoon chopped dried oregano
  or thyme
½ cup chopped green onion
1 teaspoon ground chipotle pepper
  (A pinch cayenne pepper may be
  substituted if chipotle peppers
  unavailable.)

1–2 teaspoons sun-dried sea salt, or
   to taste
Black pepper to taste

1 tablespoon organic extra-virgin
   olive oil per serving

In a soup pot, bring water just to a simmer. Turn to medium-low heat. Add bay leaf, onion, garlic, celery, cut sun-dried tomatoes, and sprouted garbanzo beans. Allow to soften and warm (about 10 minutes). Turn off heat and add diced tomatoes, zucchini, sesame seeds, parsley, basil, oregano or thyme, green onion, and hot pepper. Allow to stand and soften with the heat off for 10 minutes. Season with sea salt and pepper to taste. Add olive oil to each serving individually.

Soup can be gently warmed over low heat before serving.

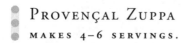

Provençal Zuppa
MAKES 4–6 SERVINGS.

This hearty soup is wonderful on a cold winter day.

3 cups fresh water
3 cloves garlic, minced
2 cups sliced leeks
1 cup minced celery
2 tablespoons dried herbes de
   Provence
1 teaspoon sun-dried sea salt
1 cup sprouted baby French lentils
   (Sprouted traditional lentils can be
   substituted.)

1½ cups shredded carrot
1½ cups quartered and thinly sliced
   zucchini
Fresh black pepper to taste
1 tablespoon organic extra-virgin
   olive oil per serving

In a large pot, bring water to a simmer at medium-high heat. Reduce the heat to medium-low and add garlic, leeks, celery, dried herbs, sea salt, and sprouted lentils. Allow to percolate for 1 to 3 minutes. Reduce to a low heat and add shredded carrots and zucchini. Allow to warm for about 5 minutes. Season with sea salt and pepper to taste, and drizzle each serving with 1 tablespoon of olive oil.

Salads and Salad Dressings

Baby Spinach Salad with Bosc Pear and Pecans

MAKES 4–6 SERVINGS.

Tender baby spinach and sweet pear slices are tossed with a simple dressing for a gorgeous salad. Use another type of pear if Bosc pears are unavailable.

1 firm Bosc pear, peeled, cored, and sliced
4 green onions, finely chopped
1 teaspoon sun-dried sea salt
4 tablespoons organic extra-virgin olive oil
2 tablespoons apple cider vinegar
1½ tablespoons balsamic vinegar (optional)

1 lemon, juiced
1 tablespoon raw honey or maple syrup
1 pound baby spinach leaves
½ cup chopped parsley and cilantro leaves
⅓ cup chopped pecans
Fresh black pepper

Toss pear and green onions with sea salt, olive oil, vinegars, lemon juice, and honey or maple syrup. Allow to marinate for 5 to 10 minutes. Add baby spinach leaves, chopped herbs, and pecans, and gently toss with salad servers. Season with additional salt and black pepper if necessary. Serve immediately.

Frisée and Shaved Fennel Salad with Ruby Grapefruit
MAKES 2–4 SERVINGS.

The frisée and endive make a wonderful contrast in texture. Additional endive or butter lettuce can be used if frisée is unavailable.

4 tablespoons organic extra-virgin
  olive oil
2 tablespoons apple cider vinegar
1 tablespoon umeboshi plum paste,
  or 2 tablespoons umeboshi
  plum vinegar
1½ tablespoons raw honey or
  agave syrup
1 teaspoon sun-dried sea salt
2 tablespoons chopped parsley

1 tablespoon chopped tarragon
2 teaspoons dried thyme
1 large head or 2 small heads frisée
  (about 6 cups)
1 fresh fennel root, sliced very thin
1 ruby red grapefruit, peeled,
  deseeded, and cut into cubes
Sun-dried sea salt to taste
Fresh cracked black pepper to taste

In a salad bowl, mix olive oil, apple cider vinegar, plum paste or vinegar, honey or agave syrup, sea salt, and chopped herbs. Break frisée into 2-inch pieces and toss along with fennel in the salad bowl with marinade until well coated.

Serve on individual plates, distributing grapefruit cubes evenly among the plates. Season with sun-dried sea salt and fresh cracked black pepper to taste.

Radicchio, Basil, and Asparagus Salad with Sun-dried Tomato and Olive Tapenade
MAKES 4–6 SERVINGS.

Colorful radicchio and fresh basil combine beautifully with al dente asparagus. A sweet and savory tapenade complements the flavor deliciously.

Asparagus
  1 bunch asparagus
  3 cups hot water
  1 lemon

A drizzle of organic extra-virgin
  olive oil
Pinch sun-dried sea salt

Tapenade
- ½ cup sun-dried tomatoes, soaked until soft and cut into thin strips
- ½ cup pitted and chopped sun-dried black olives
- 1 clove garlic, pressed or finely minced
- 3 tablespoons organic extra-virgin olive oil
- 2 tablespoons balsamic vinegar

- 1 lemon, juiced
- Pinch sun-dried sea salt, or more to taste

Salad
- 2 medium heads or 3 small heads radicchio, chopped (about 8 cups)
- ½ cup chopped basil leaves
- ¼ cup roughly chopped pine nuts
- Fresh cracked black pepper

To prepare the asparagus: Cut off the woody ends of the stems of the asparagus. In a medium pot, bring water to a boil and remove from heat. In a shallow bowl or pan, pour hot water over the asparagus and cover for 2 to 5 minutes—*no longer!* Drain off hot water. Squeeze lemon, drizzle olive oil, and sprinkle sea salt over asparagus.

To make the tapenade: In a small bowl, toss the sun-dried tomato strips, olives, garlic, olive oil, vinegar, lemon juice, and a pinch of sea salt, or to taste.

To prepare the salad: In a wide salad bowl, gently toss radicchio and basil with the tapenade. Serve marinated asparagus stalks on a bed of radicchio and basil. Sprinkle chopped pine nuts and fresh black pepper on top.

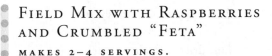

FIELD MIX WITH RASPBERRIES AND CRUMBLED "FETA"

MAKES 2–4 SERVINGS.

This salad is a celebration of the senses.

Crumbled "Feta"
- ¼ cup raw macadamia nuts
- 2 tablespoons pine nuts
- 1 tablespoon lemon juice
- 1 teaspoon lemon zest
- 1 tablespoon apple cider vinegar

- 1 teaspoon organic extra-virgin olive oil
- 1 tablespoon nutritional yeast
- Pinch dried garlic granules or powder
- Pinch sun-dried sea salt

Salad

    ½ pound young salad field mix or
        mesclun salad mix
    2–4 tablespoons organic extra-virgin
        olive oil (or less oil for a lighter
        dressing)

    2 tablespoons apple cider vinegar
    1 tablespoon raw honey, maple syrup,
        or orange juice
    Pinch sun-dried sea salt
    1 pint fresh raspberries
    Fresh cracked black pepper to taste

To make the "feta": Soak macadamia nuts in fresh water for 10 minutes. Drain off water and blot nuts dry with a clean towel. In a food processor, chop macadamia nuts and pine nuts into a fine meal. Add lemon juice and zest, apple cider vinegar, and olive oil, and pulse until well mixed. It may be necessary to scrape the walls of the food processor with a rubber spatula for a smooth consistency. Add nutritional yeast, garlic granules or powder, and sea salt, and pulse until crumbly.

To prepare the salad: In a salad bowl, toss salad mix with olive oil, vinegar, honey or maple syrup or orange juice, and sea salt. Serve on plates. Crumble macadamia feta and distribute fresh raspberries over each salad. Season with fresh black pepper to taste.

ENDIVE AND CORIANDER SALAD WITH GRAPES AND WALNUTS

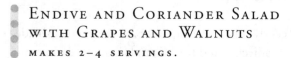

MAKES 2–4 SERVINGS.

This is a beautiful medley.

    4 green onions, finely cut
    1 cup red grapes, cut in halves
    2 teaspoons roughly crushed whole
        coriander seeds
    2–4 tablespoons good walnut or olive
        oil (or less oil for a lighter dressing)
    2 tablespoons umeboshi plum vinegar
    1 tablespoon balsamic vinegar or
        apple cider vinegar

    1 tablespoon raw honey, maple syrup,
        or organic evaporated cane juice
    Sun-dried sea salt to taste
    2 medium heads or 3 small heads
        endive
    6 delicate cilantro sprigs
    ⅓ cup chopped walnuts
    Fresh cracked black pepper to taste

In a large bowl, toss onions, grapes, and crushed coriander with oil, vinegars, sweetener, and sea salt. Separate endive leaves from the head. Gently toss with cilantro sprigs, grape mixture, and green onions.

    Serve on salad plates and sprinkle with walnuts. Season with black pepper to taste.

ARUGULA AND SUMMER MELON

MAKES 2–4 SERVINGS.

The essence of summer lies in the sweet succulence of melon and spicy fresh arugula.

1 tablespoon minced ginger

3 green onions, chopped to the top

2–4 tablespoons organic extra-virgin olive oil (use less for a lighter dressing)

1 tablespoon umeboshi plum vinegar or apple cider vinegar

1 lemon, juiced

1 tablespoon raw honey or maple syrup, or 2 tablespoons orange juice

1–2 teaspoons sun-dried sea salt, or to taste

½ pound arugula, young leaves

½ summer melon (best available— cantaloupe, canary, honeydew, galia, etc.), peeled, deseeded, and cubed

½ cup roughly chopped fresh cilantro

Pinch sun-dried sea salt

Fresh black pepper to taste

In a salad bowl, mix ginger and onions with olive oil, vinegar, lemon juice, honey or maple, and sea salt. Allow to stand 5 minutes or more to develop flavor. Toss arugula leaves in the salad bowl with marinade. Serve arugula on salad plates and top with cubed melon. Sprinkle cilantro on top of the melon. Season with a pinch of sea salt and black pepper to taste.

OAK SALAD WITH MANDARIN ORANGES AND WALNUTS

MAKES 2–4 SERVINGS.

This is a classic salad that I grew up with.

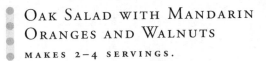

1 head red oak leaf lettuce, torn

3 tablespoons organic extra-virgin olive oil

2 tablespoons red wine vinegar or apple cider vinegar

1 teaspoon sun-dried sea salt

2 mandarin oranges or tangerines, peeled and sectioned

½ cup chopped walnuts

In a salad bowl, toss all ingredients until well coated.

Insalata Perfetta

MAKES 2–4 SERVINGS.

Insalata Perfetta è facile da fare. È fatta con lattuga, pomodoro, sedano, cipolla, olio d'oliva, aceto, e sale.

4 cups torn fresh lettuce (the freshest-looking in the market)
1 small red onion, thinly sliced
1 cup chopped celery
1 carrot, finely shredded
1–2 tomatoes, quartered and sliced
2 tablespoons dried Italian herb mixture (oregano, rosemary, thyme, marjoram)

¼ cup organic extra-virgin olive oil
2 tablespoons apple cider vinegar
2 tablespoons balsamic vinegar
1–2 teaspoons sun-dried sea salt
Fresh black pepper to taste

In a large salad bowl, combine lettuce, onion, celery, carrot, and tomatoes. Sprinkle with dried herbs, drizzle with olive oil and vinegars, and sprinkle with sea salt and fresh black pepper to taste. Toss until well coated. Allow to stand 5 to 10 minutes and serve immediately.

Perfect every time.

Horiatiki Salata

MAKES 2–4 SERVINGS.

Horiatiki is a traditional Greek country salad.

1 red bell pepper, diced
1 yellow bell pepper, diced
2 tomatoes, diced
1 cucumber, peeled and sliced
1 red onion, cut in half and sliced into thin wedges
1 cup pitted and sliced mild black olives
1 cup quartered artichoke hearts (optional)

⅓ cup chopped basil
⅓ cup chopped parsley
1 tablespoon finely chopped fresh oregano
1 teaspoon dried thyme or marjoram
¼ cup organic extra-virgin olive oil
2 lemons, juiced
1 orange, juiced
1–2 teaspoons sun-dried sea salt, or to taste

Fresh cracked black pepper to taste
1 cup Greek Herb and Olive "Feta"
  (page 314)

1 generous head of butter lettuce or
  green leaf lettuce, torn

Toss all of the vegetables and herbs with olive oil, lemon juice, orange juice, and sea salt and black pepper to taste. Allow to stand at least 15 minutes to develop flavor. Crumble "Feta" into tossed marinated vegetables. Serve on a bed of butter lettuce or green leaf lettuce.

SALAD NIÇOISE

MAKES 2–4 SERVINGS.

Salad Niçoise is a traditional French salad with fresh string beans and potatoes in a tangy marinade. Here, Jerusalem artichokes or steamed potatoes can be used.

5 green onions, minced
2 cloves garlic, finely minced
6 tablespoons organic extra-virgin
  olive oil
2 tablespoons balsamic vinegar
1 tablespoon apple cider vinegar
1 lemon, juiced
1 tablespoon prepared Dijon mustard
1 tablespoon maple syrup or raw
  honey

1–2 teaspoons sun-dried sea salt
2 cups peeled and cubed Jerusalem
  artichokes, or 2 cups cubed red-
  skinned potatoes, steamed
½ pound fresh green string beans
1 generous head butter lettuce or
  green leaf lettuce, torn
Fresh cracked black pepper to taste

In a salad bowl, mix onions and garlic with olive oil, vinegars, lemon juice, mustard, maple syrup or honey, and sea salt. Toss artichokes or potatoes with marinade. Snap off the ends of the string beans and steam just until beans turn bright green. Remove and run under cold water until the beans are cool to the touch. Toss the string beans with the artichokes or potatoes and marinade. Tear the lettuce leaves and gently toss with the marinade, artichokes or potatoes, and string beans with salad servers. Season with fresh cracked pepper to taste.

CRISP CAESAR SALAD WITH TAMARIND CAESAR DRESSING AND PINE NUT PARMESAN

MAKES 4–6 SERVINGS.

Tamarind is a tangy, sweet complement to a Caesar salad and can be found in Indian and ethnic markets. Crumble in leftover flat bread as croutons.

Pine Nut Parmesan
- ¼ cup pine nuts
- ¼ cup whole cashews or macadamia nuts
- Drizzle of organic extra-virgin olive oil or fresh water
- 2–3 tablespoons nutritional yeast

- Pinch dried garlic granules or powder
- Pinch sun-dried sea salt

Salad
- 1 large head or 2 medium heads romaine lettuce, torn
- Tamarind Caesar Dressing (page 300)

To make the pine nut parmesan: In a food processor or blender, chop pine nuts and cashews or macadamia nuts into a fine meal. Drizzle in a touch of oil or water. Pulse until moist and ground. Add nutritional yeast, dried garlic, and sea salt, and pulse until crumbly.

To make the salad: Separate romaine lettuce leaves and break into pieces. Dollop the Caesar Dressing on a few tablespoons at a time and toss with lettuce until well coated but not drenched. Serve and sprinkle with the Pine Nut Parmesan.

NEW WALDORF SALAD

MAKES 2–4 SERVINGS.

Waldorf Salad is a classic salad made famous by the kitchen of the swank Waldorf-Astoria Hotel in New York. A fresh new twist keeps this classic alive.

Dressing
- 3 tablespoons raw sesame tahini
- 1 clove garlic
- ¼ cup lemon juice

- 2 tablespoons apple cider vinegar
- 1 tablespoon organic extra-virgin olive oil

1½ tablespoons raw honey or maple
    syrup, or 2 soft dates, pitted
2 teaspoons dill
1–2 teaspoons sun-dried sea salt, or
    to taste
Fresh water as needed

Salad

1 apple, sliced
3 stalks celery, chopped
2 carrots, shredded
3 green onions, finely chopped to
    the top
½ cup raisins
½ cup chopped walnuts
¼ cup chopped parsley
1 head crisp lettuce, torn

To make the dressing: In a blender, blend tahini, garlic, lemon juice, vinegar, olive oil, honey or maple syrup or dates, dill, and sea salt, adding water 2 tablespoons at a time as necessary to blend until smooth.

To make the salad: Cut apple into quarters and cut out core and seeds. Cut into slices. Chop celery in ¼-inch pieces along the stalk. Toss together apple, celery, carrots, onions, raisins, walnuts, and parsley. Drizzle in dressing and toss. Serve on a bed of torn lettuce.

Salad Dressings

LEMON TAHINI HOUSE DRESSING
MAKES 1 PINT.

This is a great house dressing with a creamy lemon zest. Try adding fresh herbs for a delicious variation. Stores well for days.

2 tablespoons raw tahini
¼ cup sunflower seeds, soaked
    2–4 hours
½ cup lemon juice
2 teaspoons lemon zest
½ cup orange juice
2 tablespoons nama shoyu
1 tablespoon organic extra-virgin
    olive oil
1 tablespoon raw honey

1 clove raw garlic
1 tablespoon shredded or finely
    minced ginger
¼ cup parsley leaves
¼ cup cilantro leaves
Pinch sun-dried sea salt to taste
2 teaspoons dill, or ¼ cup basil leaves
    (optional for variation)
1–1¼ cups fresh water

In a blender, blend all ingredients until smooth. The dressing will be quite thick. Add up to ¼ cup more fresh water, if desired, to thin. Store in a glass jar with a lid in the refrigerator.

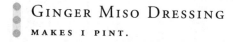 CARROT CASHEW DRESSING
MAKES 1–2 PINTS.

A delicately seasoned creamy dressing with smooth cashews and
fresh carrot juice. Buy fresh carrot juice from a juice bar or
from the market for convenience. Add ginger for a great lift.

1 cup whole raw cashews (raw cashew
  pieces can be used), soaked 1 hour
2 cups fresh carrot juice
½ cup cilantro leaves
1 clove garlic
1 tablespoon shredded or finely
  minced ginger (optional)

2 teaspoons ground coriander seeds
2 tablespoons nama shoyu
1 tablespoon apple cider vinegar or
  brown rice vinegar
Pinch sun-dried sea salt to taste
½–1 cup fresh water to thin

In a blender, blend soaked cashews, carrot juice, cilantro, garlic, ginger (if desired), coriander, nama shoyu, and vinegar until smooth. Add a pinch of sea salt to taste and fresh water, ¼ cup at a time, to thin to desired consistency.

GINGER MISO DRESSING
MAKES 1 PINT.

This dressing complements any fresh salad with a lovely lift.
Or use it to marinate vegetables or a seaweed salad.

3 tablespoons white miso
2 tablespoons peeled and shredded or
  minced fresh ginger
1 clove garlic, minced
1 green onion, chopped to the top

2 tablespoons nama shoyu
2–4 tablespoons cold-pressed sesame
  oil or organic extra-virgin olive oil
1 tablespoon maple syrup or raw
  honey

2 tablespoons umeboshi plum vinegar

¼ cup lemon juice

¼ cup orange juice

Pinch sun-dried sea salt

¼–½ cup fresh water

In a blender, blend all ingredients except water until smooth. Add water as necessary for a thinner dressing.

Store in a glass jar with a lid.

THOUSAND ISLAND DRESSING

MAKES 1 QUART.

A classic creamy tomato dressing with a touch of tangy flavor.

1 cup whole raw cashews (cashew pieces can be used), soaked 1 hour

¼ cup sun-dried tomatoes, soaked in ½ cup fresh water (5–15 minutes)

3 dates, pitted and soaked in ¼ cup fresh water (5–15 minutes)

1 cup diced tomatoes

1 clove garlic

2 tablespoons chopped cilantro

2 tablespoons chopped parsley

¼ cup lemon juice

½ cup orange juice

2 tablespoons nama shoyu

2 tablespoons apple cider vinegar

1 tablespoon organic extra-virgin olive oil

2 cups fresh water

Pinch sun-dried sea salt

In a blender, blend drained cashews, sun-dried tomatoes *and* soaking water, dates *and* soaking water, diced tomatoes, garlic, cilantro, parsley, lemon juice, orange juice, nama shoyu, vinegar, olive oil, and water until smooth. Season with a pinch of sea salt. The dressing will be nice and thick. Add more water as necessary to thin dressing.

Store in a glass jar with a lid in the refrigerator.

Sun-Fired Italian Vinaigrette
MAKES 1 PINT.

*A dynamic Italian vinaigrette that is
excellent on any crunchy salad.*

¼ cup sun-dried tomatoes
6 tablespoons organic extra-virgin
   olive oil
¼ cup apple cider vinegar
1 tablespoon balsamic vinegar
   (optional)
2 tablespoons nama shoyu

1 tablespoon raw honey or maple syrup
1 clove garlic
2 tablespoons dried Italian seasoning
Pinch sun-dried sea salt, or to taste
Pinch chili pepper, or to taste
   (optional)

Soak sun-dried tomatoes in ½ cup fresh water until soft (5–15 minutes).

In a blender, blend sun-dried tomatoes and soaking water, olive oil, apple cider vinegar, balsamic vinegar (if desired), nama shoyu, honey or maple syrup, garlic, olives, and dried seasoning until smooth. Season to taste with sea salt and chili pepper, if desired.

Balsamic Vinaigrette
MAKES 1 PINT.

*This is a tangy vinaigrette with all of the flavor of balsamic
vinegar, olive oil, and just the right seasoning. It's excellent
with romaine lettuce and tomatoes.*

6 tablespoons organic extra-virgin
   olive oil
3 tablespoons balsamic vinegar
1 tablespoon apple cider vinegar
1½ tablespoons maple syrup or
   raw honey

1 tablespoon nama shoyu
1 tablespoon white miso
1–2 cloves garlic
¼ cup chopped parsley
2 teaspoons oregano
Sun-dried sea salt to taste

In a blender, blend all ingredients until smooth.

Store in a glass jar in the refrigerator.

RASPBERRY VINAIGRETTE
MAKES I PINT.

This savory, sweet vinaigrette is gorgeous with butterleaf lettuce, shaved fennel, pine nuts or chopped macadamia nuts, and fresh raspberries.

1 pint fresh raspberries (thawed
    frozen raspberries can be used)
¼ cup organic extra-virgin olive oil
½ cup orange juice
2 tablespoons apple cider vinegar
1 tablespoon balsamic vinegar
    (optional)

1 tablespoon white miso
1 green onion, chopped to the top
2–4 tablespoons chopped parsley
1 teaspoon savory, marjoram, or
    thyme
Pinch sun-dried sea salt, or to taste

In a blender, blend all ingredients until smooth.
    Store in a glass jar with a lid in the refrigerator.

OIL-FREE VINAIGRETTE
MAKES ABOUT I PINT.

A great oil-free vinaigrette for the light side. Great with any salad.

1 cup diced tomatoes
¼ cup lemon juice
2 tablespoons apple cider vinegar
1 tablespoon nama shoyu
1 tablespoon white miso
1 tablespoon raw honey or maple syrup

1 clove garlic
¼ cup parsley
¼ cup basil
Pinch sun-dried sea salt, or to taste
Fresh black pepper to taste

In a blender, blend all ingredients until smooth.
    Store in a glass jar with a lid in the refrigerator.

TAMARIND CAESAR DRESSING
MAKES 1½ PINTS.

An authentic Caesar dressing with tamarind for a perfect sweet-sour tang. Toss with romaine lettuce and crumbled flat bread or crackers for an absolutely great salad.

¼ cup raw tahini
¼ cup pine nuts
1–2 cloves garlic
2 green onions, or ¼ medium onion
1 lemon, juiced
3 tablespoons apple cider vinegar
1½ tablespoons maple syrup or raw honey, or 2 soft dates, pitted
3 tablespoons nutritional yeast

1 teaspoon black pepper, or to taste
1 teaspoon sun-dried sea salt, or to taste
2 tablespoons tamarind paste (if tamarind is not available, use 2 dates, 1 teaspoon lemon zest, and 3 tablespoons lemon juice)
2 cups fresh water, or as necessary

In a blender, blend all ingredients until smooth. The dressing should be quite thick. Add more water to thin as desired.

Store in a glass jar with a lid in the refrigerator.

CRACKED PEPPER AND LEMON RANCH DRESSING
MAKES ABOUT 1 QUART.

Serve this zesty ranch dressing with crunchy lettuce, shredded purple cabbage, sliced cucumber, chopped celery, and cherry tomatoes.

½ cup whole raw cashews (raw cashew pieces can be used), soaked 1 hour
¼ cup pine nuts
½ cup lemon juice
1 tablespoon lemon zest
2 tablespoons apple cider vinegar
1 clove garlic

2 tablespoons nutritional yeast
1 tablespoon fresh cracked black pepper
1–2 teaspoons sun-dried sea salt, or to taste
2 cups fresh water

In a blender, blend all ingredients until smooth.

Store in a glass jar with a lid in the refrigerator.

CREAMY AVOCADO AND HERB DRESSING
MAKES 1 PINT.

Serve this simple, smooth dressing with butter lettuce, cherry tomatoes, cucumber slices, and finely sliced red onion.

1 avocado
⅓ cup lemon juice
¼ cup orange juice
2 tablespoons nama shoyu
⅓ cup parsley leaves

⅓ cup cilantro leaves
1 teaspoon coriander seed
½–1 cup fresh water
Pinch sun-dried sea salt, or to taste

In a blender, blend all ingredients and ½ cup fresh water until smooth. Season to taste with sea salt. Add an additional ½ cup water for a lighter dressing.

Store in a glass jar with a lid in the refrigerator.

RED SUMISO DRESSING
MAKES ½ CUP.

Serve this simple dressing with fresh lettuce or with soaked seaweed.

3 tablespoons red miso
2 tablespoons brown rice vinegar
1 tablespoon umeboshi plum vinegar
1 tablespoon raw honey
¼ cup fresh water

Mix all ingredients in a small bowl.

Store in a glass jar with a lid in the refrigerator.

Appetizers:
Great Beginnings

Appetizing Finger Feasts

Pesto-Stuffed Mushrooms
MAKES 12 MUSHROOMS.

These savory, marinated mushrooms stuffed with fresh walnut pesto make a welcome appetizer for any palate.

Walnut Pesto
- 3 cups basil leaves
- 1–2 cloves garlic
- 1 cup walnuts
- ¼ cup pine nuts
- 1 tablespoon organic extra-virgin olive oil (optional)
- 1 tablespoon white miso
- ½ teaspoon sun-dried sea salt

Mushrooms
- 12 medium crimini mushrooms, stems removed
- 4 tablespoons organic extra-virgin olive oil
- 3 tablespoons nama shoyu
- 2 tablespoons apple cider vinegar
- 1 clove garlic, finely minced
- Pinch sun-dried sea salt

To prepare the pesto: In a food processor, finely chop basil and garlic. Add walnuts, pine nuts, olive oil (if desired), miso, and sea salt and chop until well mixed but not completely smooth.

To prepare the mushrooms: Mix the mushrooms with olive oil, nama shoyu, apple cider vinegar, garlic, and sea salt. Allow to marinate for at least 30 minutes, occasionally turning over the mushrooms to keep well coated.

Gently squeeze the mushrooms from excess marinade. (The marinade can be saved to use again or for other recipes.) Stuff each mushroom with the walnut pesto and dehydrate at 108°F for 1 hour to warm and marry flavors before serving. Alternatively, an oven can be used to warm the mushrooms. Put the mushrooms on a baking tray in the oven set to the lowest temperature (for 30 minutes to 1 hour) with the door slightly ajar to monitor the heat.

The mushrooms can be made a day ahead of time for entertaining and warmed before serving.

Crystal Spring Rolls with Bon Bon Dipping Sauce

MAKES 6 ROLLS.

The key to these rolls is lots of fresh herbs and a fantastic dipping sauce. For variation, instead of the dipping sauce, try serving with Chili Mango Chutney (page 304).

Rolls

4 cups warm fresh water

6 spring roll rice wrappers

4 cups threaded or shredded (using a Saladacco, mandoline, grater, or peeler) zucchini (2 medium or 3 small zucchini)

4 cups threaded or shredded (using a Saladacco, mandoline, grater, or peeler) carrot (2 large or 3 medium carrots)

2 cups cilantro leaves

2 cups mint leaves (parsley leaves can be used if mint is unavailable)

4 green onions, finely chopped to the top

Bon Bon Dipping Sauce

4 tablespoons raw almond butter

2 tablespoons organic creamy peanut butter (optional for an authentic flavor)

3 tablespoons nama shoyu

2 tablespoons organic extra-virgin olive oil

2 tablespoons apple cider vinegar

1 tablespoon raw honey or maple syrup

2 soft dates, pitted

2 green onions, finely chopped

1–2 cloves garlic

1 tablespoon shredded or finely minced ginger

½ cup chopped cilantro

½ cup chopped parsley

1–2 teaspoons dried chili pepper

¼–½ cup fresh water

To prepare the rolls: Fill a wide, shallow bowl with 2 cups of the warm fresh water for softening the rice wrappers. Submerge one wrapper at a time in the water until soft. Do not oversoak, as the wrappers are delicate and become difficult to handle without breaking. The water will need to be refilled to keep warm and to provide enough water to soak the rice wrappers in.

Spread a dry dish towel on the counter. Place the wrapper flat on the towel. (Put the next wrapper in the water to soften for the next roll.) Put ⅔ cup each of zucchini and carrot in the bottom-center of the wrapper. Put ⅓ cup each of cilantro and mint leaves, and sprinkle with chopped green onion. (Make sure there is enough to go around!) Fold over the wrapper and tuck under the veggies and herbs. Fold the sides toward the middle (like wrapping a burrito). Gently roll closed as tightly as possible without breaking the wrapper. If the wrapper does break, use another softened wrapper to double-wrap it. Cover with plastic wrap to keep moist.

To prepare the dipping sauce: In a blender, blend almond and peanut butter (if using), nama shoyu, olive oil, vinegar, honey or maple syrup, dates, green onions, garlic, ginger, cilantro, and parsley until smooth, adding fresh water a little at a time as necessary to blend smooth. The sauce should be pourable, but should still be thick. Set aside half of the sauce and add chili pepper to the remaining half, blending until well mixed. (Or spice the whole batch if it tickles your fancy!)

CHILI MANGO CHUTNEY

MAKES 1½ CUPS.

Sweet mango meets spicy chili and cooling cilantro in a divine marriage. A dynamic complement served as a condiment with simple vegetables or as a side with guacamole.

1 firm ripe mango
2 tablespoons finely chopped cilantro
2 teaspoons dried chili pepper (add more to turn up the heat!)
2 teaspoons umeboshi plum paste or umeboshi plum vinegar
Pinch sun-dried sea salt
Fresh black pepper

Peel, pit, and dice the mango. The mango should be firm enough not to succumb to mush while dicing. Chop cilantro and mix in with chili pepper and umeboshi plum paste or plum vinegar. Season with sea salt and black pepper to taste.

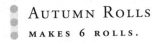

Autumn Rolls

MAKES 6 ROLLS.

*Savory mushrooms wrapped in marinated cabbage leaves are
delectable packages. Serve with the seasoned pomegranate
walnut sauce for many a compliment.*

Cabbage Wraps

6 large leaves cabbage, lightly steamed

2 tablespoons organic extra-virgin
    olive oil

2 tablespoons apple cider vinegar

Pinch sun-dried sea salt

Mushroom Filling

6 cups sliced portobello mushrooms

1 red onion, sliced

2 cloves garlic, finely minced

¼ cup organic extra-virgin olive oil

3 tablespoons nama shoyu

1 tablespoon apple cider vinegar

1 tablespoon dried oregano

2 teaspoons thyme or savory

2 teaspoons crushed or ground
    coriander seeds

Pinch sun-dried sea salt

Pomegranate Walnut Sauce

1 cup walnuts

½ cup pomegranate juice (if
    unavailable, blend the seeds of
    1–2 pomegranates in a blender and
    pour through a strainer)

1 tablespoon apple cider vinegar

1 tablespoon balsamic vinegar

2 tablespoons nama shoyu

2 teaspoons ground coriander seeds

1 teaspoon rosemary

½ cup fresh water

To prepare the rolls: Marinate the cabbage leaves in olive oil, vinegar, and sea salt.

Marinate the mushrooms in onion, garlic, olive oil, nama shoyu, vinegar, oregano, thyme
or savory, coriander, and sea salt for at least 30 minutes or until soft and well absorbed. Squeeze
the excess marinade off with clean hands or through a colander with the back of a large spoon.
Try to keep as many of the herbs with the mushrooms as possible.

Shake off the marinating cabbage leaves and lay flat with the stem ends facing you. Place a
handful of squeezed mushrooms in the bottom-center of the leaf. Fold the leaf over and tuck
under the mushrooms. Fold the sides of the leaf in (like wrapping a burrito) and roll the leaf
closed as tightly as possible. Garnish with pomegranate seeds.

To make the sauce: Soak the walnuts in 2 cups of fresh water for 1 hour. Drain and rinse. Blend
the soaked walnuts, pomegranate juice, vinegars, nama shoyu, coriander, and rosemary until

smooth, adding water a little at a time to blend into desired consistency. The sauce should be thick but able to pour.

NAPA WRAPPED ASPARAGUS
MAKES 6 ROLLS.

Seasoned al dente asparagus with lemon and dill wrapped in marinated Napa cabbage leaves makes a beautiful appetizer or side dish. Serve warm or chilled for the right season.

Napa Wrappers
    6 large Napa (or Chinese) cabbage
        leaves (long heads), marinated or
        lightly steamed
    2 tablespoons nama shoyu
    2 tablespoons umeboshi plum vinegar
    2 cloves garlic, pressed or finely
        minced

Filling
    1 bunch asparagus
    4 cups fresh water
    2 tablespoons organic extra-virgin
        olive oil
    2 lemons, juiced
    1 tablespoon lemon zest
    2 tablespoons white miso

1 tablespoon dill
Pinch sun-dried sea salt
12 basil leaves
18 mint leaves

Lemon Cashew Sauce
    ½ cup whole raw cashews
    ½ cup lemon juice
    1 tablespoon lemon zest
    1 tablespoon organic extra-virgin
        olive oil (optional)
    1 tablespoon white miso
    1 tablespoon nutritional yeast
    1½ teaspoons dill
    1 teaspoon raw honey
    ¼ cup fresh water

To prepare the Napa wrappers: Steam the cabbage leaves lightly until tender and marinate with nama shoyu, umeboshi plum vinegar, and garlic. Or marinate raw leaves for several hours or overnight until softened, turning occasionally to keep coated.

To prepare the asparagus: Cut off the woody portion of the bottom of the asparagus stems. Heat water to a simmer. Lay the asparagus in a shallow bowl and pour the hot water over the asparagus. Allow to stand for a few minutes until asparagus becomes *just* tender. Drain the water. In a small bowl, mix the olive oil, lemon juice, lemon zest, miso, dill, and sea salt. Pour over the asparagus and gently turn until well coated. Separate the marinated asparagus into six bunches.

Lay a cabbage leaf flat. Spread 2 basil leaves and 3 mint leaves on the bottom-center of each cabbage leaf. Put a bundle of marinated asparagus on top. Fold the bottom of the cabbage leaf over and tuck under the asparagus. Tightly roll the leaf shut.

To prepare the sauce: Soak the cashews in 1 cup fresh water for 30 minutes. Drain and rinse. In a blender, blend soaked cashews, lemon juice, lemon zest, olive oil (if desired), miso, nutritional yeast, dill, and honey until smooth, adding fresh water only as necessary to blend to desired consistency. The sauce should be thick but able to pour.

The sauce can be drizzled on each bundle or served on the side.

AUTUMN APPLE TIER
MAKES 4–6 TIERS.

This is a sophisticated tier with cored apple slices and a savory walnut spread. It's beautiful nestled in a bundle of decorative frisée lettuce, sunflower, or buckwheat sprouts.

2 firm apples, peeled

1 lemon

1 teaspoon sun-dried sea salt

1½ cups walnuts, soaked 1–2 hours and drained

½ cup dry walnuts

2 tablespoons white miso

1 tablespoon red miso

2 tablespoons organic extra-virgin olive oil

1 tablespoon apple cider vinegar

¼ cup chopped green onion

2 teaspoons shredded or finely minced ginger

½ cup chopped parsley

2 teaspoons lemon zest

2 teaspoons dried oregano

2 teaspoons ground coriander seeds

1 teaspoon rosemary

1 teaspoon dill

Sun-dried sea salt to taste

⅓ cup pomegranate seeds for garnish (optional)

¼ cup chopped parsley for garnish

Slice the apples across the seeds into quarter-inch slices. Cut the seeds out in a neat circle. Several can be stacked and cut at the same time. Stack the apple slices in a bowl and squeeze the lemon and sprinkle salt over them to prevent discoloration.

In a food processor, chop soaked walnuts and dry walnuts into a fine meal. Add white and red miso, olive oil, vinegar, green onion, ginger, parsley, lemon zest, oregano, coriander, rosemary, and dill and blend into a smooth paste. Season with sea salt to taste.

To assemble, each tier should have two cored apple slices. Evenly spread 3 to 4 tablespoons of the walnut spread on a cored apple slice. Stack another apple slice on top and spread 3 to 4 tablespoons on top. Garnish with pomegranate seeds (if desired) and chopped parsley.

TOMATO SUMMER STACKS
MAKES 6–8 STACKS.

This appetizer serves beautifully on a simple plate or on a leaf of fresh curly lettuce.

2 large tomatoes
1¼ cups raw macadamia nuts, soaked
    for 30 minutes (whole raw cashews
    can be substituted)
¼ cup pine nuts
1 small clove garlic
¼–½ cup lemon juice
1 teaspoon lemon zest
2 tablespoons organic extra-virgin
    olive oil

1 teaspoon sun-dried sea salt
½ cup finely chopped parsley
¼ cup finely chopped cilantro
¼ cup finely chopped basil
1 ear corn
2 green onions, finely chopped to
    the top
1 tablespoon dill

Cut the tomatoes across the width into half-inch slices. Drain the macadamia nuts. In a food processor, chop the macadamia nuts, pine nuts, and garlic into a fine meal. Add lemon juice, lemon zest, olive oil, and sea salt and blend until smooth. Add more lemon juice if necessary to blend into a smooth paste. Mix in parsley, cilantro, and basil gently or by hand. The chopped herbs should remain fairly intact so the spread does not turn green.

Cut the corn from the cob. Mix with green onions and dill.

Spread 3–4 tablespoons of the spread on a slice of tomato. Generously top with fresh corn mixture, pressing it a bit into the spread. Make sure there is enough to go around! These are fantastic.

PEA MOLE AND FRESH FIGS ON JICAMA

MAKES 6–8 SERVINGS.

Sweet pea mole with fresh figs is an absolute delicacy.

1½ cups cilantro leaves

2 cups petite peas (fresh, or frozen
 and thawed)

¼ cup lime juice

1 tablespoon lime zest

1–2 tablespoons olive oil (optional)
 (the mole is lighter without olive oil)

1 teaspoon fresh ground black pepper

1 teaspoon sun-dried sea salt, or
 to taste

1 jicama, peeled and sliced

1 pint quartered fresh figs

In a food processor, finely chop cilantro. Add peas, lime juice and zest, and olive oil (if desired), and pulse thoroughly, but not until smooth. It should have a nice texture. Season with pepper and sea salt to taste.

Spread 3–4 tablespoons pea mole on each jicama slice. Top with three or four fig quarters. Voilà.

LAYERED PÂTÉ TERRINE

MAKES 6–8 SERVINGS.

This is delicious served with sliced vegetables and crackers.

Top Layer (Red)

1 cup whole raw cashews, soaked for
 15 minutes

1 cup sun-dried tomatoes, soaked
 until soft

1 cup chopped red bell pepper

1 clove garlic

2 tablespoons red miso

2 tablespoons organic extra-virgin
 olive oil

Pinch cayenne pepper (optional)

½–1 teaspoon sun-dried sea salt, or
 to taste

Middle Layer (White)

2 cups whole raw cashews, soaked for
 15 minutes

1 cup raw macadamia nuts, soaked
 for 15 minutes

⅓ cup lemon juice

2 tablespoons organic extra-virgin
 olive oil

2 tablespoons nutritional yeast

½ teaspoon sun-dried sea salt, or
 to taste

Bottom Layer (Green)
  1 cup walnuts, soaked for 15 minutes
  ½ cup whole raw cashews, soaked for
    15 minutes
  1 clove garlic
  ½ cup chopped green onion
  2 packed cups spinach leaves

  2 cups basil leaves
  1 cup parsley leaves
  ⅓ cup pine nuts
  Sun-dried sea salt to taste
  2 tablespoons red miso
  2 tablespoons organic extra-virgin
    olive oil

To prepare the top layer: Drain and rinse the cashews. Spread on a dry towel and blot dry.

In a food processor, chop soaked cashews into a fine meal. Add softened sun-dried tomatoes and bell pepper, garlic, miso, olive oil, cayenne (if desired), and sea salt and blend until smooth. It may be necessary to scrape the sides of the food processor with a rubber spatula. Press the spread down to blend smooth. Stash in the refrigerator until ready to use.

To prepare the middle layer: Drain and rinse the cashews and macadamia nuts. Spread on a dry towel and blot dry.

In a food processor, chop the nuts into a fine meal. Add lemon juice and olive oil and blend into a smooth paste. It may be necessary to scrape the sides of the food processor with a rubber spatula. Press the spread down to blend smooth. Add nutritional yeast and sea salt and blend until smooth and mixed. Stash in the refrigerator until ready to use.

To prepare the bottom layer: Drain and rinse the walnuts and cashews. Spread on a dry towel and blot dry.

In a food processor, finely chop the garlic, green onion, spinach leaves, basil leaves, and parsley. Add walnuts, cashews, pine nuts, and sea salt and grind as smooth as possible. Add miso and olive oil and blend until smooth. It may be necessary to scrape the sides of the food processor with a rubber spatula. Press the spread down to blend smooth. Stash in the refrigerator until ready to use.

To assemble: Oil an 8- by 9-inch-long rectangular bread pan or ceramic dish with a bit of olive oil. Line the pan with plastic wrap. The oil will help the wrap to stay flush to the pan. It is best to allow the spreads to chill for several hours in the refrigerator and become firm before spreading so that they can hold their own. Evenly spread the red layer into the plastic-lined pan. Spread the white layer evenly on top of the red layer. This is best done in two or three sections to avoid mixing the layers. Spread the green layer evenly over the white layer. This is best done in two or three sections to avoid mixing the layers. Fold the plastic wrap over the top of the terrine to cover. Allow to chill in the pan for several hours or overnight before serving.

To serve: Unwrap the plastic from the pan, but leave it in place atop the terrine. Place a serving plate upside-down on the pan, making sure the plastic wrap is out of the way. Deftly, flip the pan over onto the plate. Slide the pan away gently, so as not to disturb the terrine. Peel off the plastic wrap. Slice in 1- to 1½-inch slices (use a wet knife to avoid sticking) and lay flat on a plate. Serve with sliced vegetables like carrots, celery, and jicama and crackers. A masterpiece!

Seed and Nut Cheeses

See Chapter 17 for the delicious benefits of seed and nut cheeses.

Making Seed and Nut Cheeses

MAKES 2–4 SERVINGS.

For every cup of nuts or seeds, use 2 teaspoons miso and just enough water to cover them (about 1¼ cups).

Equipment

1 quart or half-gallon widemouthed
    glass jar
1 cup seeds and/or nuts
About 5 cups fresh water
12- by 12-inch screen, cheesecloth,
    or silk screen (Screen and silk
    screen can be washed and used
    again and again. Cheesecloth is
    only good for one use.)

Rubber band
2 teaspoons unpasteurized miso, or
    1 cup Rejuvelac (a "starter" for
    good culturing; see page 235)
Blender or food processor
Large spoon (a slatted spoon with
    holes works best)
2 bowls

In the glass jar, soak seeds/nuts in water for 4–12 hours. Cover the mouth of the jar with the screen or cheesecloth, and secure with a rubber band. Drain off the water. Fill the jar with fresh water to rinse the seeds/nuts and drain again.

    In a blender or food processor, combine seeds/nuts with miso or Rejuvelac and just enough

continued

water to cover them. Pulse until the seeds/nuts are pulverized but not blended smooth. The ideal finished texture is quite like cottage cheese. The right texture is important for successful pressing.

Wash the glass jar thoroughly with hot water. Return the blended seeds/nuts to the glass jar and cover the mouth of the jar with the screen or cheesecloth, securing it with a rubber band. Be sure that there are several inches of space left at the top of the jar to avoid a mess, as the cheese will expand and grow as it ferments. Place the jar in a warm place (between 85° and 95°F) undisturbed for 6–12 hours. On top of the refrigerator, near a warm stove, or in a dehydrator set at a very low temperature are all good places. Do not leave for longer than 12 hours, as the cheese is likely to become rancid and spoil. During this time the cheese will ferment and separate. The top layer of the cheese may be a darker color. This is fine. It is just the result of oxygen breaking it down. (This happens with fruit if it is cut open and left exposed to the air.) The bulk of the cheese will rise to the top of the jar. It will appear to have air bubbles in it from fermenting. The liquid whey will separate to the bottom of the jar. The whey on the bottom may be fairly clear or darker in color.

With a large spoon, scoop some cheese onto the screen, cheesecloth, or silk screen. Squeeze and wring the cheese firmly over a bowl to collect the whey. Place finished cheese in second bowl. The texture of the pressed cheese should be crumbly and fairly dry.

The cheese is ready to be used. It can also be stored to keep fresh for several days. To store for lasting freshness, seal the cheese from oxygen—a glass or plastic container with a sealing lid is the best choice. Pack the cheese firmly in the container. Press a piece of plastic wrap over the top of the cheese and seal with the lid. These measures are taken to limit the exposure of the cheese to air. It should keep fresh for at least a week.

Autumn Harvest Cheese

MAKES ABOUT 3 CUPS.

*This cheese is excellent wrapped in generous spinach leaves or
steamed cabbage leaves or served with Essene bread and pear slices.*

1½ cups walnuts, fermented
  into cheese (see directions on
  pages 311–312)
1½ cups pumpkin seeds, fermented
  into cheese (see directions on
  pages 311–312)
1 cup finely shredded carrot
2 cloves garlic, minced
⅔ cup minced red onion
¼ cup finely chopped parsley leaves
2 teaspoons dried rosemary

2 teaspoons dried thyme or marjoram
2 teaspoons dried oregano
2 teaspoons ground coriander seeds
2 tablespoons walnut oil or organic
  extra-virgin olive oil
2 teaspoons maple syrup or raw
  honey
1 tablespoon nama shoyu
Pinch cayenne pepper
Sun-dried sea salt to taste
Fresh black pepper to taste

In a bowl, mix together prepared walnut and pumpkin seed cheeses, carrot, garlic, red onion,
parsley, rosemary, thyme or marjoram, oregano, coriander, oil, maple syrup or honey, nama
shoyu, and cayenne pepper. Season with sea salt and pepper to taste.

Provençal Fromage

MAKES 3 CUPS.

*France is the land of cheese, and Provence is the region of kind
herbs. This cheese is excellent in a layered vegetable torta with
marinated zucchini and haricot verts, red onion, and shaved fennel. Or serve with celery and fresh figs.*

½ cup pine nuts
2 cloves garlic
2 teaspoons dried thyme
2 teaspoons dried marjoram
2 teaspoons dried rosemary
½ teaspoon dried lavender

½ teaspoon ground fennel seeds, or
  2 tablespoons herbes de Provence
1 cup walnuts, fermented into cheese
  (see directions on pages 311–312)
1 cup cashews, fermented into cheese
  (see directions on pages 311–312)

½ cup sunflower seeds, fermented into
  cheese (see directions on pages
  311–312)
¼ cup lemon juice
2 tablespoons apple cider vinegar
3 tablespoons organic extra-virgin
  olive oil

Fresh water, if necessary, to blend
2 teaspoons raw honey (optional)
1–2 teaspoons sun-dried sea salt
Fresh black pepper to taste

In a food processor, finely chop pine nuts, garlic, and herbs. Add prepared cheeses, lemon juice, apple cider vinegar, olive oil, and honey (if desired) and blend into a smooth paste. It may be necessary to add a bit more oil or a few tablespoons of fresh water to blend well. Season with sea salt and pepper to taste.

GREEK HERB AND OLIVE "FETA"
MAKES 4 CUPS.

Serve this savory blended cheese with a Greek salad with
bell peppers, tomatoes, red onion, and cucumbers or in
a Mediterranean quiche.

1½ cups whole raw cashews,
  fermented into cheese (see
  directions on pages 311–312)
1 cup sunflower seeds, fermented into
  cheese (see directions on pages
  311–312)
½ cup pine nuts, fermented into
  cheese (see directions on pages
  311–312)
1 cup mild black olives, pitted and
  sliced
½ cup minced red onion

2 cloves garlic, minced
¼ cup chopped parsley
2 tablespoons chopped dried oregano
2 teaspoons dried thyme or marjoram
2 teaspoons dried tarragon
½ cup lemon juice
2 tablespoons nutritional yeast
2–4 tablespoons organic extra-virgin
  olive oil (optional) (For a lighter
  cheese, use less olive oil.)
2 teaspoons sun-dried sea salt, or
  to taste

In a large bowl, mix together prepared cheeses, olives, onion, garlic, parsley, oregano, thyme or marjoram, tarragon, lemon juice, nutritional yeast, and olive oil (if using), and season with sea salt to taste.

MACADAMIA NUT RICOTTA

MAKES 2 CUPS.

*This delectable cheese is gorgeous as a creamy dip or layered in
a terrine with marinated mushrooms and zucchini and
Sun-Dried Tomato Marinara (page 355).*

¼ cup pine nuts
1 clove garlic, pressed or finely
    minced
2 cups raw macadamia nuts,
    fermented into cheese (see
    directions on pages 311–312)
½ cup lemon juice

2 tablespoons organic extra-virgin
    olive oil (optional) (For a lighter
    cheese, do not use olive oil.)
Fresh water, if necessary, to blend
3 tablespoons nutritional yeast
1–2 teaspoons sun-dried sea salt,
    or to taste

In a food processor, finely chop pine nuts and garlic. Add prepared macadamia nut cheese,
lemon juice, and olive oil (if using), and blend until smooth. It may be necessary to add a few
tablespoons of fresh water to blend well. Add as little water as possible in order to keep a nice
thick consistency. Add nutritional yeast and season with sea salt to taste.

CASHEW CREAM CHEESE

MAKES 2 CUPS.

*All of the decadence of cream cheese from a simple cashew cheese
base. This is superb as a layer in an open-faced sandwich with
Bread and Butter Pickles (page 316) or cucumber slices.*

2 cups whole raw cashews, fermented
    into cheese (see directions on
    pages 311–312)
¼ cup lemon juice

2–4 tablespoons organic extra-virgin
    olive oil
Fresh water, if necessary, to blend
1 teaspoon sun-dried sea salt

In a food processor, blend prepared cashew cheese, lemon juice, olive oil, and sea salt into a
smooth cream. It may be necessary to add a few tablespoons of fresh water to blend super-
smooth.

BREAD AND BUTTER PICKLES
MAKES 2 CUPS.

*Sweet fresh cucumber pickles are a treat for an open-face
sandwich or to top a crunchy salad. Peeling the cucumbers
helps a quicker pickle. Keeps fresh for weeks.*

  2 cucumbers, peeled and sliced
  4 tablespoons apple cider vinegar
  3 tablespoons raw honey or organic evaporated cane juice
  1 tablespoon whole coriander seeds
  2 teaspoons sun-dried sea salt

Mix the apple cider vinegar, honey or evaporated cane juice, coriander seeds, and sea salt.
Toss with cucumbers. Put in a clean glass jar with a lid. Allow to stand 2–7 days in the refrigerator for best results before serving.

ALMOND MISO CHEESE
MAKES 2 CUPS.

*This cheese is delicate and tasty as a spread with flax crackers
or in a sushi roll with marinated shiitake mushrooms and
slivered snap peas.*

  2 cups almonds, fermented into
    cheese (see directions on pages
    311–312)
  2 tablespoons white miso

  1½ tablespoons umeboshi plum paste
  1 clove garlic, minced
  2 teaspoons minced fresh ginger

In a food processor, blend together the almond cheese, miso, umeboshi plum paste, garlic, and
ginger until fairly smooth.

Spring Lemon and Dill Sesame Cheese
MAKES 2 CUPS.

This cheese is delicious served with dehydrated falafel,
tomatoes, and cucumber.

1 clove garlic, minced
1½ tablespoons dried dill
¼ cup chopped parsley
¼ cup chopped cilantro
2 teaspoons chopped tarragon
2 green onions, finely chopped
2 cups sesame seeds, fermented into
    cheese (see directions on pages
    311–312)

¼ cup lemon juice
1 tablespoon lemon zest
2 tablespoons nutritional yeast
2 tablespoons raw tahini
1 tablespoon sesame oil or organic
    extra-virgin olive oil
1 teaspoon sun-dried sea salt, or
    to taste

In a food processor, chop all ingredients until well mixed.

Dips, Spreads, and Salsas

Traditional Hummus
MAKES 2–4 SERVINGS.

Traditional hummus with garlic, parsley, lemon, and creamy
tahini. Good for all times.

1 cup garbanzo beans
1–2 cloves garlic
1 cup fresh parsley leaves
4–6 tablespoons raw sesame tahini
⅓ cup lemon juice

2 tablespoons organic extra-virgin
    olive oil or sesame oil (optional)
2 teaspoons sun-dried sea salt, or a
    pinch more to taste

In a glass jar with a mesh or screen covering, soak garbanzo beans in 3 cups filtered water for
6–8 hours.

    Drain off soak water and rinse and drain again. Allow to stand upside-down, at an angle, to
drain (in a dish rack or in the sink).

Rinse and drain in the morning and evening for 2–4 days, until the beans sprout tails that are as long as the beans.

In a food processor, chop sprouted garbanzo beans to a pulp. Put chopped beans in a strainer and generously rinse until the starch is drained away and the rinse water is clear. Additionally, the beans can be blanched or steamed after being rinsed.

In the food processor, finely chop garlic and parsley. Add rinsed garbanzo beans, tahini, lemon juice, and olive oil (if using), and blend until creamy. Season with sea salt to taste.

SPINACH AND PINE NUT HUMMUS WITH OLIVES
MAKES 2–4 SERVINGS.

A lovely integration of delicate spinach and savory pine nuts. Baby spinach leaves are best to use as they are much more tender.

2 cups sprouted garbanzo beans, rinsed or blanched/steamed
2 cups chopped spinach leaves
½ cup basil leaves
2 tablespoons chopped chives
2 tablespoons plus ⅓ cup pine nuts
1 clove garlic
2 tablespoons organic extra-virgin olive oil

2 teaspoons apple cider vinegar
Splash balsamic vinegar
¼ cup lemon juice
1–2 teaspoons sun-dried sea salt, or to taste
½ cup pitted and chopped mild black olives

In a food processor, chop sprouted garbanzo beans to a pulp. Put chopped beans in a strainer and generously rinse until the starch is drained away and the rinse water is clear. Additionally, the beans can be blanched or steamed after being rinsed.

In a food processor, finely chop spinach, basil, chives, and 2 tablespoons of the pine nuts. Set aside. Blend rinsed beans, garlic, ⅓ cup pine nuts, olive oil, vinegars, lemon juice, and sea salt until creamy.

Mix the olives into the hummus with the chopped spinach, basil, chives, and pine nuts.

FALAFEL BALLS
MAKES 12 BALLS.

Roll balls out of ¼ cup of any hummus mixture and place on nonstick sheets on dehydrator trays. Dehydrate at 108°F for 12–20 hours or until a crust has formed. (Climate, temperature, and humidity all affect dehydrating time.) Alternatively, the falafel balls can be dried on a cookie sheet or in a casserole dish in the oven set at the lowest temperature for 4–6 hours until a crust forms. Leave the door slightly ajar if necessary to regulate the temperature. The falafel balls are best with a crust on the outside and moist inside.

Store in a resealable bag or a covered container in the refrigerator.

ALMOND RIM PÂTÉ
MAKES 2 CUPS.

A simple almond pâté complemented by green onions,
ginger, and a touch of sweetness.

2 cups almonds, soaked
3 tablespoons minced fresh ginger
3 green onions, chopped to the top
1 clove garlic
¼ cup nama shoyu
2 large soft dates, pitted, or 1½
    tablespoons brown rice syrup,
    maple syrup, or raw honey

Soak almonds in 3 cups fresh water for overnight (6–12 hours). Drain and rinse.

In a food processor, grind almonds, ginger, green onions, and garlic into a fine meal. Add nama shoyu and dates or sweetener and blend until smooth.

LOWER EAST SIDE SPREAD
MAKES 4 CUPS.

*Fennel seeds, fresh black pepper, and oregano are reminiscent of
sausage spices from the Lower East Side of New York. Superb
served with fresh bell peppers or dehydrated into sausages.*

1½ cups sunflower seeds, soaked
1½ cups pumpkin seeds, soaked
2 cloves garlic
⅔ cup chopped red onion
1½ tablespoons fennel seeds
2 tablespoons oregano

1½ cups chopped broccoli (include
   the stem)
2 tablespoons raw tahini (optional)
2 teaspoons fresh black pepper
2 teaspoons sun-dried sea salt, or
   more to taste

Soak the sunflower seeds and the pumpkin seeds together in 4 cups fresh water for 2–4 hours.
Drain and rinse.

In a food processor, chop garlic, onion, fennel, and oregano. Add broccoli, soaked sunflower and pumpkin seeds, and tahini. Blend into a smooth paste. Season with pepper and
sea salt.

Alternatively, in a Champion, Green Power, or Oscar juicer with the "blank" plate, push
through soaked sunflower and pumpkin seeds, garlic, onion, and chopped broccoli. Finely
chop oregano. Mix in fennel seeds, oregano, and tahini. Season with salt and pepper.

BENNE TAPENADE
MAKES 2–4 SERVINGS.

*Tapenade is a dish common to warm Italian and Mediterranean
regions. So many olives with so many flavors. A variety of olives
can be blended for different flavors.*

1 cup pitted sun-dried black olives
1 cup pitted mild green olives
2 tablespoons organic extra-virgin
   olive oil
Pinch sun-dried sea salt

In a food processor or blender, blend pitted olives, olive oil, and sea salt until smooth.

VARIATION FOR SUN-SEASONED TAPENADE:
Soak sun-dried tomatoes in 2 cups fresh water until softened for 5–15 minutes. In a blender or food processor, blend softened sun-dried tomatoes, pitted olives, olive oil, and sea salt. This tapenade can be left with a bit of texture or blended until smooth. Add more oil as necessary to blend.

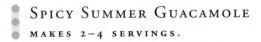

SPICY SUMMER GUACAMOLE
MAKES 2–4 SERVINGS.

Spicy guacamole is a cornerstone of any heat lover's house.

2 ripe avocados
¼ cup lemon juice
1 clove garlic, pressed or minced
2 green onions, finely chopped
1–2 teaspoons dry chipotle pepper or chili pepper
Pinch cayenne pepper
1 tomato, seeded and diced
1 medium cucumber, peeled, seeded, and diced

1 medium red bell pepper, minced
3 tablespoons finely chopped cilantro leaves
3 tablespoons finely chopped parsley leaves
2 tablespoons finely chopped basil leaves
1 teaspoon cumin seeds
1 teaspoon sun-dried sea salt, or to taste

In a large bowl, mash the avocado with a fork. Add lemon juice and mash some more. Mix in garlic, green onions, and hot pepper. Mix in tomato, cucumber, bell pepper, herbs, and cumin. Gently mash together and season with sea salt.

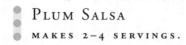

Plum Salsa
MAKES 2–4 SERVINGS.

Plums are both sweet and tangy, and make an excellent base for a
salsa. Choose plums that are neither too firm nor too mushy.

3 red or purple plums, peeled and
 diced
1 tomato, seeded and diced
1 clove garlic, finely minced
1 serrano hot pepper, finely minced
 (use more for some heat!)
3 green onions, finely chopped to top
¼ cup finely chopped cilantro

1 lemon, juiced
1 teaspoon lemon zest
1 tablespoon apple cider vinegar
1 tablespoon organic extra-virgin
 olive oil (optional)
Pinch fresh ground black pepper
Sun-dried sea salt to taste

Mix all ingredients together. Allow to stand for at least 10 minutes for flavors to develop.

Roma Olive Salsa
MAKES 2–4 SERVINGS.

Roma tomatoes with sweet flesh and very few seeds are great for
salsa. The olives lend a savory, rich body to the salsa with a
twist of capers and a good, balanced heat.

4 Roma tomatoes, seeded and diced
½ cup pitted and chopped black
 olives
1 lemon, juiced
2 tablespoons balsamic vinegar or
 apple cider vinegar
2 cloves garlic, minced
1 serrano pepper, minced
Pinch cayenne pepper
2 tablespoons finely chopped cilantro

2 tablespoons finely chopped parsley
1 tablespoon finely chopped basil
3 tablespoons capers
1 tablespoon organic extra-virgin
 olive oil (optional) (The oil gives
 this salsa more body; for a lighter
 salsa, omit the oil.)
Sun-dried sea salt to taste
Fresh ground black pepper to taste

Mix all ingredients together, seasoning to taste with sea salt and pepper. Allow to stand for at
least 10 minutes for flavors to develop.

Starfruit Salsa

MAKES 2–4 SERVINGS.

Starfuit, also called carambola, is excellent for salsa with a mildly sweet flavor.

2 starfruits, diced (about 2 cups)
1 yellow tomato, diced (Red tomato can be substituted.)
½ cup pitted and chopped mild green olives
3 green onions, finely chopped to top
½ red Anaheim pepper, minced

¼ habanero pepper, minced
Pinch chili powder
1 lime, juiced
2 tablespoons finely chopped cilantro
2 tablespoons finely chopped parsley
Sun-dried sea salt to taste
Fresh black pepper to taste

Mix all ingredients together, seasoning with sea salt and pepper to taste.

New Sushi

Traditional Rolls

Sushi is a fine art of food from the Far East that can be handled by anyone with a little practice. A sheet of nori seaweed is used to roll various delicious ingredients and cut into delectable morsels of dynamic flavor and texture. Practically anything can be rolled into a sushi roll for an elegant presentation. Finely sliced vegetables and decorative greens make a delicacy of this simple art.

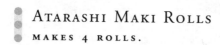 ATARASHI MAKI ROLLS
MAKES 4 ROLLS.

This traditionally rolled sushi is filled with a creamy sesame spread,
crisp cucumber slices, snow peas, scallions, and decorative sprouts
and greens. Serve with Ume Ponzu Dipping Sauce (page 344).

4 sheets nori

Sesame Spread
    2 cups sunflower seeds
    1 large clove garlic

2 tablespoons chopped ginger
¼ cup sesame seeds
3 tablespoons raw tahini
3 tablespoons white miso
2 tablespoons nama shoyu

¼ cup lemon juice

3 tablespoons nutritional yeast

¼ cup poppy seeds

Vegetables

1 cucumber

12 snow peas or snap peas

2 green onions (optional)

Several leaves of green leaf lettuce

To make the sesame spread: Soak sunflower seeds in 3 cups fresh water for 2–6 hours. Drain and rinse. Spread the rinsed seeds on a dry towel and blot dry or allow to air-dry for a bit to maintain a nice thick consistency for the spread.

In a food processor, finely chop the garlic and add the ginger. Add the sunflower seeds and sesame seeds and grind until as smooth as possible. Add tahini, miso, nama shoyu, and lemon juice and grind into a smooth paste. It may be necessary to scrape the sides of the food processor with a rubber spatula and continue to grind. Add nutritional yeast and poppy seeds and grind until well mixed.

To prepare the vegetables: Peel the cucumber and cut in half lengthwise. Scoop out the seeds. Cut the cucumber in half and slice into thin pieces.

Snap off the stems of the snow peas or snap peas. Slice the peas lengthwise into thin strips. Cut off the bottoms and a few inches of the tops of the green onions. Slice the green onions lengthwise into thin strips.

To roll the sushi: See "Rolling and Cutting Sushi Rolls" on page 326.

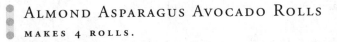

ALMOND ASPARAGUS AVOCADO ROLLS
MAKES 4 ROLLS.

In these rolls, a simple smooth almond spread is complemented by asparagus spears and avocado slices. Serve with White Ginger Dipping Sauce (page 343) or simply with nama shoyu and pickled ginger.

4 sheets nori

1 avocado, cut into slices

Almond Spread

3 cups almonds

4 tablespoons ginger

2 green onions

3 tablespoons red miso

2 tablespoons nama shoyu

2 tablespoons raw honey or brown
    rice syrup, or 3–4 soft dates, pitted

1 tablespoon apple cider vinegar or
    brown rice vinegar

Asparagus
    8 spears asparagus
    4 cups hot water

To make the almond spread: Soak almonds in 4 cups fresh water overnight or for 6–8 hours. Drain and rinse. Lay the almonds on a dry towel and blot dry or allow to air-dry.

Rolling and Cutting Sushi Rolls

A bamboo rolling mat is an essential tool for perfect traditional rolls. The mat enables rolling a tight roll without ripping the delicate nori sheet.

To roll traditional sushi rolls, the nori sheet is place on the bamboo mat. Smear 3–4 tablespoons of the spread or pâté evenly across the bottom third of the nori sheet, leaving 1 inch of nori sheet exposed at the bottom. Next, lay a portion of the prepared vegetables over the spread. Be sure to place them horizontally. For a nice touch, extend the vegetables ½ inch past the edge of the nori sheet for decorative end pieces. Cut or tear greens lengthwise and lay three or four pieces across the spread and vegetables. Allow the decorative ends of the greens to extend past the sheet.

Fold the bottom of the sheet up and over the ingredients. Tuck the edge under the ingredients and roll a little farther by hand. Next, wrap the mat over the roll and begin rolling. Grip the roll, protected by the bamboo mat, with your left hand and gently tug the top of the mat with your right hand to tighten the roll. Wet the top edge of the nori sheet with a little water and roll shut. Hold the roll in the mat for a moment until the moistened edge seals.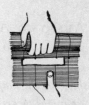

To cut traditional sushi rolls, use a sharp serrated knife. Begin cutting in the center of the roll and then move out to the edges, making 1-inch to 1½-inch pieces. Hold the roll together so that the insides do not come out. Use an even sawing motion with gentle pressure. Run the knife under fresh water between cuts to keep it clean and free from sticking.

In a food processor, finely chop ginger and green onions. Add almonds and grind into a fine meal. Add miso, nama shoyu, honey or brown rice syrup or dates, and vinegar and blend into a smooth paste. It may be necessary to scrape the sides of the food processor with a rubber spatula and continue to blend until smooth.

To prepare the asparagus: Cut off the bottoms of the asparagus. Heat the water to a boil and remove from flame and allow to cool a moment. In a shallow bowl or pan, pour the hot water over the asparagus and allow to warm for 3–5 minutes or until asparagus turns bright green. Do not soak too long. The asparagus should be al dente and crunchy.

To roll the sushi: See "Rolling and Cutting Sushi Rolls" on page 326.

SUSHI PICKLED GINGER
MAKES 1 CUP.

Traditional pickled ginger is a refreshing palate cleanser.
Serve with sushi rolls for an authentic experience.

4 tablespoons raw honey or organic evaporated cane juice
3 tablespoons brown rice syrup
1 tablespoon nama shoyu
2 teaspoons sun-dried sea salt
1 cup peeled and finely sliced ginger

Mix together raw honey or evaporated cane juice, brown rice syrup, nama shoyu, and sea salt.
Toss with sliced ginger. Put marinating ginger in a clean glass jar with a lid. Allow to marinate for at least 1 day, or for 2–3 days for best results before serving. The pickled ginger will keep fresh for weeks.

PACIFIC RIM ROLLS
MAKES 4 ROLLS.

This is a classic infusion of Asian flavor with miso ginger spread, daikon radish, green onions, and pea shoots. Serve with Red Sesame Dipping Sauce (page 345) or nama shoyu with wasabi and pickled daikon.

4 sheets nori

Miso Ginger Spread
  2 cups almonds
  ¼ cup ginger
  2 green onions
  1 cup parsley leaves
  3 tablespoons red miso
  2 tablespoons white miso
  2 tablespoons raw tahini
  1 tablespoon raw honey or brown
    rice syrup

2 tablespoons umeboshi plum paste,
    or 4 umeboshi plums
1 cup sesame seeds

Vegetables
  1 small daikon radish
  1 carrot
  2 green onions
  2 cups pea shoots or sunflower
    sprouts

To make the miso ginger spread: Soak almonds in 4 cups fresh water overnight or for 6–8 hours. Drain and rinse. Lay on a dry towel and blot dry or allow to air-dry to avoid a soggy spread.

In a food processor, finely chop ginger, green onions, and parsley. Add almonds and chop into a fine meal. Add red and white miso, tahini, honey or brown rice syrup, and umeboshi plum paste or umeboshi plums. Blend until smooth. It may be necessary to scrape the sides of the food processor with a rubber spatula and continue to blend for a thoroughly smooth spread. Add sesame seeds and blend until well mixed.

To prepare the vegetables: Peel daikon radish and carefully slice into delicate matchsticks by hand or with a mandoline (see Chapter 12). Peel the carrot. Cut in half and slice into delicate matchsticks by hand or with a mandoline. Cut off the bottom and a few inches of the top of the green onions. Slice lengthwise into thin strips.

To roll the sushi: See "Rolling and Cutting Sushi Rolls" on page 326.

EAST MEETS WEST ROLLS
MAKES 4 ROLLS.

These rolls beautifully integrate the flavors of a walnut, Asian apple-pear, avocado, and greens. Serve with Spring Persimmon Dipping Sauce (page 345) and Leek and Miso Pickles (page 330).

4 sheets nori
1 Asian apple-pear (or any firm pear)
1 avocado
1 head frisée lettuce or endive

Walnut Spread
3 cups walnuts
2 cloves garlic
1 small shallot, or ¼ red onion

1 cup parsley leaves
2 tablespoons dried oregano
2 stalks celery, chopped
2 tablespoons red miso
3 soft dates, pitted
2 tablespoons organic extra-virgin
  olive oil
Pinch sun-dried sea salt

Cut the apple-pear into slices and cut away the seeds and core. Cut the avocado in half. Chop the blade of a chef's knife into the avocado pit. Turn the knife to cleanly remove the pit without fuss. Cut the avocado into slices while still in the skin. Gently peel away the skin or scoop out the sliced flesh with a spoon. Set aside for rolling.

To make the walnut spread: Soak walnuts in 4 cups fresh water for 1 hour. Drain and rinse. Lay on a dry towel and blot dry or allow to air-dry to avoid a soggy spread.

In a food processor, finely chop garlic, shallot or onion, parsley, oregano, and celery. Add walnuts, miso, dates, and olive oil and blend into a smooth paste. It may be necessary to scrape the sides of the food processor with a rubber spatula and continue to blend for a smooth spread. Season with sea salt.

To roll the sushi: See "Rolling and Cutting Sushi Rolls" on page 326.

Leek and Miso Pickles
MAKES 2 CUPS.

These simple pickles, made from miso and leeks, are an excellent condiment for sushi plates or to serve with flat bread and a spread or pâté.

2 cups finely sliced leeks
¼ cup white miso
¼ cup red miso

Slice leeks very thinly. Gently mix with miso and press into a container with a cover or jar with a lid. Allow to stand in the refrigerator for 2–7 days. Keeps fresh for weeks.

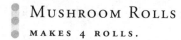

Mushroom Rolls
MAKES 4 ROLLS.

Savory marinated mushrooms give these sushi rolls a divine texture. The mushrooms are complemented by a simple cashew spread for a delightful balance. Serve with White Citrus Miso Dipping Sauce (page 344) or nama shoyu.

4 sheets nori

Marinated Mushrooms
2 portobello mushrooms
3 tablespoons organic extra-virgin
   olive oil
3 tablespoons nama shoyu
1 tablespoon umeboshi plum vinegar
1 clove garlic, pressed or minced

Spread
2½ cups cashews
2 tablespoons ginger
1 small clove garlic
½ cup cilantro leaves
2 tablespoons white miso
¼ cup lemon juice
2 tablespoons nutritional yeast

To marinate the mushrooms: Remove the stems and thinly slice the mushrooms. Mix together olive oil, nama shoyu, umeboshi plum vinegar, and garlic. Toss mushrooms in mixture until well coated and allow to marinate for 30 minutes or until savory and soft. The mushrooms can be marinated for a day or two and stored in the refrigerator. Before using the mushrooms, squeeze by hand or press through a strainer to squeeze out excess marinade.

To prepare the spread: Soak cashews in 3 cups fresh water for 30 minutes. Drain and rinse.

In a food processor, finely chop ginger, garlic, and cilantro. Add cashews and grind into a fine meal. Add miso and lemon juice and blend into a smooth spread. It may be necessary to scrape the sides of the food processor with a rubber spatula and continue to blend for an even, smooth spread. Blend in nutritional yeast until well mixed.

To roll the sushi: See "Rolling and Cutting Sushi Rolls" on page 326.

WILD RICE CAVIAR AND SHIITAKE MUSHROOM ROLLS
MAKES 4 ROLLS.

In these rolls, succulent shiitake mushrooms are complemented by the nutty flavors of wild rice and arame. Serve with Miso Wasabi Dipping Sauce (page 343), Ume Ponzu Dipping Sauce (page 344), or nama shoyu with a side of pickled ginger.

4 sheets nori

Marinated Shiitake Mushrooms
4 cups thinly sliced shiitake
   mushrooms
3 tablespoons sesame oil
2 tablespoons nama shoyu
2 tablespoons umeboshi plum vinegar
2 tablespoons shredded or finely
   minced ginger
Pinch sun-dried sea salt

Wild Rice Caviar
2½ cups long-grain wild rice for
   sprouting (yields 2½ cups)
1½ cups dry hijiki
1 clove garlic
2 tablespoons dulse flakes
2 tablespoons organic extra-virgin
   olive oil
2 tablespoons umeboshi plum paste,
   or 4 umeboshi plums
1 tablespoon raw honey or brown rice
   syrup
2 tablespoons nutritional yeast

To marinate the mushrooms: Mix together the sliced mushrooms, sesame oil, nama shoyu, umeboshi plum vinegar, ginger, and sea salt. Toss mushrooms in mixture until well coated. Allow to marinate for at least 30 minutes or until soft and savory. The mushrooms can be marinated a day or two in advance and stored in the refrigerator. Before using the mushrooms in the rolls, squeeze by hand or press through a strainer to wick away excess marinade. The marinade can be used again or served as a dipping sauce.

To make the wild rice caviar: In a glass jar covered by screen or mesh and secured by a rubber band, soak long-grain wild rice in 4 cups fresh water overnight or for 6–12 hours. Drain and rinse. Allow to stand upside down at a 45-degree angle to drain. Rinse and drain two to three times a day for 2–5 days until rice is soft and has split open.

Soak hijiki in 3 cups warm fresh water until soft (about 10–20 minutes). Drain off soak water.

In a food processor, chop sprouted wild rice, hijiki, garlic, dulse flakes, olive oil, umeboshi plum paste or plums, honey or brown rice syrup, and nutritional yeast. The mixture should be well chopped with some texture. Be careful not to blend into a paste.

To roll the sushi: See "Rolling and Cutting Sushi Rolls" on page 326.

NEAR EAST SUSHI ROLLS
MAKES 4 ROLLS.

Flavors of the Near East and Mediterranean mingle in these delicate sushi rolls. Serve with White Citrus Miso Dipping Sauce (page 344) or nama shoyu.

4 nori sheets
1 cup Jerusalem artichoke matchsticks, or 1 cucumber, sliced into matchsticks
16 romaine lettuce heart leaves

Sun-Dried Chutney
1 cup sun-dried tomatoes
½ cup pitted and chopped black olives

½ cup pitted and chopped green olives
4 dates, pitted and chopped
2 tablespoons organic extra-virgin olive oil
Pinch sun-dried sea salt
Pinch cayenne pepper (optional)

Near East Spread

2½ cups sunflower seeds
1 cup chopped zucchini
1 clove garlic
½ cup chopped green onion
1 cup chopped basil
½ cup chopped cilantro
½ cup chopped parsley

½ cup pine nuts
¼ cup raw tahini
2 tablespoons white miso
¼ cup lemon juice
1 teaspoon lemon zest
½ cup sesame seeds
3 tablespoons nutritional yeast
Pinch sun-dried sea salt

To make the sun-dried chutney: With a pair of kitchen scissors, cut the sun-dried tomatoes into small pieces. Soak the pieces in 1½ cups fresh water until soft (about 5–15 minutes). Drain off soak water and save for other recipes, if desired.

In a food processor, mix the softened sun-dried tomato pieces, olives, and dates with olive oil, sea salt, and cayenne pepper (if desired). The texture should have some body but be well chopped and mixed. It may be necessary to pulse chop a few times in the food processor for good consistency. Be careful not to blend into a paste.

To make the Near East spread: Soak the sunflower seeds in 3 cups fresh water for 1–4 hours. Drain and rinse. Lay the rinsed seeds out on a dry towel and blot dry or allow to air-dry to avoid a soggy spread.

In a food processor, finely chop zucchini, garlic, green onion, basil, cilantro, and parsley. Add sunflower seeds, pine nuts, tahini, miso, lemon juice, and lemon zest and blend into a smooth paste. It may be necessary to scrape the sides of the food processor with a rubber spatula and continue to blend for an even, smooth spread. Add sesame seeds, nutritional yeast, and sea salt, and mix well.

To roll the sushi: See "Rolling and Cutting Sushi Rolls" on page 326.

Hand Rolls and Cone Rolls

SESAME MISO CONE ROLLS
MAKES 8 CONE ROLLS.

*These gorgeous sushi cone rolls are filled with a simple sesame
miso spread, delicate matchsticks, and decorative greens.
Serve with Miso Wasabi Dipping Sauce (page 343)
or simply with nama shoyu.*

4 sheets nori, cut in half
1 carrot
½ avocado, sliced
4–8 green lettuce leaves

Sesame Miso Spread
¼ cup raw tahini
3 tablespoons white miso

1 tablespoon raw honey, maple syrup,
  or brown rice syrup
3–4 tablespoons lemon juice
2 tablespoons shredded or finely
  minced ginger
¼ cup finely chopped green onion
4 tablespoons sesame seeds

Peel the carrot and slice into matchsticks by hand or with a mandoline (see Chapter 12). Cut
the avocado in half and remove the pit. Slice into eight slices and gently peel away the skin or
scoop out the flesh with a spoon. Clean the lettuce leaves and break or cut into 4-inch pieces.
Be sure there are eight pieces with pretty outer edges for decorative rolls.

To make the sesame miso spread: In a bowl, mix tahini, miso, honey or syrup, and lemon juice
into a smooth paste. Add ginger, green onion, and sesame seeds. Mix well. The spread should
be quite thick. Add a few more tablespoons of sesame seeds if the spread is too runny.

To roll the cone roll: See "Rolling Cone Rolls" on page 335.

Rolling Cone Rolls

Cone rolls can be rolled by hand without a mat. To roll cone rolls, cut the nori sheet in half. Lay the longer edge of the sheet flush to you from left to right. Smear 3 to 4 tablespoons of the pâté or spread on a 45-degree angle from the bottom center of the nori sheet to the top left-hand corner. Lay the prepared vegetables and decorative greens or sprouts in the same fashion. Fold the bottom left-hand corner over the ingredients toward the top center of the sheet and tuck the edge under the ingredients. Following the natural shape of a cone, roll the sheet toward the center and to the right edge. The tip of the cone should hinge from a point at the bottom center. Moisten the bottom right-hand corner with water to seal the cone. Hold for a moment until dry.

NOUVEAU CONE ROLLS

MAKES 8 CONE ROLLS.

These decorative cone rolls offer a dynamic balance of flavor. Sunflower sprouts or decorative lettuce leaves add a lovely touch. Serve with White Ginger Dipping Sauce (page 343), or Spring Persimmon Dipping Sauce (page 345), or nama shoyu and pickled ginger.

4 nori sheets, cut in half
1 Asian apple-pear (or any firm pear)
8 sprigs cilantro (small upper stems and leaves)
8 sprigs parsley (small upper stems and leaves)
1 cup sunflower sprouts, or 8 small leaves delicate green lettuce

Walnut Spread
¾ cup walnuts
2 tablespoons raw tahini

2 tablespoons red miso
2 teaspoons raw honey, maple syrup, or brown rice syrup
1 tablespoon apple cider vinegar
1 tablespoon umeboshi plum paste or 1 umeboshi plum, chopped
3 tablespoons shredded or finely minced ginger
¼ cup finely chopped green onion
Pinch sun-dried sea salt

Cut the Asian apple-pear into thin slices. Discard the core and seeds. Set aside apple-pear slices, cilantro, parsley, and sunflower sprouts or lettuce for rolling.

To make the walnut spread: Finely chop the walnuts. This can be done by hand or in a food processor. In a bowl, mix chopped walnuts, tahini, miso, honey or syrup, apple cider vinegar, umeboshi plum paste or plum, ginger, and green onion. Season with sea salt. The spread should be quite thick.

To roll the cone roll: see "Rolling Cone Rolls" on page 335.

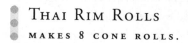

THAI RIM ROLLS
MAKES 8 CONE ROLLS.

These Thai rolls make a gorgeous package of just the right herbs and textures. Serve with Spring Persimmon Dipping Sauce (page 345) or nama shoyu.

4 sheets nori
½ cup thinly sliced red bell pepper
1 cucumber
1 carrot
½ avocado
8 sprigs cilantro
8 sprigs fresh mint
8 sprigs parsley

Thai Spread

4 tablespoons raw almond butter
2 tablespoons white miso
4 umeboshi plums, chopped, or
   3 tablespoons umeboshi plum paste
1 tablespoon apple cider vinegar
1 tablespoon nama shoyu
2 teaspoons raw honey or brown
   rice syrup
1 clove garlic, finely minced
3 tablespoons shredded or finely
   minced ginger
½ cup finely chopped green onion
Pinch cayenne pepper (optional)
3–4 tablespoons sesame seeds

Peel the cucumber and cut in half lengthwise. Scoop out the seeds with a spoon. Cut the cucumber in half and slice into thick matchsticks. Peel the carrot. Continue to peel the carrot into delicate ribbons to the core. Cut the avocado into slices while still in the skin. Gently peel away the skin or scoop out the sliced flesh with a spoon. Set aside prepared vegetables and herbs for rolling.

To make the Thai spread: Mix together almond butter, miso, umeboshi plums or paste, apple cider vinegar, nama shoyu, and honey or brown rice syrup. Mix in garlic, ginger, green onion, cayenne pepper (if desired), and sesame seeds. The spread should be quite thick. If the spread is too thin, add 2 or more tablespoons of sesame seeds.

To roll the cone roll: See "Rolling Cone Rolls" on page 335.

ALTRO MARE HAND ROLLS
MAKES 8 CONE ROLLS.

Flavors reminiscent of the Near East and the Mediterranean are evenly balanced in these delicious hand rolls. Serve with White Ginger Dipping Sauce (page 343) or simply with nama shoyu.

4 sheets nori, cut in half
1 cucumber
8 sun-dried tomato halves
8–16 leaves basil
8 sprigs parsley
8 leaves of romaine hearts

Mushrooms
8 crimini mushrooms
2 tablespoons olive oil
2 tablespoons nama shoyu

Altro Spread
¼ cup pine nuts
2 tablespoons raw tahini
2 tablespoons white miso
1 tablespoon apple cider vinegar
½ cup chopped mild black olives
1 clove garlic, finely minced
¼ cup finely minced green onion
2 tablespoons nutritional yeast
2–4 tablespoons sesame seeds

Peel the cucumber and cut in half lengthwise. Scoop out the seeds with a spoon. Cut the cucumber in half and slice into thick matchsticks. With a pair of kitchen scissors, cut the sun-dried tomato halves into strips. Soak in 1 cup fresh water until soft (about 5–10 minutes). Drain the soak water. Set aside prepared vegetables, herbs, and greens for rolling.

To prepare the mushrooms: Finely slice the mushrooms and marinate in olive oil and nama shoyu for 20–30 minutes or until savory and soft. Before rolling, squeeze the mushrooms by hand or press in a strainer to wick away excess marinade. The extra marinade can be used for dipping if desired.

To make the altro spread: Finely chop the pine nuts. Mix with tahini, miso, apple cider vinegar, olives, garlic, green onion, and nutritional yeast. The spread should be quite thick. Add a few tablespoons of sesame seeds if it is too thin.

To roll the cone roll: See "Rolling Cone Rolls" on page 335.

SESAME INSIDE-OUT ROLLS
MAKES 2 ROLLS.

These inside-out rolls, filled with delicate matchsticks and decorative greens, make a spectacular presentation. Serve with Ume Ponzu Dipping Sauce (page 344) or simply with nama shoyu.

2 sheets nori
1 carrot
1 cucumber
4–6 leaves green or red leaf lettuce

Sesame Inside-Out Spread
¼ cup raw tahini
3 tablespoons white miso

2 teaspoons raw honey or brown rice syrup
½ cup finely chopped green onion
2 tablespoon shredded or finely minced ginger
2 cups sesame seeds
2–4 tablespoons nutritional yeast

Peel the carrot and cut into matchsticks by hand or with a mandoline (see Chapter 12). Peel the cucumber. Cut in half lengthwise. Scoop out the seeds with a spoon. Cut into matchsticks by hand or with a mandoline. Set aside prepared vegetables and lettuce leaves for rolling.

To make the sesame spread: Mix together tahini, miso, honey or brown rice syrup, green onion, and ginger. Mix in sesame seeds and nutritional yeast. The spread should be very thick and on the dry side to hold its shape for rolling. Add a few more tablespoons of sesame seeds if the spread is not thick enough.

To roll the inside-out roll: See "Rolling Inside-Out Rolls" on page 339.

Rolling Inside-Out Rolls

To roll an inside-out roll, wrap the bamboo mat in plastic wrap to avoid sticking. To do this, place a piece of plastic wrap two times as wide as the bamboo mat on the counter. Place the mat in the middle of the plastic wrap and fold the wrap around the mat to cover it completely.

Next, evenly smear 3–4 tablespoons of pâté or spread (specifically prepared for an inside-out roll) on the top two thirds of a nori sheet. Be sure the spread or pâté reaches the sides and top edges. Gently turn the nori sheet over and place it spread-side-down onto the wrapped bamboo mat.

Lay the prepared vegetables across the bottom third of the nori sheet. Next, place the greens across the vegetables. Extend the decorative edges of the greens a half inch past the nori sheet for decorative end pieces.

Fold the bottom of the sheet up and over the ingredients. Tuck the edge under the ingredients and begin to roll. Next, wrap the mat over the roll and begin rolling. Grip the roll, protected by the bamboo mat, with your left hand and gently tug the top of the mat with your right hand to tighten the roll. Hold the roll in the mat for a moment to set.

Cut the roll as explained in "Rolling and Cutting Sushi Rolls" on page 326, but be especially careful, as inside-out rolls are fairly delicate.

ALMOND AND BLACK SESAME INSIDE-OUT ROLLS

MAKES 2 ROLLS.

In these gorgeous rolls, almonds are offset by black sesame seeds.
Serve with Miso Wasabi Dipping Sauce (page 343), Red Sesame
Dipping Sauce (page 345), or simply with nama shoyu.

2 sheets nori
1 carrot
1 cucumber
½ avocado
4–6 leaves red or green leaf lettuce

Almond and Black Sesame Spread
1 cup almonds
2 tablespoons shredded ginger
1 clove garlic
3 soft dates, pitted

3 tablespoons red miso

2 tablespoons raw almond butter

1 tablespoon umeboshi plum paste
(optional)

1 cup black sesame seeds

½ cup white sesame seeds

Peel the carrot and cut into matchsticks by hand or with a mandoline (see Chapter 12). Peel the cucumber and cut in half lengthwise. Scoop out the seeds with a spoon. Cut into matchsticks by hand or with a mandoline. Slice the avocado while still in the skin. Scoop out the slices with a spoon or peel away the skin with a paring knife. Set aside vegetables and lettuce for rolling.

To make the almond and black sesame spread: Soak almonds in 2 cups fresh water overnight or for 6–12 hours. Drain and rinse. Spread the almonds out on a dry dish towel and blot dry with another towel or allow to air-dry to ensure a dry consistency for the spread.

In a food processor, grind almonds, ginger, and garlic into a fine meal. Add the dates, miso, almond butter, and umeboshi plum paste (if desired), and blend as smooth as possible. Add ¾ cup black sesame seeds and ¼ cup white sesame seeds and blend again until as smooth as possible. It may be necessary to scrape the sides of the processor with a rubber spatula and continue for a smooth, even paste. Add more sesame seeds if necessary to achieve a thick, fairly dry spread.

After smearing the spread on the nori and before placing vegetables on it, sprinkle with remaining black and white sesame seeds.

To roll the inside-out roll: See "Rolling Inside-Out Rolls" on page 339.

AVOCADO AND ASPARAGUS INSIDE-OUT ROLLS

MAKES 2 ROLLS.

Al dente asparagus spears, avocado slices, almond miso spread, and black sesame seeds make these rolls a feast of textures. Serve with White Ginger Dipping Sauce (page 343), Miso Wasabi Dipping Sauce (page 343), or simply with nama shoyu and pickled daikon.

2 sheets nori
½ avocado
4–8 spears asparagus
3 cups water
4 sprigs parsley
4 sprigs cilantro

Sesame Miso Spread
2 tablespoons raw almond butter
2 tablespoons raw tahini

2 tablespoons white miso
1 tablespoon red miso
1 tablespoon lemon zest
½ cup finely chopped green onion
2 tablespoons shredded or minced ginger
2 tablespoons nutritional yeast
¾ cup white sesame seeds
¾ cup black sesame seeds

Scoop out the avocado flesh or peel away the skin. Cut off the tough bottoms of the asparagus spears. Heat the water to a simmer. In a shallow bowl or pan, pour the hot water over the asparagus spears and allow to stand for a few minutes until the stalks turn bright green and tender. Drain the water. Set aside the avocado, asparagus, and herbs for rolling.

To make the sesame miso spread: Mix almond butter, tahini, white and red miso, lemon zest, green onion, ginger, nutritional yeast, ½ cup of the white sesame seeds, and ½ cup of the black sesame seeds. The spread should be thick and on the dry side. Add a few more tablespoons of sesame seeds to dry out the spread (only if necessary).

After smearing the spread on the nori sheet and before placing vegetables on it, sprinkle with remaining white and black sesame seeds.

To roll the inside-out roll: See "Rolling Inside-Out Rolls" on page 339.

CUCUMBER ROLLS
MAKES 6–12 PIECES.

These light rolls are wrapped with thinly sliced cucumber instead of nori. A sharp knife and a steady hand are necessary for neat cucumber rolls. Serve with Red Sesame Dipping Sauce (page 345) or White Citrus Miso Dipping Sauce (page 344).

2 large cucumbers
2 carrots
1 avocado
1 cup thinly sliced red bell pepper
1 green onion, thinly sliced
4 sprigs fresh parsley
6–12 toothpicks

Peel the cucumbers and cut off the ends. Cut the cucumbers in half across the seeds. Using a sharp knife, carve a thin "sheet" of cucumber, rotating the cucumber against the blade of the knife. Create an uninterrupted piece, stopping only when you reach the seeds. Repeat with the other cucumber pieces. Set aside.

Peel the carrots. Thread carrot with a Saladacco (see Chapter 12) or peel to the core with a peeler to create delicate ribbons. Cut the avocado in half. Chop the blade of a chef's knife into the avocado pit. Twist the knife to neatly extract the pit. Cut into slices while still in the skin. Scoop out the slices with a spoon or peel away the skin.

Lay the cucumber sheets on a cutting board. Place avocado slices across the bottom of each cucumber sheet. Lay a bunch of carrot threads or ribbons, slices of red pepper, and green onion across the avocado slices. Top with a sprig of fresh parsley. Fold the close end of the cucumber sheet over the vegetables and tuck the edge under. Gently roll the cucumber skin closed. Pierce the roll with evenly spaced toothpicks to hold together for cutting. With a sharp serrated knife, cut the cucumber roll between the toothpicks.

Dipping Sauces

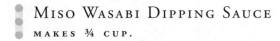

MISO WASABI DIPPING SAUCE
MAKES ¾ CUP.

In this dynamic dipping sauce, the hot kick of wasabi is balanced by savory red miso.

    2 teaspoons wasabi powder
    ¼ cup fresh water
    2 tablespoons red miso
    2 tablespoons nama shoyu
    ¼ cup fresh orange juice
    Pinch sesame seeds or minced green
        onion for garnish (optional)

Mix all of the ingredients together until smooth. Allow to stand 5–10 minutes to develop flavor. Serve in dipping bowls and garnish, if desired, with sesame seeds or green onion.

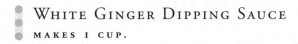

WHITE GINGER DIPPING SAUCE
MAKES 1 CUP.

This light dipping sauce is great with any sushi roll.

    3 tablespoons white miso
    2 tablespoons shredded or finely
        minced ginger
    1 lemon, juiced
    1 orange, juiced
    2 tablespoons umeboshi plum vinegar

1 tablespoon raw honey, maple syrup,
    or brown rice syrup
2–4 tablespoons fresh water as
    necessary to thin
Pinch sesame seeds or minced green
    onion for garnish (optional)

Mix all of the ingredients together until smooth. For a thinner sauce, add a few tablespoons of fresh water. Serve in dipping bowls and garnish, if desired, with sesame seeds or minced green onion.

Ume Ponzu Dipping Sauce
MAKES ½ CUP.

*There is a dynamic balance between umeboshi plums
and vinegar in this light ponzu sauce.*

¼ cup nama shoyu
3 tablespoons umeboshi plum vinegar
2 tablespoons umeboshi plum paste
2 teaspoons maple syrup or brown
   rice syrup
Pinch sesame seeds or minced green
   onion for garnish (optional)

Mix all of the ingredients together until smooth. Serve in dipping bowls and garnish, if desired,
with sesame seeds or minced green onion.

White Citrus Miso Dipping Sauce
MAKES 1 CUP.

*This creamy dipping sauce adds a delightful
flavor to any sushi roll.*

2 tablespoons raw tahini
2 tablespoons white miso
2 tablespoons lemon juice
2 tablespoons orange juice
2 tablespoons umeboshi plum vinegar
1 tablespoon shredded or finely
   minced ginger

2 tablespoons minced green onion
2 teaspoons raw honey, brown rice
   syrup, or agave syrup
2–4 tablespoons fresh water or more
   for desired consistency
Pinch sesame seeds or minced green
   onion for garnish

Mix or blend all of the ingredients until smooth. Add a touch more water for a thinner sauce.
Serve in dipping bowls and garnish with sesame seeds or minced green onion.

Red Sesame Dipping Sauce
MAKES 1 CUP.

*This savory creamy dipping sauce enhances
the flavor of any sushi roll.*

3 tablespoons raw tahini

3 tablespoons red miso

1 clove garlic

2 tablespoons chopped green onion

1 tablespoon shredded or finely
minced ginger

2 umeboshi plums, or 1 tablespoon
umeboshi plum paste

½ cup orange juice

¼ cup fresh water or more for desired
consistency

Pinch of sesame seeds or minced
green onion for garnish

In a blender, blend all ingredients until smooth. Add a few more tablespoons of fresh water if a thinner consistency is desired. Serve in dipping bowls and garnish with sesame seeds or minced green onion.

Spring Persimmon Dipping Sauce
MAKES MORE THAN 1 CUP.

*Sweet succulent persimmons are complemented by tangy umeboshi
plums and vinegar for a dynamic dipping sauce.*

1 ripe persimmon

1 tablespoon shredded or finely
minced ginger

2 umeboshi plums, or 1 tablespoon
umeboshi plum paste

2 tablespoons umeboshi plum vinegar

2 tablespoons nama shoyu

1 tablespoon brown rice vinegar or
apple cider vinegar

¼ cup fresh water as necessary

2 tablespoons minced green onion for
garnish (optional)

Peel the delicate skin from the persimmon. Remove any seeds or firm parts. In a blender, blend persimmon, ginger, umeboshi plums or paste, umeboshi plum vinegar, nama shoyu, and brown rice or apple cider vinegar until smooth. Add a little water as necessary for desired consistency. Serve in dipping bowls and garnish, if desired, with minced green onion.

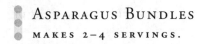

26

Vegetable Sides and Accompaniments

Asparagus Bundles
MAKES 2–4 SERVINGS.

Al dente asparagus spears tied with threaded vegetables
make a simple and gorgeous presentation.

1 bunch asparagus spears
6 cups hot water
2 tablespoons organic extra-virgin
   olive oil
1 lemon, juiced
1 teaspoon lemon zest

2 teaspoons crushed coriander seeds
1 teaspoon sun-dried sea salt
1 beet or 1 carrot, or the flexible
   green leaves of a green onion
Fresh cracked black pepper to taste

Cut off the tough ends of the asparagus. Bring water to a boil, turn off heat, and allow to cool a moment. Place asparagus spears in a shallow pan and pour hot water over them. Allow to stand for 5 minutes or so, until asparagus becomes just tender. Drain the asparagus and toss with olive oil, lemon juice, lemon zest, coriander seeds, and sea salt. Allow to marinate at least 10 minutes.

Spiralize the beet with a Saladacco (see Chapter 12) into threads. Alternatively, peel a carrot and continue to peel to the core into peeled ribbons.

Gather 4–6 spears asparagus and tie into a bundle with 6–8 threads beet or a few peels of carrot ribbon. Tie threaded beet into a square knot or bow. Season with cracked fresh black pepper.

LEMONGRASS ASPARAGUS BUNDLES WITH LEMON CASHEW SAUCE
MAKES 2–4 SERVINGS.

These seasoned asparagus spears are tied with lemongrass. Serve with Lemon Cashew Sauce for drizzling or dipping.

1 bunch asparagus
6 cups hot water
4 long blades fresh lemongrass (If fresh lemongrass is unavailable, the flexible green leaves of a green onion can be used.)
2 tablespoons organic extra-virgin olive oil
1 lemon, juiced
2 teaspoons lemon zest
2 teaspoons raw honey or maple syrup

1 teaspoon sun-dried sea salt
2 teaspoons dried lemongrass

Lemon Cashew Sauce
½ cup cashews
¼ cup lemon juice
2 teaspoons lemon zest
1 tablespoon apple cider vinegar
2 tablespoons nama shoyu
1½ teaspoons raw honey or maple syrup

Cut off the tough ends of the asparagus. Bring water to a boil, turn off heat, and allow to cool a moment. Place asparagus spears and blades of lemongrass in a shallow pan and pour hot water over them. Allow to stand for 5 minutes or so, until asparagus becomes just tender. Drain the asparagus and toss with olive oil, lemon juice, lemon zest, honey or maple syrup, sea salt, and lemongrass. Allow to marinate at least 10 minutes.

Gather 4–6 spears asparagus and tie into a bundle with a blade or two of lemongrass.

To make the lemon cashew sauce: Soak cashews in 1 cup fresh water for 30 minutes. Drain and rinse.

In a blender, blend cashews, lemon juice, lemon zest, apple cider vinegar, nama shoyu, and honey or maple syrup until smooth. It may be necessary to add another tablespoon or two of lemon juice or fresh water to blend to desired consistency. The sauce should be fairly thick but pourable. Drizzle sauce over asparagus bundles or serve in a dipping bowl.

Szechuan Snow Peas

MAKES 2–4 SERVINGS.

This spicy dish of sweet snow peas can also be made with sugar snap peas. Any dried spicy pepper can be used if Szechuan pepper is not available.

4 cups fresh snow peas
1 clove garlic, pressed or finely
    minced
2 tablespoons organic extra-virgin
    olive oil or sesame oil
1½ tablespoons umeboshi plum
    vinegar, brown rice vinegar, or
    apple cider vinegar

2 tablespoons nama shoyu
2 teaspoons raw honey, maple syrup,
    or brown rice syrup
2 teaspoons Szechuan pepper
Generous pinch cayenne pepper

Snap off the tough end of the peas. In a bowl, mix garlic, olive oil, vinegar, honey or syrup, and peppers. Toss peas with marinade until well coated. Allow to stand at least 20 minutes to develop flavor, tossing occasionally.

Steamed Garlic Green Beans

MAKES 2–4 SERVINGS.

This simple dish of fresh green beans and garlic gets its kick from chipotle or chili pepper.

4 cups fresh green beans
2 cloves garlic, pressed
3 tablespoons organic extra-virgin
    olive oil
2 tablespoons nama shoyu
1–2 teaspoons chipotle pepper or
    dried chili pepper, or to taste

Snap off the stem end of the string beans. Steam the green beans lightly, just until they turn bright green and tender. Immediately toss with pressed garlic, olive oil, nama shoyu, and pepper.

Steamed Sesame Ginger Broccoli

MAKES 2–4 SERVINGS.

This simple broccoli dish has a fortune of good flavor. It works great as a side dish to an Asian-inspired main course.

4 cups broccoli florets
1½ tablespoons minced ginger
1 clove garlic, pressed or minced
2½ tablespoons organic extra-virgin
  olive oil or sesame oil

2 tablespoons nama shoyu
1 tablespoon umeboshi plum vinegar
  (optional)
⅓ cup sesame seeds
Pinch sun-dried sea salt, or to taste

Steam the broccoli lightly, just until it turns bright green and is still crunchy. Mix together the ginger, garlic, oil, nama shoyu, and vinegar. Immediately toss the broccoli with the marinade and sesame seeds until well coated. Season with sea salt.

Sweet Summer Corn and Squash

MAKES 2–4 SERVINGS.

Delicate summer squash and sweet crunchy corn need little more than some fresh herbs and olive oil to make the perfect meal accompaniment.

2 young zucchinis
2 ears fresh corn, cut from the cob
8 cherry tomatoes, cut in half
2 green onions, finely chopped to
  the top
3 tablespoons organic extra-virgin
  olive oil

¼ cup chopped parsley
¼ cup chopped cilantro
2 teaspoons dried dill
1 teaspoon sun-dried sea salt, or
  to taste

Cut the zucchinis into quarters and then into ½-inch pieces. Steam lightly, just until tender. Alternatively, to avoid steaming, thinly slice the zucchinis. Set aside. Cut the corn from the cob and cut the tomatoes in half. Toss zucchini together with the corn, tomatoes, green onions, olive oil, parsley, cilantro, dill, and sea salt. If using raw zucchini, allow to marinate for at least 20 minutes.

Steamed Artichokes and Aioli Sauce
Makes 2 servings.

*Drizzle creamy seasoned Aioli Sauce over these classic steamed
artichokes for a side dish with wonderful flavor and texture.*

2 artichokes

Aioli Sauce
½ avocado
3 tablespoons olive oil
¼ cup lemon juice
1 tablespoon apple cider vinegar
1 tablespoon raw honey or maple
   syrup

1 tablespoon nama shoyu
1 tablespoon prepared mustard
   (optional)
1 clove garlic
¼ cup chopped parsley
2 tablespoons chopped basil
Fresh water, as needed
Pinch sun-dried sea salt, or to taste

Steam the artichoke hearts for 30–40 minutes until tender. Test doneness by pulling out a leaf.
It should come out easily and be tender to the teeth.

To make the aioli sauce: In a blender, blend avocado, olive oil, lemon juice, apple cider vinegar,
honey or maple syrup, nama shoyu, mustard (if desired), garlic, parsley, and basil until smooth.
Add fresh water a few tablespoons at a time to blend to desired consistency. Season with sea
salt. The sauce should be quite thick and smooth.

Steamed Simple Greens
Makes 2–4 servings.

*A simple dish like this is a snap to prepare. Use whatever
type of kale is freshest at the market.*

2 tablespoons organic extra-virgin
   olive oil
1 tablespoon flax oil
1 clove garlic, pressed or finely
   minced

1 bunch kale (red kale, curly kale,
   or dinosaur kale)
2 tablespoons nama shoyu
Pinch sun-dried sea salt, or to taste

Mix olive oil, flax oil, garlic, and nama shoyu together. Chop the greens and steam lightly, just until they turn bright green and tender. Immediately toss in a bowl with the oils, garlic, and nama shoyu until well coated. Season with sea salt.

Savory Almond Spinach
MAKES 2–4 SERVINGS.

*I can eat a bowl of this creamy fresh spinach
and herbs all by myself!*

  1 bunch spinach
  ½ cup chopped parsley
  2 tablespoons almond butter
  1 tablespoon flax oil
  2 tablespoons nama shoyu
  1 lemon, juiced
  1 clove garlic, pressed or minced

Clean the spinach and remove any large stems.

In a food processor, finely chop the spinach and parsley. Mix almond butter, flax oil, nama shoyu, lemon juice, and garlic by hand or in a blender. Pour the almond sauce over the spinach and toss together until well coated. Allow to stand for a few minutes to absorb flavor.

Steamed Beets and Snow Peas
MAKES 2–4 SERVINGS.

*In this side dish, steamed beets and sweet snow peas
complement each other nicely. Serve on a fresh lettuce
leaf for a beautiful presentation.*

  ¼ cup finely chopped parsley
  2 tablespoons organic extra-virgin
    olive oil
  2 tablespoons apple cider vinegar
  2 teaspoons raw honey or maple
    syrup (optional)

  1 clove garlic, pressed or finely minced
  2 teaspoons crushed coriander seeds
  1 teaspoon sun-dried sea salt
  3 cups cubed beets
  2 cups snow peas or snap peas
  ½ cup chopped green onion

Mix together the parsley, olive oil, apple cider vinegar, honey or maple syrup, garlic, coriander seeds, and sea salt.

Steam the beets just until a fork can pierce the cubes. Run under cold water until cool to the touch. Snap off the stem ends of the snow peas or snap peas. Toss together the beets, snow peas or snap peas, and green onion, and marinate until well coated. The flavor develops after standing for a few minutes or stored in the refrigerator overnight.

THREE PRETTY PEAS
MAKES 2–4 SERVINGS.

This side dish is a delightful medley of sweet and crunchy green peas.

- 1 cup haricot verts or young green beans
- 1 lemon, juiced
- 2 tablespoons organic extra-virgin olive oil

- 1 teaspoon sun-dried sea salt
- 1½ cups petits pois
- 1½ cups snow peas or snap peas
- Fresh black pepper to taste (optional)

Snap off the stem ends of the haricot verts and cut in half. In a bowl, toss haricot verts with lemon juice, olive oil, and sea salt. Allow to marinate for at least 20 minutes. Toss in petite peas and snow peas or snap peas until well coated. Season, if desired, with fresh black pepper to taste.

STEAMED MISO CARROT AND BURDOCK
MAKES 2–4 SERVINGS.

Burdock is one of the best root vegetables for healthy blood. If fresh burdock is unavailable, dried burdock can be found in the macrobiotic section of a good market or in Asian markets.

- 2 cups burdock, peeled and cut into matchsticks
- 2 cups carrots, cut into matchsticks
- 2 tablespoons white miso

- 1 tablespoon raw almond butter or raw tahini
- 1 tablespoon nama shoyu
- 2 teaspoons apple cider vinegar

2 teaspoons flax oil (optional)

2 teaspoons brown rice syrup, raw
   honey, or maple syrup

1 clove garlic, pressed or finely minced

1 tablespoon grated or finely minced
   ginger

Steam the burdock matchsticks for about 10 minutes just until tender (the thickness of the matchsticks will determine steaming time). If you can gauge it, add the carrot matchsticks to the steaming basket for the last few minutes. Otherwise, steam the carrots separately to avoid overcooking.

In a medium bowl, mix together miso, almond butter or tahini, nama shoyu, apple cider vinegar, flax oil (if desired), brown rice syrup, garlic, and ginger. Add the steamed burdock and carrot matchsticks and turn over until well coated.

Keeps well and absorbs flavor when refrigerated overnight.

STEAMED LEEKS AND TENDER CABBAGE
MAKES 2–4 SERVINGS.

This is an unbelievably simple, but delicious, dish. Who knew cabbage could be so tasty? Chinese Cabbage, also called Napa cabbage, is the best choice. This type of cabbage is already tender and needs less time to steam.

3 cups roughly chopped cabbage
   (savoy, or Chinese or Napa)

1½ cups leeks

2 tablespoons organic extra-virgin
   olive oil

1 tablespoon flax oil

3 tablespoons umeboshi plum vinegar

1 tablespoon nama shoyu

Steam the cabbage and leeks together just until tender, 2–4 minutes. Toss with oils, umeboshi plum vinegar, and nama shoyu.

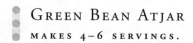
Carrots and Currants
MAKES 2–4 SERVINGS.

*The sweetness of finely shredded carrots is set off by currants and
complemented by crunchy chopped walnuts. A few herbs in all
of the right places make this a well-placed side dish.*

3 cups finely shredded carrots
½ cup currants or raisins
½ cup chopped walnuts
½ cup chopped parsley
1 teaspoon dill
1½ tablespoons nama shoyu
2 teaspoons flax oil

Toss carrots with currants or raisins, walnuts, parsley, dill, nama shoyu, and flax oil until well
coated. Serve on a pretty lettuce leaf for a delectable presentation.

Green Bean Atjar
MAKES 4–6 SERVINGS.

*This is an authentic South African dish of fresh
green string beans preserved in spiced oil.*

6–8 cups water
2 pounds fresh green string beans
2 tablespoons sun-dried sea salt
1 cup organic extra-virgin olive oil
1½ tablespoons curry powder

1 teaspoon turmeric (optional)
1½ tablespoons chopped hot chili
  pepper
1 tablespoon chopped garlic
2 teaspoons crushed coriander seeds

Boil water and allow to cool slightly. Place beans in a deep bowl and pour enough hot water to
cover. Allow to stand 2 minutes. Drain and rinse. Return beans to bowl and add sea salt. Mix
until salt dissolves. Cover with plastic wrap or a plate and allow to set for 2 hours. Drain beans
and squeeze to remove excess moisture. Pack beans in a quart jar. Mix oil and spices in a bowl.
Pour over beans. Cover the jar. Place jar in the refrigerator for at least 2 hours or up to 2 days
before serving.

SPAGHETTI SQUASH AND SUN-DRIED TOMATO MARINARA

MAKES 4 SERVINGS.

*Golden spaghetti squash has the texture of delicate pasta. Serve
with savory Sun-Dried Tomato Marinara for a delicious
combination of flavor and texture.*

Spaghetti Squash
- 1 spaghetti squash
- 3 tablespoons organic extra-virgin olive oil
- Pinch sun-dried sea salt

Sun-Dried Tomato Marinara
- 1 cup sun-dried tomatoes
- 4 Roma tomatoes, or 3 large tomatoes
- 1 clove garlic
- 1 cup fresh basil leaves
- ½ cup fresh Italian parsley leaves
- ½ teaspoon chipotle peppers, or pinch cayenne pepper (optional)
- 1 tablespoon dried Italian seasoning
- 2 tablespoons olive oil (optional)
- 1 tablespoon honey or maple syrup
- 1 teaspoon apple cider vinegar or lemon juice
- Sun-dried sea salt to taste
- Ground fresh black pepper to taste

To make the spaghetti squash: Peel the spaghetti squash and cut in half across the seeds. Scoop out the seeds. Cut each half into quarters. Steam the squash for 10–15 minutes until tender enough to pierce with a fork. Put the squash in a bowl and drizzle with olive oil and a pinch of sea salt and mash with a fork.

To make the Sun-Dried Tomato Marinara: Soak sun-dried tomatoes in just enough fresh water to cover them until soft (about 5–15 minutes). Drain and rinse. Set aside. Cut tomatoes in half and scoop out seeds. Dice the tomatoes. Set aside.

In a food processor, finely chop garlic and herbs. Add sun-dried tomatoes, olive oil (if desired), honey or maple syrup, and apple cider vinegar or lemon juice, and chop in pulses. Do not blend until smooth; leave a touch of texture.

In a bowl, fold together sun-dried-tomato mixture with diced tomatoes. Season with sea salt and pepper to taste.

Serve Sun-Dried Tomato Marinara over squash.

27

Classic and New Entrées

STUFFED EGGPLANT MANICOTTI WITH SUN-DRIED TOMATO AND BASIL MARINARA

MAKES 10–12 STUFFED MANICOTTI ROLLS.

In this dish, thinly sliced marinated eggplant is stuffed with rich macadamia nut ricotta and topped with savory sun-dried tomato and basil marinara. Serve warm for an authentic experience.

Eggplant Manicotti

1 eggplant

1½ tablespoons sun-dried sea salt

⅓ cup lemon juice

2 tablespoons organic extra-virgin olive oil

1 clove garlic, minced

Pinch sun-dried sea salt

Macadamia Nut Ricotta

1 cup macadamia nuts

½ cup whole raw cashews (raw cashew pieces can be used)

¼ cup pine nuts

⅓ cup lemon juice

2 tablespoons organic extra-virgin olive oil (optional)

1 clove garlic, minced

3 tablespoons nutritional yeast

1 teaspoon sun-dried sea salt, or to taste

Sun-Dried Tomato and Basil Marinara
- 1 cup sun-dried tomatoes
- 6 Roma tomatoes, or 4 large tomatoes
- 1 clove garlic
- ¼ cup finely minced red onion
- 1 cup fresh basil leaves
- ½ cup fresh Italian parsley leaves
- Sprig oregano and rosemary, or dried Italian seasoning
- 2 tablespoons olive oil
- 1 tablespoon maple syrup or raw honey
- 1 teaspoon apple cider vinegar or lemon juice
- 1–2 teaspoons sun-dried sea salt, or to taste
- ½ teaspoon chipotle pepper, or pinch cayenne pepper (optional)

To prepare the eggplant manicotti: Peel the eggplant. Slice thinly across the seeds into 10–12 slices. Toss the eggplant slices with sea salt. Marinate for 1 hour. The bitter juices will wick away from the eggplant. Gently squeeze the eggplant, and marinate the slices in lemon juice, olive oil, garlic, and sea salt for 1–2 hours. Gently squeeze the slices to wick away excess marinade before rolling.

To make the macadamia nut ricotta: Soak ¾ cup of the macadamia nuts and cashews together in 3 cups fresh water for 20 minutes. Drain and rinse.

In a food processor, chop remaining ¼ cup of dry macadamia nuts and pine nuts into a fine meal. Set aside. Reserve a few tablespoons for garnish. Chop soaked macadamia nuts and cashews into a fine meal. Add lemon juice, olive oil, and garlic and blend until as smooth as possible. Add a few tablespoons of fresh water to aid in blending smooth. The ricotta should be fairly smooth and thick. Add the ground dry macadamia nuts and pine nuts and nutritional yeast and blend until well mixed. Season with sea salt.

To stuff the manicotti: Spoon 2–4 tablespoons of ricotta onto each marinated slice of eggplant and roll into a manicotti-shaped roll (like a cannoli). The manicotti can be served "fresh" like this or dehydrated for 2–4 hours at 108°F to warm and set and to marry flavors and texture.

To make the sun-dried tomato and basil marinara: Soak the sun-dried tomatoes in 1 cup fresh water until soft (5–15 minutes). Drain and rinse. Set aside. Cut the tops out of the tomatoes. Cut the tomatoes in halves and scoop out the seeds with a spoon. Dice the tomatoes. Set aside.

In a food processor, finely chop garlic, red onion, and herbs. Add sun-dried tomatoes, olive oil, maple syrup or honey, and apple cider vinegar or lemon juice and chop in pulses. Do not blend until smooth; leave a touch of texture.

In a bowl, fold together sun-dried-tomato mixture with diced tomatoes. Season with sea salt and, if desired, chipotle or cayenne pepper. Spoon a generous amount of marinara over each serving of manicotti.

Garnish with reserved ground macadamia nuts and pine nuts.

PORTOBELLO-STUFFED RAVIOLI WITH WALNUT PESTO
MAKES 10–12 RAVIOLI.

Savory marinated mushrooms fill these succulent eggplant ravioli.
Fresh Walnut Pesto complements these ravioli nicely.

Eggplant Ravioli
  1 eggplant
  1 tablespoon sun-dried sea salt
  ⅓ cup lemon juice
  2 tablespoons organic extra-virgin
     olive oil
  1 clove garlic, minced
  1 teaspoon sun-dried sea salt

Marinated Portobellos
  2½ cups diced portobello mushrooms
  1 clove garlic, minced
  2 tablespoons organic extra-virgin
     olive oil
  2 tablespoons nama shoyu
  1 tablespoon apple cider vinegar
  1 teaspoon raw honey or maple syrup

Ricotta and Tomatoes
  1 cup macadamia nuts
  ¼ cup lemon juice
  2–4 tablespoons fresh water
  2 tablespoons nutritional yeast
  1 teaspoon sun-dried sea salt
  1 tomato

Walnut Pesto
  ½ cup walnuts
  2 cups fresh basil
  1–2 cloves garlic
  ¼ cup pine nuts
  ½ cup organic extra-virgin olive oil
  ⅓ cup lemon juice
  2 tablespoons white miso
  1 teaspoon sun-dried sea salt, or
     to taste

To prepare the eggplant ravioli: Peel the eggplant. Thinly slice across the seeds into 10–12 slices. Toss the eggplant with sea salt and marinate for 1 hour. The bitter juice of the eggplant will wick away. Gently squeeze the slices to remove excess liquid. Marinate the slices in lemon juice, olive oil, garlic, and sea salt for 1–2 hours. Gently squeeze the slices to wick away excess marinade before folding.

To prepare the marinated portobellos: Slice the mushrooms and toss them with the garlic, olive oil, nama shoyu, apple cider vinegar, and honey or maple syrup. Allow to marinate 30–60 minutes until savory and soft. The longer the better. The mushrooms can be marinated a day in advance and stored in the refrigerator.

Squeeze the mushrooms by hand or press in a strainer to wick away excess marinade before mixing with ricotta and tomatoes.

To prepare the ricotta and tomatoes: Soak macadamia nuts in 2 cups fresh water for 20 minutes. Drain and rinse.

In a food processor, chop macadamia nuts into a fine meal. Add lemon juice and a few tablespoons of fresh water and blend into a fairly smooth cream. Add nutritional yeast and season with sea salt. Cut the top out of the tomato and cut in half. Scoop the seeds out with a spoon. Dice the tomato. Mix together the squeezed mushrooms, ricotta, and diced tomato.

To stuff the ravioli: Put 2–3 tablespoons of mushroom-ricotta mixture in the center of each piece of marinated eggplant. Fold the eggplant slice in half to make a ravioli. Place the ravioli on dehydrator sheets and dehydrate at 108°F for 4–8 hours. The ravioli should not be dried through and through.

To prepare the walnut pesto: Soak walnuts in 1 cup fresh water for 1 hour. Drain and rinse.

In a food processor, finely chop basil and garlic. Add walnuts and pine nuts and chop into a fine meal.

In a bowl, mix the meal with olive oil, lemon juice, and miso. Season with sea salt. The pesto should be thick and have some texture, but it should be pourable. Add a few tablespoons of fresh water or olive oil if the pesto is too thick. Spoon pesto over each serving of ravioli. Serve with a slice of lemon.

BUTTERNUT ANGEL HAIR WITH PUTTANESCA SAUCE
MAKES 2–4 SERVINGS.

This finely threaded butternut squash perfectly complements the Puttanesca Sauce.

Angel Hair
- 1–2 squashes with a generous neck
- 6 tablespoons organic extra-virgin olive oil
- 2 tablespoons dried Italian seasoning
- 1½ teaspoons sun-dried sea salt

Puttanesca Sauce
- 1 cup sun-dried tomatoes
- 2 cloves garlic
- ¼ cup chopped red onion
- ½ cup chopped basil
- 1 cup pitted olives

2 tablespoons organic extra-virgin
  olive oil
1 tablespoon apple cider vinegar
1½ tablespoons raw honey or maple
  syrup
2 tablespoons dried Italian seasoning,
  or 2 teaspoons oregano, 1 teaspoon
  marjoram, 1 teaspoon savory,
  1 teaspoon thyme, and 1 teaspoon
  rosemary

3 tomatoes
1–2 teaspoons sun-dried sea salt

Pine Nut Parmesan

¼ cup pine nuts
¼ cup raw cashews
½ small clove garlic
2 tablespoons nutritional yeast
2 tablespoons lemon juice
½ teaspoon sun-dried sea salt

To make the angel hair: Peel the butternut squash(es). Using a Saladacco (see Chapter 12), slice the neck of the squash into fine, thin threads. Toss the threads with olive oil, Italian seasoning, and sea salt. Spread the marinated butternut threads on dehydrator trays and dehydrate at 108°F for 8–12 hours until dry but not brittle. If a dehydrator is not available, simply serve fresh.

To make the puttanesca sauce: Soak the sun-dried tomatoes in 1½ cups fresh water until soft (5–15 minutes). Drain the soak water and set aside.

In a food processor, finely chop garlic, red onion, and basil. Add sun-dried tomatoes, olives, olive oil, apple cider vinegar, honey or maple syrup, and dried herbs and blend until well mixed. Set aside.

Cut the tops out of the tomatoes. Cut the tomatoes in half and scoop out the seeds with a spoon. Cut tomatoes into pieces. Finely chop in pulses in the food processor, but do not blend smooth.

Spoon the sauce over each serving of angel hair. Mix the sun-dried tomato and olive mixture with the fresh tomatoes. Season with sea salt. The sauce should be quite thick and hearty.

To make the pine nut parmesan: In a food processor, grind pine nuts, cashews, garlic, nutritional yeast, lemon juice, and sea salt into a fine meal.

Sprinkle each serving with Pine Nut Parmesan.

ZUCCHINI LINGUINI WITH CRIMINI MUSHROOMS AND ALFREDO CREAM SAUCE

MAKES 2–4 SERVINGS.

Smooth alfredo cream sauce complements delicately peeled zucchini tossed with succulent marinated crimini mushrooms for an outstanding palette of flavor and texture.

Marinated Mushrooms

2½ cups sliced crimini mushrooms
3 tablespoons organic extra-virgin olive oil
2 tablespoons nama shoyu
2 teaspoons apple cider vinegar
1–2 cloves garlic, minced

Alfredo Sauce

1½ cups whole raw cashews (raw cashew pieces can be used)
½ cup pine nuts
6 tablespoons organic extra-virgin olive oil
⅓ cup lemon juice
1–2 cloves garlic
3 tablespoons nutritional yeast
⅔–1 cup fresh water as needed
1–2 teaspoons sun-dried sea salt
¼ cup finely chopped parsley

Zucchini Linguini

4 zucchini

Garnish

¼ cup chopped parsley
1 tablespoon paprika
2 teaspoons black pepper

To make the marinated mushrooms: Toss the mushrooms with olive oil, nama shoyu, apple cider vinegar, and minced garlic. Allow to marinate for at least 30 minutes to an hour. The longer, the better. The mushrooms can be prepared a day in advance and stored in the refrigerator. Pour the marinating mushrooms through a strainer to remove excess marinade before serving. Reserve the marinade for other uses, if desired.

To make the alfredo sauce: Soak cashews in 2 cups fresh water for 30 minutes. Drain and rinse.

In a blender, blend cashews, pine nuts, olive oil, lemon juice, garlic, nutritional yeast, and ⅔ cup of the water into a smooth cream. The sauce should be thick but pourable. Add more water as necessary for desired consistency. Fold in finely chopped parsley.

To make the zucchini linguini: Peel the skin from the zucchini and discard. Continue to peel the zucchini to the core with a peeler. Keep turning the zucchini as you peel to create delicate linguini ribbons.

Cover each serving of zucchini with marinated mushrooms. Gently toss to mix. Spoon alfredo sauce over each serving. Garnish with a sprinkling of chopped parsley, paprika, and black pepper.

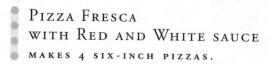

PIZZA FRESCA WITH RED AND WHITE SAUCE
MAKES 4 SIX-INCH PIZZAS.

Fresh flat bread pizza crusts are delectably layered with a creamy white sauce and a savory red sauce for a symphony of flavor and texture.

Pizza Crusts
- 1 cup whole spelt, whole kamut, or spring wheat berries for sprouting (yields 1½ cups)
- 1 clove garlic
- ½ cup flaxseeds
- ½ cup minced red onion
- ½ cup shredded carrot
- ½ cup diced red bell pepper or shredded beet
- ¼ cup chopped basil
- ¼ cup chopped parsley
- 1 teaspoon rosemary
- 1 teaspoon oregano
- 1 tablespoon organic extra-virgin olive oil
- 1 teaspoon sun-dried sea salt, or to taste

White Sauce
- ⅔ cup macadamia nuts
- ½ cup whole raw cashews
- 2 tablespoons pine nuts
- 1 clove garlic
- ⅓ cup lemon juice
- 2 tablespoons organic extra-virgin olive oil
- 3 tablespoons nutritional yeast
- 1 teaspoon sun-dried sea salt, or to taste
- ¼ cup fresh water as necessary

Red Sauce
- ⅔ cup sun-dried tomatoes
- 1¼ cups seeded and diced tomatoes
- ¼ cup chopped basil
- ¼ cup chopped parsley
- 2 teaspoons dried oregano
- 1 teaspoon dried rosemary
- 1 clove garlic
- 2 tablespoons minced red onion

1½ tablespoons apple cider vinegar

1 tablespoon organic extra-virgin
    olive oil

2 teaspoons raw honey or maple
    syrup

1 teaspoon sun-dried sea salt, or
    to taste

Topping

½ cup minced red onion

1 tomato, diced

¼ cup finely shredded carrot

⅓ cup chopped basil

To make the pizza crusts: Sprout spelt, kamut, or wheat berries. In a wide-mouth glass jar covered with screen and secured with a rubber band, soak 1 cup whole spelt, kamut, or soft spring wheat berries in 3 cups fresh water overnight (about 6–12 hours). Drain and rinse. Allow to stand, draining upside down at a 45-degree angle. Rinse and drain two times a day until the sprouting tails are as long as the grain (about 2–4 days).

Grind sprouted grain and garlic. This can be done in a masticating or triturating juicer with the homogenizing "blank" plate (see "Juicing at Home," page 205). They can also be ground in a few batches in the food processor, adding a little fresh water as necessary to blend into a smooth paste.

Soak flaxseeds in 1 cup fresh water for 15 minutes or until saturated. The flaxseeds should absorb most or all of the water. With clean, wet hands, thoroughly mix in a bowl the ground sprouted grain and garlic with the soaked flaxseeds, red onion, carrot, bell pepper or beet, basil, parsley, rosemary, oregano, olive oil, and sea salt.

Press mixture into round ¼-inch-thick flats on nonstick sheets. Dehydrate for 12–20 hours at 108°F or until a dry crust forms. Flip over the flats to dry the underside for 1–2 hours. (Climate, temperature, and humidity all affect dehydrating time.) The flats can be dried to a crisp or left a little moist.

Store in a zip-lock bag in a cool dry place, in the refrigerator, or in the freezer until ready to use.

To make the white sauce: Soak macadamia nuts and cashews together in 2 cups fresh water for 30 minutes. Drain and rinse.

In a food processor, blend macadamia nuts and cashews with pine nuts, garlic, lemon juice, olive oil, nutritional yeast, sea salt, and fresh water, 2 tablespoons at a time, until smooth. The sauce should be thick and smooth. Add a touch more water if necessary to aid in blending. Set aside.

To make the red sauce: Soak sun-dried tomatoes in 1 cup fresh water to soften (5–15 minutes). Drain soak water and set aside.

In a food processor, finely chop diced tomatoes. Do not blend smooth. Set aside. Finely chop the basil, parsley, oregano, rosemary, garlic, and onion. Add sun-dried tomatoes, apple cider vinegar, olive oil, honey or maple syrup, and sea salt, and chop well. Mix in chopped diced tomatoes by hand.

To assemble the pizza: Cut the pizza crusts into 8 pieces. Arrange the pieces in their original shape on a plate. Spread 5–6 tablespoons of the white sauce on the pizza crust. Spread 5–6 tablespoons of the red sauce on the white sauce. Top each pizza with minced red onion, diced tomato, shredded carrot, and chopped basil.

Variation:
For Pesto Pizza with Fresh Tomatoes and Mushrooms, use Walnut Pesto (page 358) and Marinated Mushrooms (page 361) and sliced fresh tomatoes. Top with Pine Nut Parmesan (page 360).

Lotus Manitok
MAKES 2–4 SERVINGS.

Manitok wild rice is a traditional food of the Chippewa Indians. This wild rice dish has a nutty flavor seasoned in a savory marinade. Serve on a bed of field greens or mesclun salad.

2 cups long-grain wild rice for
 sprouting (yields 3 cups)
½ cup chopped green onion
½ cup minced red onion
1 clove garlic, minced
½ cup chopped parsley
¼ cup chopped cilantro
3 tablespoons organic extra-virgin
 olive oil

¼ cup lemon juice
2 tablespoons raw honey or maple
 syrup
3 tablespoons nama shoyu
1½ cups diced tomato
1 avocado, diced

To sprout the long-grain wild rice: Soak long-grain wild rice in 4 cups fresh water in a glass jar with a screen covering, secured by a rubber band, overnight (about 6–12 hours). Drain and rinse. Allow the jar to drain upside down on a 45-degree angle. Rinse and drain two to three times a day until the wild rice is soft and split open (about 2–5 days).

Toss the sprouted wild rice with green onion, red onion, garlic, parsley, cilantro, olive oil, lemon juice, honey or maple syrup, and nama shoyu. Allow to marinate for 20 minutes to 2 hours to marry flavors. Gently toss in tomato and avocado. Serve on a bed of field greens or mesclun salad with a slice of fresh lemon.

AUTUMN WILD RICE
MAKES 4–6 SERVINGS.

This is a feast of texture and flavor, compliments of the autumn harvest. Serve this wild rice with Rosemary Crisps (page 451).

2 cups long-grain wild rice for
  sprouting (yields 3 cups)
2 carrots
2 cloves garlic, minced
1 cup minced red onion
½ cup pitted and chopped dates
1 cup finely sliced fennel root
2 ears fresh corn, cut from the cob
½ cup minced celery
1 cup chopped walnuts
½ cup shelled pistachio nuts or
  pumpkin seeds
½ cup chopped parsley

2 tablespoons oregano
1½ tablespoons coriander seeds
1 tablespoon rosemary
2 teaspoons savory or marjoram
4 tablespoons organic extra-virgin
  olive oil
3 tablespoons apple cider vinegar
2 tablespoons nama shoyu
1 tablespoon red miso
1 tablespoon raw honey or maple
  syrup
Sun-dried sea salt to taste
Fresh black pepper to taste

To sprout the long-grain wild rice: Soak long-grain wild rice in 4 cups fresh water in a glass jar with a screen covering, secured by a rubber band, overnight (about 6–12 hours). Drain and rinse. Allow the jar to drain upside down on a 45-degree angle. Rinse and drain two to three times a day until the wild rice is soft and split open (about 2–5 days).

Peel the carrots. Continue to peel into delicate ribbons to the core. Toss the wild rice with carrot ribbons, garlic, red onion, dates, fennel, corn, celery, walnuts, pistachio nuts or pumpkin seeds, parsley, oregano, coriander, rosemary, and savory or marjoram.

Mix together olive oil, apple cider vinegar, nama shoyu, miso, and raw honey or maple syrup. Mix with wild rice mixture and season to taste with sea salt and pepper.

East-West Long Rice

MAKES 4–6 SERVINGS.

This dish is an integration of dynamic flavors and textures.
Serve on a bed of baby bok choy, tat soi, or delicate greens
with pea shoots or sunflower sprouts.

2 cups long-grain wild rice for
sprouting (yields 3 cups)
1 cucumber
1 carrot
1 cup dry wakame
1 cup chopped green onion
½ cup sesame seeds

Marinated Shiitake Mushrooms

2 cups sliced shiitake mushrooms
2 tablespoons cold-pressed sesame oil
or organic extra-virgin olive oil
2 tablespoons nama shoyu
1 tablespoon umeboshi plum vinegar

Marinade

2 tablespoons white miso
2 tablespoons red miso
¼ cup lemon juice
2 tablespoons cold-pressed sesame oil
or organic extra-virgin olive oil
1½ tablespoons umeboshi plum
paste, or 3 umeboshi plums, pitted
and chopped
1½ tablespoons brown rice syrup or
raw honey
1 tablespoon shredded or finely
minced ginger
1 clove garlic, minced
1 avocado, cubed

To sprout the long-grain wild rice: Soak long-grain wild rice in 4 cups fresh water in a glass jar with a screen covering, secured by a rubber band, overnight (about 6–12 hours). Drain and rinse. Allow the jar to drain upside down on a 45-degree angle. Rinse and drain two to three times a day until the wild rice is soft and split open (about 2–5 days).

Peel the cucumber and cut in half lengthwise. Scoop out the seeds with a spoon. Slice the cucumber into fairly thin cucumber moons. Peel the carrot. Continue to peel the carrot into delicate ribbons to the core. With a pair of kitchen scissors, cut the wakame into pieces. Soak the cut wakame in 1 cup fresh water until soft (about 5–10 minutes). Drain the soak water.

To marinate the mushrooms: Toss shiitake mushrooms with sesame or olive oil, nama shoyu, and umeboshi plum vinegar. Allow to marinate at least 30 minutes to 1 hour. The longer, the better. The mushrooms can be prepared a day in advance and stored in the refrigerator. Pour off the excess marinade before tossing with wild rice.

To make the marinade: In a bowl, mix miso, lemon juice, sesame or olive oil, umeboshi plum paste or umeboshi plums, brown rice syrup or raw honey, ginger, and garlic.

Toss the wild rice with green onion, sesame seeds, cucumber, carrot ribbons, wakame, marinated shiitake mushrooms, and marinade. Gently fold in cubed avocado before serving.

LAYERED NUEVA CORNTILLAS
MAKES 4 SERVINGS.

These crunchy corn tortillas are topped with almond spread,
chunky guacamole, and Papaya-Macadamia-Chipotle Salsa.
Serve with "sour cream" sauce on the side.

Corntillas
1 cup buckwheat
¼ cup almonds
2 ears fresh corn, cut from the cob
1 clove garlic
⅓ cup parsley leaves
⅓ cup cilantro leaves
1 teaspoon coriander seeds
Pinch sun-dried sea salt

Seasoned Almond Spread
1 cup almonds
⅓ cup lemon juice
1 clove garlic
¼ cup minced red onion
2 teaspoons cumin seeds
2 teaspoons coriander seeds
1 teaspoon marjoram or thyme
1 teaspoon paprika
Pinch cayenne pepper
Sun-dried sea salt to taste

Chunky Guacamole
2 avocados
¼ cup lemon juice
1 clove garlic, minced
¼ cup finely chopped parsley
¼ cup chopped cilantro
1 teaspoon sun-dried sea salt, or
   to taste

Papaya-Macadamia-Chipotle Salsa
1 papaya
1 small tomato
¼ cup chopped raw macadamia nuts
2 limes, juiced
1 tablespoon minced fresh ginger
1 clove garlic, finely minced
2–3 green onions, finely chopped
1–2 teaspoons dried chipotle pepper
   or dried chili pepper
¼ cup finely chopped cilantro
Pinch sun-dried sea salt

"Sour Cream" Sauce
- ½ cup whole raw cashews (raw cashew pieces can be used)
- 2 tablespoons pine nuts
- ⅓ cup lemon juice
- 2 tablespoons apple cider vinegar
- Pinch sun-dried sea salt
- ¼ cup chopped mixed parsley and cilantro for garnish

To make the corntillas: Soak buckwheat in 3 cups fresh water overnight (about 6–12 hours). Drain and rinse until the rinse water runs clear. Soak almonds in 1 cup fresh water overnight (about 6–12 hours). Drain and rinse.

Grind the buckwheat, almonds, corn, garlic, parsley, and cilantro. This can be done in a masticating or triturating juicer (see "Juicing at Home," page 205). It can also be done a few batches at a time in a food processor, adding a little fresh water as necessary to blend into a smooth paste.

With clean, wet hands, thoroughly mix in a bowl the ground buckwheat mixture with the coriander and sea salt.

Press mixture into thin, round flats on nonstick sheets. Dehydrate at 108°F for 12–20 hours or until dry. Flip over and dry the underside for an hour or two until crunchy. (Climate, temperature, and humidity all affect dehydrating time.)

Store in a zip-lock bag in a cool dry place, in the refrigerator, or in the freezer until ready to use.

To make the seasoned almond spread: Soak almonds in 2 cups fresh water overnight (about 6–12 hours). Drain and rinse.

In a food processor, chop almonds into a fine meal. Add lemon juice, garlic, red onion, cumin, coriander, marjoram or thyme, paprika, and cayenne pepper and blend into a smooth paste. Season to taste with sea salt. It may be necessary to scrape the sides of the food processor with a rubber spatula and continue to blend until smooth. Add a touch more lemon juice to aid in blending if necessary. The spread should be thick and smooth.

This spread keeps well and can be made a day in advance.

To make the chunky guacamole: Cut the avocados in half. Chop the blade of a chef's knife into the pit of the avocado. Twist the knife to neatly remove the pit. With a paring knife, crosshatch the avocado halves (like a checkerboard). Scoop the avocado into a bowl. Add lemon juice, garlic, parsley, cilantro, and sea salt and mash with a fork. Do not mash to a cream. The guacamole should be slightly chunky.

To make the Papaya-Macadamia-Chipotle Salsa: Cut the papaya in half. Scoop out the seeds with a spoon. With a paring knife, peel the papaya. Finely dice the papaya. Cut the top out of the tomato and finely dice. Mix the diced papaya and tomato with chopped macadamia nuts, lime juice, ginger, garlic, green onions, cilantro, chipotle pepper, and sea salt.

This salsa keeps well and can be made a day in advance.

To make the "sour cream" sauce: Soak cashews in 1 cup fresh water for 30 minutes. Drain and rinse.

In a blender, blend cashews, pine nuts, lemon juice, apple cider vinegar, and sea salt into a smooth cream. It may be necessary to add 2 tablespoons fresh water to aid in blending. The sauce should be thick but pourable.

To layer the corntillas: Spread ¼ cup of almond spread evenly on each corntilla. Top and spread with chunky guacamole. Top with a good amount of salsa. Garnish with chopped fresh herbs. Serve "sour cream" sauce in a dipping bowl on the side.

Serve immediately so corntillas do not get soggy.

INDONESIAN VEGETABLE PAD THAI IN COCONUT SAUCE
MAKES 4–6 SERVINGS.

This dish is a delectable integration of flavor and texture, and the divine coconut sauce completes it. Add a touch more spice for some heat!

Pad Thai Threads
- 4 zucchini
- 4 carrots
- Meat of 1 young coconut (optional)
- 8 tablespoons cold-pressed sesame oil or organic extra-virgin olive oil
- 2 tablespoons oregano
- 2 cloves garlic, minced
- 1 tablespoon shredded or finely minced ginger

Marinated Shiitake Mushrooms and Eggplant
- 3 cups sliced shiitake mushrooms
- 2 cups diced eggplant
- 1 cup minced sweet onion
- 6 tablespoons organic extra-virgin olive oil
- ¼ cup nama shoyu
- ¼ cup lemon juice
- ¼ cup orange juice
- Pinch sun-dried sea salt

Vegetables and Herbs
3 tomatoes
1 sweet onion
1 cucumber
1 red bell pepper
1 cup chopped basil
1 cup chopped cilantro
1 cup chopped parsley
1 avocado, cubed

Coconut Sauce
2½ cups fresh coconut meat
2 tablespoons raw tahini
2 cloves garlic
2 green onions, chopped
2 tablespoons shredded or finely
   minced ginger
4 dates, pitted

¼ cup lemon juice
¼ cup lime juice
¼ cup orange juice
3 tablespoons nama shoyu
2 tablespoons umeboshi plum vinegar
1 tablespoon umeboshi plum paste, or
   2 umeboshi plums, pitted
2 tablespoons white miso
2 tablespoons red miso
2 tablespoons organic extra-virgin
   olive oil
2 tablespoons curry powder
1 tablespoon coriander seeds
1–2 teaspoons chili powder, or to
   taste (optional)
Sun-dried sea salt to taste
⅓ cup chopped cilantro for garnish

To make the pad thai threads: Slice the zucchini and carrots into threads with a Saladacco (see Chapter 12). Alternatively, the zucchini and carrots can be peeled into delicate ribbons with a vegetable peeler. Thinly slice the coconut meat, if desired, into noodle-like strips. Toss the threads gently with sesame oil or olive oil, oregano, garlic, and ginger. Spread threads on dehydrator sheets and dehydrate at 108°F for 8–12 hours until dry but not crispy. The threads can be used marinated and fresh if a dehydrator is not available.

To marinate the shiitake mushrooms and eggplant: Toss mushrooms, eggplant, and onion with olive oil, nama shoyu, lemon juice, orange juice, and sea salt. Allow to marinate for 30 minutes to 1 hour. The longer, the better. The mushrooms can be prepared a day in advance and stored in the refrigerator. Gently squeeze the mushrooms by hand or press through a strainer to wick away excess marinade before tossing with pad thai threads and vegetables.

To prepare the vegetables and herbs: Cut the top out of the tomatoes. Cut each tomato into 12 wedges. Drain the water from the coconut and crack open (see page 199). Cut off the top and bottom of the sweet onion. Cut the onion in half and then into thin slices. Peel the cucumber. Cut in half lengthwise and scoop out the seeds with a spoon. Cut into fairly thin slices. Cut the red bell pepper in half. Remove the stem and seeds and cut into slices. Finely chop the herbs.

Cut the avocado in half. Chop the blade of a chef's knife into the pit of the avocado. Twist the knife to remove the pit neatly. With a paring knife, cut each half into a crosshatch (like a checkerboard) to make neat cubes. Scoop out the cubes.

To make the coconut sauce: In a blender, blend coconut meat, tahini, garlic, green onions, ginger, dates, lemon juice, lime juice, orange juice, nama shoyu, umeboshi plum vinegar, umeboshi plum paste or plums, miso, olive oil, curry powder, coriander, and chili powder (if desired) until smooth. Season to taste with sea salt. The sauce should be thick and smooth but pourable.

Gently toss the pad thai threads with the coconut sauce and the vegetables, marinated mushrooms, eggplant, noodles, and herbs. Garnish with chopped cilantro.

NORI DIM SUM DUMPLINGS WITH CORIANDER CASHEW DIPPING SAUCE
MAKES 18 DUMPLINGS.

Lovely dumplings stuffed with a delectable medley of flavor.
Perfect with Mandarin Ginger Relish (page 373).

2 sheets nori

Olive Melanzana Stuffing
½ cup pitted and chopped black olives
½ cup pitted and chopped green olives
1 cup finely diced eggplant
1 clove garlic, minced
1 tablespoon shredded or finely
   minced ginger
½ cup minced sweet onion
1 tablespoon dried oregano
¼ cup chopped parsley
¼ cup chopped cilantro
2 tablespoons organic extra-virgin
   olive oil

2 tablespoons white miso
1½ tablespoons brown rice vinegar or
   apple cider vinegar
1 tablespoon raw honey or maple syrup
1 tablespoon umeboshi plum paste,
   or 2 umeboshi plums, pitted and
   chopped

Coriander-Cashew Dipping Sauce
½ cup whole raw cashews
2 cloves garlic
1½ teaspoons shredded or finely
   minced ginger
¼ cup chopped cilantro
1 tablespoon coriander seeds

¼ cup lemon juice

1 teaspoon lemon zest

2 tablespoons cold-pressed sesame
  oil or organic extra-virgin
  olive oil

1 tablespoon white miso

1 tablespoon nama shoyu

1 tablespoon apple cider vinegar

2 teaspoons raw honey or maple syrup

2 teaspoons umeboshi plum paste, or
  1 umeboshi plum, pitted

Pinch curry powder (optional)

Cut each nori sheet into nine even pieces.

To make the Olive Melanzana Stuffing: Toss olives and eggplant with garlic, ginger, sweet onion, oregano, parsley, cilantro, olive oil, miso, vinegar, honey or maple syrup, and umeboshi plum paste or umeboshi plums. Allow to marinate for 30 minutes to 1 hour.

To make the Coriander-Cashew Dipping Sauce: Soak cashews in 1 cup fresh water for 30 minutes. Drain and rinse.

In a blender, blend cashews, garlic, ginger, cilantro, coriander seeds, lemon juice, lemon zest, sesame or olive oil, miso, nama shoyu, apple cider vinegar, honey or maple syrup, umeboshi plum paste or plum, and, if desired, curry powder. Add a few tablespoons of fresh water as needed to blend smooth.

To assemble the dumplings: Do one of the following:

1. Place about 2 tablespoons of the olive melanzana stuffing in the center of each piece of nori. Fold two corners together to form a triangle. Wet the edges of the nori to seal.
2. Place about 1½ tablespoons of the olive melanzana stuffing in the center of each piece of nori. Wet the edges of the nori piece. Bring together all four corners to form a packet. Press together the wet edges on each side to seal.

The dumplings can be served "fresh" as is, or dehydrated for 2–4 hours to set and warm.

MANDARIN GINGER RELISH

MAKES I CUP.

A sweet oriental relish, lively with the zest of ginger and tang of umeboshi plums. Tangerines can be substituted if mandarin oranges are not available.

2 mandarin oranges
2 green onions, finely chopped to
    the top
1 tablespoon minced ginger
2 tablespoons sesame seeds

1–2 umeboshi plums, or 1 tablespoon
    umeboshi plum paste
1½ tablespoons umeboshi plum
    vinegar or apple cider vinegar
1 tablespoon white miso

Peel mandarin oranges and remove the seeds and excess white pith. With a sharp serrated knife, carefully cut orange slices into small pieces.

Finely chop green onions and ginger and mix in with sesame seeds.

Chop umeboshi plum well and mix in.

Make a paste with vinegar and miso and gently mix in. Allow to stand for at least 15 minutes to develop flavor.

Stores well.

Layered Vegetable Torta and Quiche

PROVENÇAL TORTA

MAKES 6–8 SERVINGS.

This layered vegetable torta with fresh herbs, vegetables, and marinated mushrooms is married with a savory pâté in this dish.

Vegetable Layer
- 1 large eggplant, or 3 cups finely sliced zucchini
- 2 tomatoes

Marinated Mushrooms
- 4 cups sliced crimini mushrooms
- ¼ cup organic extra-virgin olive oil
- 2 tablespoons nama shoyu
- 1 clove garlic, minced
- ¼ cup lemon juice
- 2 tablespoons dried herbes de Provence or savory herb blend
- Pinch sun-dried sea salt

Provençal Pâté
- 1½ cups almonds
- 1 cup cashews
- 1 clove garlic
- ½ cup chopped green onions
- 1 cup parsley leaves
- ½ cup basil leaves
- 1 tablespoon dried savory or thyme
- 2 teaspoons dried rosemary
- 1 teaspoon fennel seeds
- ½ cup pine nuts
- ¼ cup lemon juice
- 1 teaspoon lemon zest
- 3 tablespoons nama shoyu
- 1 tablespoon raw honey
- ¼ cup nutritional yeast
- Pinch sun-dried sea salt, or to taste

Garnish
- ¼ cup chopped parsley and basil

To prepare the vegetable layer: Peel the eggplant and slice across the seeds into ¼-inch slices. Steam the eggplant slices for a few minutes or just until tender. Alternatively, to avoid steaming, use sliced zucchini. Cut the tops out of the tomatoes. Slice across the seeds and set aside.

To marinate the mushrooms: Toss mushrooms with olive oil, nama shoyu, garlic, lemon juice, dried herbs, and sea salt. Allow to marinate for at least 20–30 minutes until savory and soft. The mushrooms can be marinated a day in advance and stored in the refrigerator.

To make the Provençal Pâté: Soak the almonds in 3 cups fresh water overnight (about 6–12 hours). Drain and rinse. Soak cashews in 1½ cups fresh water for 30 minutes. Drain and rinse.

In a food processor, finely chop garlic, green onions, parsley, basil, savory or thyme, rosemary, and fennel seeds. Add almonds, cashews, and pine nuts and chop into a fine meal. Add lemon juice, lemon zest, nama shoyu, and honey and blend into a smooth pâté. It may be necessary to scrape the sides of the food processor with a rubber spatula and continue to blend for an even, smooth spread. Add nutritional yeast and blend until smooth. Season with sea salt.

To assemble the torta: For best results, use an 8-by-10-inch torte pan with a removable bottom. Alternatively, the torta can be assembled in a traditional pie plate or a casserole dish (or, with confidence, on a platter).

Lay the steamed eggplant slices or zucchini in the bottom of the pan or dish. Spread the Provençal pâté evenly over the eggplant. Squeeze the mushrooms by hand or press through a strainer to remove excess marinade. Spread the mushrooms evenly over the pâté and press down with your palm or the back of a spoon for a firm torta that will serve well. Lay the slices of tomato over the mushrooms. Press the torta down gently so it will set together nicely. Garnish with chopped fresh herbs.

For best results, allow to set in the refrigerator for at least an hour. Cut into pieces and serve with a spatula. This torta can be warmed in the dehydrator, set at 108°F for an hour, or in the oven set on the lowest temperature with the door slightly ajar.

SUN-FIRED TOMATO LASAGNA TERRINE
MAKES 6–8 SERVINGS.

This is an award-winning masterpiece of delectable flavors and texture with delicate zucchini noodles, marinated portobello mushrooms, macadamia nut ricotta, and sun-fired tomato marinara.

Marinated Mushrooms
4 portobello mushrooms
2 cloves garlic
2 green onions
4–6 leaves fresh basil
4–6 tablespoons olive oil
4 tablespoons nama shoyu
2 tablespoons lemon juice or apple cider vinegar
Sun-dried sea salt to taste
Ground fresh black pepper to taste

Zucchini "Noodles"
4 young summer squash (zucchini)
¼ cup lemon juice
½ teaspoon sun-dried sea salt

Macadamia Nut Ricotta
1½ cups macadamia nuts
¼ cup pine nuts
2–4 tablespoons nutritional yeast
1 teaspoon sun-dried sea salt, or to taste
4 tablespoons lemon juice
1 small clove garlic, finely minced
2 tablespoons organic extra-virgin olive oil (optional)
4–6 tablespoons filtered water, as necessary
1 ear sweet white corn (optional, when in season)

Sun-Fired Tomato Marinara
1½ cups sun-dried tomatoes
6 Roma tomatoes, or 4 large tomatoes
1 clove garlic
2–4 green onions, chopped
1 cup fresh basil leaves
½ cup fresh Italian parsley leaves

½ teaspoon chipotle pepper or pinch cayenne pepper (optional)

2 tablespoons dried Italian seasoning, or 1 sprig oregano and rosemary

2 tablespoons organic extra-virgin olive oil (optional)

1 tablespoon raw honey or maple syrup

1 teaspoon apple cider vinegar or lemon juice

Sun-dried sea salt to taste

Ground fresh black pepper to taste

To marinate the mushrooms: Remove stems and wipe mushrooms clean with a dry towel. Cut in half and thinly slice. Mince garlic and green onions. Chiffonade the basil.

In a bowl, toss together mushrooms, garlic, green onions, basil, olive oil, nama shoyu, lemon juice or apple cider vinegar, and sea salt and black pepper to taste. Set aside and allow to marinate for at least 20 minutes to 1 hour. The longer the mushrooms marinate, the more savory the flavor. They can be prepared a day ahead of time and keep well covered in the refrigerator for several days.

To make the zucchini "noodles": Cut the ends off the zucchini and cut in half to make two shorter pieces. Slice as thin as possible lengthwise. This can be done by hand or with a mandoline (see Chapter 12). Marinate zucchini strips with lemon juice and sea salt. Set aside and allow to marinate while preparing the remainder of the dish.

To make the Macadamia Nut Ricotta: Soak 1 cup of the macadamia nuts in 1½ cups fresh water for 20–30 minutes. Drain and rinse. In a food processor, grind soaked macadamia nuts, the remaining ½ cup dry macadamia nuts, and pine nuts into a fine meal. Add nutritional yeast and sea salt, and chop in pulses until well mixed. Set aside a few tablespoons of the nut meal for garnish. Add lemon juice, garlic, and olive oil, adding 2 tablespoons of water at a time as necessary to blend until smooth.

When fresh corn is in season and, if desired, cut the kernels from one fresh ear of corn and fold corn into the ricotta. This adds to the texture and flavor. Set aside. Keep refrigerated to store.

To make the Sun-Fired Tomato Marinara: Soak sun-dried tomatoes in just enough fresh water to cover them until soft (5–15 minutes). Set aside. Cut tomatoes in half and scoop out seeds. Dice tomatoes. Set aside.

In a food processor, finely chop garlic, green onions, and herbs. Add drained sun-dried tomatoes, olive oil, honey or maple syrup, and apple cider vinegar or lemon juice and chop in pulses. Do not blend smooth; leave a touch of texture.

In a bowl, fold together sun-dried tomato mixture with diced tomatoes. Season with sea salt and pepper to taste. Set aside.

To assemble the lasagna: Drain marinating zucchini slices and gently squeeze or blot with a clean towel. Neatly arrange on a serving platter or in a casserole dish. Spread macadamia nut ricotta evenly over the zucchini "noodles." Squeeze mushrooms by hand or press through a strainer to wick away excess marinade for a well-set lasagna. Save the marinade for other recipes, if desired. Arrange mushrooms evenly and gently press into the ricotta. Gently press the marinara through a strainer to remove excess juice. Save juice for other uses, if desired. Spoon marinara over mushrooms and smooth out. Garnish with nut meal.

Allow to stand 30 minutes to marry flavors. The flavor improves with time and can stand up to 1 day before serving. Keeps well.

MEDITERRANEAN PESTO TORTA
MAKES 6–8 SERVINGS.

*This layered fresh torta has its delicious ingredients in all of the
right places. It is excellent served with a Caesar salad.*

Marinated Onions
- 1 red onion
- 2 tablespoons organic extra-virgin olive oil
- 1 tablespoon nama shoyu
- 1 tablespoon apple cider vinegar
- Pinch sun-dried sea salt

Pesto-Olive Tapenade
- 2 cups walnuts
- 2 cups fresh basil leaves
- 1 cup parsley leaves
- 2 cloves garlic
- ½ cup pine nuts
- ½ cup pitted black olives
- ½ cup pitted green olives
- 2 tablespoons organic extra-virgin olive oil
- 1 tablespoon apple cider vinegar
- 2 tablespoons white miso
- 2 tablespoons nutritional yeast
- Pinch sun-dried sea salt
- 4 cups sliced zucchini
- 1½ cups chopped artichoke hearts
- 2 tomatoes, sliced across the seeds
- ¼ cup chopped herbs (basil, parsley, cilantro) for garnish

To marinate the onions: Thinly slice onion. Marinate with olive oil, nama shoyu, apple cider vinegar, and sea salt. Allow to stand for 20 minutes until savory and softened.

To make the pesto olive tapenade: Soak walnuts in 3 cups fresh water for 1 hour. Drain and rinse.

In a food processor, finely chop basil, parsley, and garlic. Add walnuts and pine nuts and chop into a fine meal. Add olives, olive oil, apple cider vinegar, and miso and blend until smooth. It may be necessary to scrape the sides of the food processor with a rubber spatula and continue to blend until smooth. Add nutritional yeast and blend until smoth. Season with sea salt. In a bowl, fold the zucchini slices into the tapenade.

To assemble the torta: Press the pesto olive tapenade mixture into the bottom of a pie or torte pan or a casserole dish. Alternatively, press the mixture into a circle or square on a platter. Spread the artichoke hearts evenly over the tapenade. Layer the tomato slices on top of the artichoke hearts and gently press.

Drain the marinade from the onions. The marinade can be saved for other recipes, if desired. Layer the marinated onions on the tomatoes. Garnish with chopped herbs.

Allow torta to set for at least an hour in the refrigerator to set and serve well. Slice and serve with a spatula. It keeps fresh for several days, and the flavors are more mature the day after it is prepared.

PORTOBELLO MUSHROOM AND SPINACH QUICHE
MAKES 6–8 SERVINGS.

Meaty portobello mushrooms and fresh spinach combine to make a delicious seasoned filling, wrapped in a savory walnut buckwheat crust.

Walnut Buckwheat Crust
¾ cup whole buckwheat groats
2 cloves garlic
½ cup chopped red onion
½ cup chopped parsley
1 cup chopped carrot
1 cup chopped celery
½ cup walnuts
1 tablespoon ground coriander seeds
1 teaspoon sun-dried sea salt

Portobello Mushrooms
2 portobello mushrooms
3 tablespoons organic extra-virgin olive oil
2 tablespoons nama shoyu
2 cloves garlic, finely minced

Filling
½ cup whole cashews
¼ cup pine nuts

¼ cup lemon juice

2 tablespoons olive oil

2 tablespoons nama shoyu

3 tablespoons nutritional yeast

Pinch sun-dried sea salt

3 cups chopped spinach or baby
  spinach

½ cup chopped basil

To make the walnut buckwheat crust: Soak whole buckwheat groats in 2 cups fresh water for 2–8 hours. Drain and rinse in a colander or strainer until the water runs clear. It may be necessary to rinse several times until rinse water runs clear.

In a food processor, finely chop garlic, red onion, and parsley. Add carrot and celery and finely chop. Add walnuts and finely chop. Add drained buckwheat, coriander seeds, and sea salt and chop until well mixed. Press evenly into a pie plate. Dehydrate at 108°F for 12–20 hours or until a crust forms.

To prepare the portobello mushrooms: Remove the stems of the mushrooms. Cut in half and then into thin slices. Toss with olive oil, nama shoyu, and garlic and allow to marinate for at least 30 minutes or until savory and soft. The mushrooms can be marinated a day in advance and stored in the refrigerator; their flavor will only improve with time.

To make the filling: Soak cashews in 1 cup fresh water for 30 minutes. Drain and rinse.

In a food processor, grind drained cashews and pine nuts into a fine meal. Add lemon juice, olive oil, and nama shoyu and blend until smooth. Add nutritional yeast and sea salt and blend until well mixed.

Squeeze the mushrooms by hand or press through a strainer to wick away excess marinade. Save the marinade to use for other recipes, if desired. Fold in spinach, basil, and marinated mushrooms with cashew filling.

To assemble the quiche: Press the mixture firmly into walnut buckwheat crust and smooth with the back of a spoon or a rubber spatula.

Serves best after setting for an hour in the refrigerator. Keeps fresh for several days.

SUMMER CORN AND BROCCOLI QUICHE
MAKES 6–8 SERVINGS.

This truly delicious quiche is made with fresh sweet corn, herbs, broccoli, fresh seed cheese, and a savory almond corn crust.

Almond-Corn Crust
1¼ cups almonds
1 ear fresh corn, cut from the cob
½ cup minced celery
½ cup chopped carrot
1 cup parsley leaves
1 cup cilantro leaves
1 tablespoon coriander seeds
1 teaspoon sun-dried sea salt

Filling
1 cup chopped broccoli florets (The broccoli can be steamed lightly and then marinated.)

1 clove garlic, minced
¼ cup lemon juice
2 tablespoons organic extra-virgin olive oil
3 tablespoons nama shoyu
2½ cups Basic Seed Cheese (page 311–312), or 2½ cups sunflower seeds
½ cup chopped green onion
1 cup chopped parsley leaves
1 cup chopped cilantro leaves
2 ears fresh corn, cut from the cob
4 tablespoons nutritional yeast
Pinch sun-dried sea salt, or to taste

To make the almond-corn crust: Soak almonds in 2 cups fresh water overnight (about 6–12 hours). Drain and rinse.

In a food processor, chop almonds into a fine meal. Add corn and chop until well mixed. Set aside. Finely chop celery, carrots, parsley, and cilantro. Add almond-corn mixture, coriander seeds, and sea salt, and blend until as smooth as possible. It may be necessary to scrape the sides of the food processor with a rubber spatula and continue to blend for a smooth consistency.

Press the almond-corn dough evenly into a 10-inch pie plate. Dehydrate at 108°F for 12–20 hours or until a crust forms.

To make the filling: Toss the chopped broccoli with garlic, lemon juice, olive oil, and nama shoyu. Allow to marinate for at least an hour. This can be done several hours in advance or the day before (when preparing the crust) and stored in the refrigerator. Reserve marinade for later use. If soaked sunflower seeds are substituting for Basic Seed Cheese, soak sunflower seeds in 3 cups fresh water for 4–6 hours. Drain and rinse.

In a food processor, finely chop green onion, parsley, and cilantro. Add Basic Seed Cheese or sunflower seeds. Blend until well mixed. Drain the marinade from the broccoli directly into the food processor with the herbs and cheese or sunflower seeds. Add ½ cup of the fresh corn and blend until smooth. It may be necessary to scrape the sides of the food processor with a rubber spatula and continue to blend until smooth.

In a bowl, mix seed cheese or sunflower seed filling with nutritional yeast, broccoli, and remaining fresh corn. Season with sea salt.

Press the filling into the pie crust and smooth with a rubber spatula.

This quiche serves well right away or after being chilled for an hour. Keeps fresh for several days. Serves beautifully with wedges of fresh tomato.

NEW SHEPHERD'S PIE
MAKES 6–8 SERVINGS.

This New Shepherd's Pie is perfect for a hearty appetite. Steamed cauliflower replaces white potatoes for newfound nutrition. Serve warm for an authentic experience.

Mushroom Layer
- 3 cups sliced crimini mushrooms
- 3 tablespoons organic extra-virgin olive oil
- 2 tablespoons nama shoyu
- 1 clove garlic, minced
- 2 cups shredded carrot
- 1 cup minced celery
- ½ cup minced red onion
- ½ cup chopped parsley
- 1 ear fresh corn, cut from the cob (optional)

Cauliflower Layer
- 2 cups chopped cauliflower
- 1 cup whole raw cashews
- 1 cup peeled and chopped zucchini
- 3 tablespoons organic extra-virgin olive oil
- 2 tablespoons white miso
- 1 clove garlic
- 2 teaspoons rosemary
- Pinch sun-dried sea salt, or to taste

Pinch paprika and fresh black pepper for garnish

To make the mushroom layer: Toss crimini mushrooms with olive oil, nama shoyu, and garlic. Allow to marinate for at least 30 minutes or until savory and soft. The longer, the better. The mushrooms can be marinated a day in advance and stored in the refrigerator.

Mix the marinated mushrooms with carrot, celery, red onion, and parsley. Add fresh corn if available for a sweet crunchy texture.

To make the cauliflower layer: Steam the cauliflower for a few minutes or until soft enough for a fork to pierce. Set aside. Soak cashews in 2 cups fresh water for 1 hour. Drain and rinse. Set aside.

In a food processor, chop cashews into a fine meal. Add cauliflower, zucchini, olive oil, miso, garlic, rosemary, and sea salt and blend until smooth. It may be necessary to scrape the sides of the food processor with a rubber spatula and continue to blend until smooth.

To assemble the pie: Evenly spread the mushroom mixture in the bottom of a 6-by-6-inch or 6-by-8-inch casserole dish. Smooth out with a rubber spatula. Spread the blended cauliflower-zucchini mixture evenly over the vegetables. Smooth with a rubber spatula. Sprinkle with paprika and fresh black pepper for garnish.

Warm in the dehydrator at 108°F for 1–2 hours, or in the oven, set on the lowest temperature with the door slightly ajar, for 30 minutes to 1 hour.

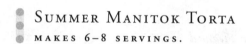

SUMMER MANITOK TORTA
MAKES 6–8 SERVINGS.

*In this torta, fresh summer tomatoes, pea molé, herbs, and avocado
are layered in a nutty wild rice crust. It's great with a crunchy
salad and Sweet and Spicy Tomato Cucumber Relish (page 383).*

Wild Rice Crust
   1½ cups long-grain wild rice for
      sprouting (yields 2½ cups)
   1 clove garlic
   ½ cup green onion
   1 cup parsley leaves
   1 cup cilantro leaves
   2 tablespoons nama shoyu
   2 soft dates, pitted
   Pinch sun-dried sea salt

Pea Molé
   1½ cups cilantro leaves
   2 cups peas, fresh or frozen and
      thawed
   1 tablespoon lemon zest
   3 tablespoons lemon juice
   1 teaspoon black pepper, or to taste
   ½ teaspoon sun-dried sea salt, or to
      taste

   1 avocado
   3 tomatoes
   ¼ cup chopped parsley and cilantro,
      for garnish

SWEET AND SPICY TOMATO CUCUMBER RELISH

MAKES 2 CUPS.

Sweet with ripe tomatoes and a dab of honey, and spicy with
fresh mustard seeds. Allow to stand for an hour or more
to let the flavors mature.

2 Roma tomatoes

1 cucumber

1 clove garlic

2 green onions, finely chopped

1 tablespoon raw honey or maple
   syrup

1 tablespoon apple cider vinegar

1 tablespoon ground mustard seeds

2 teaspoons ground cumin seeds

Pinch cayenne pepper

¼ teaspoon sun-dried sea salt

Fresh black pepper to taste

Cut tomatoes in half and remove seeds. Dice into small pieces. Peel cucumber. Scoop the
seeds out with a spoon and mince the cucumber into small pieces. Finely mince garlic and
onion and mix in with honey or maple syrup, vinegar, mustard seeds, cumin seeds, cayenne,
sea salt, and pepper to taste.

Allow to stand at least 20 minutes to develop flavor. Keeps well.

To make the wild rice crust: Sprout long-grain wild rice. Soak wild rice in 3 cups fresh water for
8–12 hours. Drain and rinse two to three times a day until the rice is soft and split (about 2–5
days).

In a food processor, finely chop garlic, green onion, parsley, and cilantro. Add sprouted wild
rice, nama shoyu, dates, and sea salt, and finely chop. Press evenly into a 10-inch pie plate.

Dehydrate at 108°F for 12 hours or until a crust forms. Alternatively, dry the crust in the
oven, set at the lowest temperature with the door slightly ajar for 4–8 hours or until a crust has
formed. This crust can be used without dehydrating for a moister texture.

To make the pea molé: In a food processor, finely chop cilantro. Add peas, lemon zest, and
lemon juice and chop in pulses until well mixed but not smooth. Season with black pepper and
sea salt.

To assemble the torta: Cut the avocado in half. For neat slices, chop the blade of a chef's knife into the pit. Twist the knife to neatly extract the pit. Slice the avocado while still in its skin. Scoop the slices out or peel away the skin. Lay the avocado in the bottom of the wild rice crust. Press the avocado with a rubber spatula or the back of the spoon for an even layer.

Spread the pea mole evenly over the avocado slices. Cut the tops out of the tomatoes. Slice the tomatoes across the seeds. Arrange the tomato slices over the pea mole. Cut a few of the slices in half and place the halves around the perimeter of the crust for a nice presentation. Sprinkle with chopped herbs for garnish.

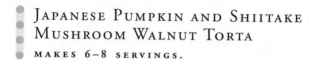

JAPANESE PUMPKIN AND SHIITAKE MUSHROOM WALNUT TORTA
MAKES 6–8 SERVINGS.

A gorgeous layered torta with butternut squash, a savory walnut
tapenade, marinated shiitake mushrooms, and fresh corn.
Delicious served with Apricot Ginger Chutney (page 385).

Marinated Mushrooms
- 3 cups thinly sliced shiitake mushrooms
- 3 tablespoons organic extra-virgin olive oil
- 3 tablespoons nama shoyu
- 2 tablespoons shredded or finely minced ginger

- ½ cup parsley leaves
- 2 tablespoons red miso
- 1 tablespoon organic extra-virgin olive oil
- 1 tablespoon apple cider vinegar
- 2 teaspoons raw honey or maple syrup
- Pinch sun-dried sea salt, or to taste

Walnut Tapenade
- 2 cups walnuts
- 1 clove garlic
- ½ cup chopped red onion
- ½ cup basil leaves

- 1 kabocha squash (1 kuri squash or butternut squash if kabocha is unavailable)
- 2 ears fresh corn, cut from the cob (optional)

To marinate the mushrooms: Toss mushrooms with olive oil, nama shoyu, and ginger. Allow to marinate for at least 30 minutes or until soft and savory. The longer, the better. The mushrooms can be marinated the day before and stored in the refrigerator.

APRICOT GINGER CHUTNEY

MAKES 1 CUP.

A refreshing sweet chutney spiced with ginger and fennel seeds.
Great as a condiment served with hot and spicy dishes or
as a complement to salsa.

1 cup diced apricots
1 tablespoon minced fresh ginger
2 teaspoons fennel seed
Pinch sun-dried sea salt

In a small bowl, mix ingredients together. Allow to stand for at least 10 minutes to develop
flavor.

To make the walnut tapenade: Soak walnuts in 3 cups fresh water for 1–2 hours. Drain and rinse.

In a food processor, finely chop garlic, red onion, basil, and parsley. Add walnuts and chop into a fine meal. Add miso, olive oil, apple cider vinegar, and honey or maple syrup and blend until well mixed but not entirely smooth. Season with sea salt.

To prepare the kabocha squash: Peel the squash and slice into ¼-inch pieces. Steam the squash until a fork can easily pierce the slices (about 4–8 minutes).

To assemble the torta: Layer steamed squash in a casserole dish, on a pie plate, or on a platter. Press together with the back of a fork or with clean fingers. Spread the walnut tapenade evenly over the squash. If using corn, spread the corn evenly over the tapenade and press in gently with clean fingers or a rubber spatula.

Squeeze the mushrooms by hand or through a strainer to wick away excess marinade. Spread the mushrooms evenly over the tapenade and corn. Smooth or press the mushrooms with a rubber spatula or clean fingers.

The torta can be served warm from a dehydrator set at 108°F for an hour or in an oven set at the lowest temperature with the door slightly ajar for 30 minutes to an hour. Keeps well in the refrigerator for several days.

Winter Wild Rice Quiche
MAKES 6–8 SERVINGS.

*This hearty nutty quiche with sprouted long-grain wild rice
and winter squash is perfect for a winter's day.*

Wild Rice Crust
1½ cups long-grain wild rice for
    sprouting (yields 2 cups)
½ cup chopped carrot
½ cup minced celery
1 clove garlic
1 tablespoon dried oregano
2 teaspoons dried rosemary
1 teaspoon celery seeds
1 teaspoon sun-dried sea salt

Squash and Beet
1 medium beet
½ cup finely sliced fennel
2 cups peeled and sliced butternut or
    delicata squash
1 cup sliced leeks
1 clove garlic, minced
1 tablespoon shredded or finely
    minced ginger
½ cup minced red onion
2 tablespoons organic extra-virgin
    olive oil
1 tablespoon nama shoyu

2 tablespoons raw honey or maple
    syrup
½ teaspoon black pepper

Pumpkin Seed Topping
1½ cups pumpkin seeds
1 tablespoon shredded or finely
    minced ginger
1 clove garlic
½ cup parsley leaves
3 tablespoons hulled hemp seeds, or
    2 tablespoons raw tahini
2 tablespoons white miso
1 teaspoon raw honey or maple syrup
2 teaspoons savory or marjoram
2 teaspoons coriander seeds
Pinch chipotle pepper or chili pepper
Pinch sun-dried sea salt

Garnish
3 tablespoons dry pumpkin seeds
    (optional)
¼ cup chopped parsley (optional)
¼ cup pomegranate seeds (optional)

To make the wild rice crust: Sprout long-grain wild rice. Soak wild rice in 3 cups fresh water for 8–12 hours. Drain and rinse two to three times a day until rice is split open and soft (about 2–5 days).

In a food processor, finely chop carrot, celery, garlic, oregano, rosemary, and celery seeds. Add sprouted wild rice and sea salt, and finely chop. It may be necessary to scrape the sides of the food processor with a rubber spatula and continue to chop for a thorough consistency. Press the wild rice mixture evenly into a 10-inch pie plate.

Dehydrate at 108°F for 12 hours or until a crust has formed. Alternatively, dry the crust in the oven, set at the lowest temperature with the door slightly ajar for 4–8 hours or until a crust has formed. This crust can be used without dehydrating for a moister texture.

To prepare the squash and beet: Peel the beet and thinly slice. Steam the beet slices for a few minutes or until a fork can easily pierce the slices. Lay the beet slices in the bottom of the prepared wild rice crust. Layer sliced fennel on top of the sliced beet.

Steam the squash and leeks for a few minutes or until a fork can easily pierce the squash slices. Set aside.

In a bowl, mix garlic, ginger, red onion, olive oil, nama shoyu, honey or maple syrup, and black pepper. Gently toss the steamed squash and leeks with this marinade. Layer the squash slices and leeks on the beet and fennel. Press down to form a nice layer with clean fingers or a rubber spatula.

To make the pumpkin seed topping: Soak pumpkin seeds in 2 cups fresh water for 2–4 hours. Drain and rinse. Lay seeds out on a dry towel and blot dry or allow to air-dry for a good consistency.

In a food processor, finely chop ginger, garlic, and parsley. Add pumpkin seeds and chop into a fine meal. Add hemp seeds or tahini, miso, honey or maple syrup, savory or marjoram, and coriander seeds. Chop until well mixed. This mixture should have a crumbly texture and not be entirely smooth. Season with chipotle pepper or chili pepper and sea salt. Spread the pumpkin seed mixture over the squash. Garnish, if desired, with pumpkin seeds, parsley, and pomegranate seeds.

This quiche is delicious served warm. Warm in the dehydrator at 108°F for an hour or in the oven, set at the lowest temperature with the door slightly ajar, for 30 minutes to 1 hour.

NEW CHICK PEA SPANAKOPITA
MAKES 6–8 SERVINGS.

This savory seasoned spanakopita is made with a crunchy chick pea crust and fresh layers of spinach, tomato, red bell pepper, zucchini, herbs, and avocado.

Chick Pea Crust
1¾ cups chick peas (garbanzo beans)
    for sprouting (yields 2½ cups)
2 cloves garlic
1 cup parsley leaves
3 tablespoons raw tahini
¼ cup lemon juice
2 teaspoons lemon zest
1 teaspoon sun-dried sea salt, or
    to taste

Vegetable Layers
4 cups chopped spinach
1 medium zucchini, thinly sliced
½ cup chopped basil
½ cup chopped parsley
½ cup chopped cilantro
2 teaspoons oregano
¼ cup organic extra-virgin olive oil

3 tablespoons lemon juice
Pinch sun-dried sea salt
2 avocados
3–4 tomatoes, sliced

Lemon Tahini Sauce
¼ cup raw tahini
½ cup lemon juice
Juice of 1 orange
2 teaspoons lemon zest
1 clove garlic
2 tablespoons nama shoyu
1 soft date, pitted
Pinch sun-dried sea salt, or to taste

Garnish
¼ cup chopped black olives
    (optional)
2 tablespoons sesame seeds (optional)

To make the chick pea crust: Sprout the chick peas. In a glass jar, covered with screen or mesh secured by a rubber band, soak chick peas in 3 cups fresh water overnight (about 6–12 hours). Drain and rinse two times a day until the sprouted tails are as long as the bean (about 2–3 days).

In a food processor, finely chop garlic and parsley. Add sprouted chick peas, tahini, lemon juice, and lemon zest and blend until smooth. It may be necessary to scrape the sides of the food processor with a rubber spatula and continue to blend until smooth. Season with sea salt. Press the chick pea mixture into a 10-inch pie plate or, alternatively, press the mixture into a 10-inch round, flat patty on a platter. Dehydrate at 108°F for 12–20 hours or until the crust has a crunchy texture.

To prepare the vegetable layers: Toss together the spinach, zucchini, fresh herbs (set aside a pinch or two for garnish), oregano, olive oil, lemon juice, and sea salt. Evenly distribute the spinach-zucchini mixture in the bottom of the crust or spread evenly over the flat crust.

Cut the avocados in half. Chop the blade of a chef's knife into the pits of the avocados and twist to neatly remove the pits. Cut the avocados into slices while still in the skin. Scoop out the slices or peel away the skin. Layer the avocado slices evenly over the spinach-zucchini mixture. Press the avocado slices with a rubber spatula or clean fingers to form a neat layer.

Cut out the tops of the tomatoes. Slice across the seeds. Layer the tomato slices on the avocados.

Garnish, if desired, with chopped olives, sesame seeds, and reserved fresh chopped herbs.

To make the lemon tahini sauce: Blend tahini, lemon juice, orange juice, lemon zest, garlic, nama shoyu, and date until smooth. Season with sea salt. This sauce should be thick but pourable. Add a few tablespoons of fresh water only if necessary to blend to desired consistency. Serve sauce in a small cup or a dipping bowl with a small spoon.

28

Burgers and Patties

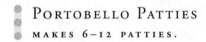

Portobello Patties
MAKES 6–12 PATTIES.

These savory patties are made from portobello mushrooms and just the right amount and type of seasoning. Serve with a salad or as an open-faced sandwich with avocado and tomato.

2 cups walnuts
4 cups chopped portobello
   mushrooms or crimini mushrooms
3 tablespoons organic extra-virgin
   olive oil
3 tablespoons nama shoyu
1 tablespoon apple cider vinegar
2 cloves garlic
1 cup chopped red onion

½ cup chopped basil
½ cup chopped parsley
1 tablespoon dried oregano
2 cups chopped zucchini
½ cup chopped celery
2 tablespoons nutritional yeast
   (optional)
1–2 teaspoons sun-dried sea salt

Soak walnuts in 4 cups fresh water for 2–4 hours. Drain and rinse.

Chop portobello mushrooms. Toss with olive oil, nama shoyu, and apple cider vinegar. Allow to marinate at least 30 minutes. The mushrooms can be marinated a day in advance and stored in the refrigerator.

In a food processor, finely chop garlic, onion, basil, parsley, and oregano. Add soaked walnuts, chopped zucchini, and celery, and chop finely. It may be necessary to scrape the sides of the food processor with a rubber spatula and continue to chop for a smooth consistency. Drain off the marinade from the mushrooms. Add marinated mushrooms and chop in a few pulses to mix, but do not blend smooth. There should be a savory texture to the mixture. Add nutritional yeast, if desired, and season with sea salt.

Form patties out of ½ cup to 1 cup of mixture. Place patties on nonstick sheets or plastic wrap. Dehydrate at 108°F for 12–20 hours or until a crust has formed. Flip over the patties and return to the dehydrator without the nonstick sheets or plastic wrap to dry the underside for an hour or two. (Climate, temperature, and humidity all affect dehydrating time.) Alternatively, the patties can be dried on a cookie sheet or in a casserole dish in the oven set at the lowest temperature for 4–6 hours until a crust forms. Flip the patties over for an hour to dry the underside. Leave the door slightly ajar if necessary to regulate the temperature.

The patties are best with a crust on the outside and moist inside for savory texture. The patties can also be dried thoroughly for longer storage and spritzed with fresh water to moisten before serving.

Store in a resealable bag or a covered container in the refrigerator.

ALMOND BURGERS
MAKES 4–8 BURGERS.

Fresh almond burgers have a great texture and taste. Serve with a salad or as an open-faced sandwich with Sweet Pickle Relish (page 392).

2 cups almonds	2 tablespoons white miso
4 green onions	2 tablespoons nama shoyu
1 clove garlic	1 tablespoon maple syrup or raw
1 tablespoon chopped ginger	honey
2 cups chopped carrot	

Sweet Pickle Relish
MAKES 1 CUP.

*A sweet and tangy relish reminiscent of the days of old. The
flavors develop after sitting overnight or for several hours.*

1 cucumber
3 tablespoons apple cider vinegar
2 tablespoons raw honey or
   organic evaporated cane juice

2 teaspoons whole coriander seeds
1 teaspoon sun-dried sea salt

Peel cucumber, cut in half, and scoop out the seeds with a spoon. Finely dice cucumber. Mix
in apple cider vinegar, honey or evaporated cane juice, whole coriander seeds, and sea salt.
Allow to stand 4-6 hours or overnight to marry the flavors.

Soak almonds in 4 cups fresh water overnight (about 6–12 hours). Drain and rinse.

In a food processor, finely chop green onion, garlic, ginger, and carrot. Add soaked almonds, miso, nama shoyu, and maple syrup or honey and finely chop. It may be necessary to
scrape the sides of the food processor with a rubber spatula and continue to chop for a thorough consistency. The mixture should be moist and well ground.

Form patties out of ½ cup to 1 cup of mixture. Place patties on nonstick sheets. Dehydrate
at 108°F for 12–20 hours or until a crust has formed. Flip over the patties and return to the
dehydrator without the nonstick sheets to dry the underside for an hour or two. (Climate, temperature, and humidity all affect dehydrating time.) Alternatively, the patties can be dried on a
cookie sheet or in a casserole dish in the oven set at the lowest temperature for 4–6 hours until a crust forms. Flip the patties over for an hour to dry the underside. Leave the door slightly
ajar if necessary to regulate the temperature.

The patties are best with a crust on the outside and moist inside. The patties can also be
dried thoroughly for longer storage and spritzed with fresh water to moisten before serving.

Store in a zip-lock bag or a covered container in the refrigerator.

SUN AND MOON BURGERS

MAKES 12–18 BURGERS.

These savory, moist burgers are balanced with all the right flavors. Serve topped with Tomatillo Sweet Pepper Relish (page 394).

2 cups sunflower seeds
1 cup flaxseeds
2 cloves garlic
4 green onions
1 cup parsley leaves
1 cup cilantro leaves
2 ears fresh corn, cut from the cob
2 stalks celery, chopped
1 carrot, chopped

1 cup whole dulse leaves, or ⅓ cup dulse flakes
4 dates, pitted
1 tablespoon coriander seeds
1 tablespoon fennel seeds
2 tablespoons white miso
¼ cup nutritional yeast
Pinch cayenne pepper
Pinch sun-dried sea salt

Soak sunflower seeds in 3 cups fresh water for 2–4 hours. Drain and rinse. Soak flaxseeds in 2 cups fresh water for 15–20 minutes or until saturated. The flaxseeds will absorb most or all of the water.

In a food processor, finely chop garlic, green onions, parsley, and cilantro. Add corn, celery, carrot, dulse, dates, coriander seeds, and fennel seeds, and chop well. Add sunflower seeds, flaxseeds, and miso, and chop well. Add nutritional yeast, cayenne pepper, and sea salt.

Form patties out of ½ cup to 1 cup of mixture. Place patties on nonstick sheets. Dehydrate at 108°F for 12–20 hours or until a crust has formed. Flip over the patties and return to the dehydrator without the nonstick sheets to dry the underside for an hour or two. (Climate, temperature, and humidity all affect dehydrating time.) Alternatively, the burgers can be dried on a cookie sheet or in a casserole dish in the oven set at the lowest temperature for 4–6 hours until a crust forms. Flip the patties over for an hour to dry the underside. Leave the door slightly ajar if necessary to regulate the temperature.

The patties are best with a crust on the outside and moist inside. The patties can also be dried thoroughly for longer storage and spritzed with fresh water to moisten before serving.

Store in a zip-lock bag or a covered container in the refrigerator.

Tomatillo Sweet Pepper Relish
MAKES 2 CUPS.

Tomatillos are a sweet and tangy nightshade fruit that look like small, firm green tomatoes. They go beautifully here with sweet bell peppers, capers, and green olives.

6 tomatillos
1 small yellow bell pepper, minced
   (Red bell pepper may be
   substituted.)
3 tablespoons pitted green olives
3 tablespoons capers
1 clove garlic, finely minced

1 tablespoon apple cider vinegar
2 teaspoons raw honey or agave
   syrup
2 tablespoons nama shoyu
2 teaspoons ground cumin seeds
½ teaspoon dried chipotle pepper
Fresh black pepper to taste

Dice tomatillos. Remove stem and seeds from the yellow pepper and finely mince. Finely chop olives and mix in with capers. Finely mince garlic and mix in with vinegar, honey or agave syrup, and nama shoyu. Season with cumin seeds, chipotle peppers, and black pepper to taste. Allow to stand for at least 15 minutes to develop flavor. Keeps well.

Shiitake Mushroom Burgers
MAKES 8–12 BURGERS.

*Succulent shiitake mushrooms complete these burgers.
Serve with a salad.*

1 cup almonds
1 cup pumpkin seeds
4 cups chopped shiitake mushrooms
3 tablespoons organic extra-virgin
   olive oil
2 tablespoons nama shoyu
1 tablespoon umeboshi plum vinegar

4 green onions
1 clove garlic
1 cup parsley leaves
2 cups chopped eggplant
1 tablespoon ground coriander seeds
Sun-dried sea salt to taste

Soak the almonds and pumpkin seeds together in 4 cups fresh water overnight (about 6–12 hours). Drain and rinse.

Toss mushrooms with olive oil, nama shoyu, and umeboshi plum vinegar. Allow to marinate for 30 minutes to an hour or until savory and soft. The mushrooms can be marinated a day in advance and stored in the refrigerator.

In a food processor, finely chop green onions, garlic, parsley, and eggplant. Add drained almonds, pumpkin seeds, and coriander seeds, and finely chop. Add a few tablespoons of the excess marinade from the mushrooms and scrape the sides of the food processor with a rubber spatula for a thorough consistency. Drain the excess marinade from the mushrooms. Add the mushrooms and chop in a few pulses to mix. The mixture should not be blended smooth and should have some texture. Season with sea salt to taste.

Form patties out of ½ cup to 1 cup of mixture. Place patties on nonstick sheets on dehydrator trays. Dehydrate at 108°F for 12–20 hours or until a crust has formed. Flip over the patties and return to the dehydrator without the nonstick sheets to dry the underside for an hour or two. (Climate, temperature, and humidity all affect dehydrating time.) Alternatively, the patties can be dried on a cookie sheet or in a casserole dish in the oven set at the lowest temperature for 4–6 hours until a crust forms. Flip the patties over for an hour to dry the underside. Leave the door slightly ajar if necessary to regulate the temperature.

The patties are best with a crust on the outside and moist inside. The patties can also be dried thoroughly for longer storage and spritzed with fresh water to moisten before serving.

Store in a zip-lock bag or a covered container in the refrigerator.

Lower East Side Patties
MAKES 4–8 PATTIES.

Authentic New York Lower East Side flavorings—garlic, oregano, fennel seeds, and black pepper—deck these patties.

1 cup sunflower seeds
1 cup pumpkin seeds
2 cups broccoli
1 cup chopped red onion
1 clove garlic
1 cup parsley leaves
1½ tablespoons dried oregano

1½ tablespoons fennel seeds
2 teaspoons black pepper
¼ cup lemon juice
2 tablespoons organic extra-virgin
  olive oil
1–2 teaspoons sun-dried sea salt, or to
  taste

Soak sunflower seeds and pumpkin seeds together in 4 cups fresh water for 2–4 hours. Drain and rinse.

In a food processor, finely chop broccoli, onion, garlic, parsley, oregano, and fennel seeds. Add drained sunflower and pumpkin seeds, black pepper, lemon juice, and olive oil and blend until smooth. It may be necessary to scrape the sides of the food processor with a rubber spatula and continue to blend for a smooth consistency. Season with sea salt.

Form patties out of ½ cup to 1 cup of mixture. Place patties on nonstick sheets. Dehydrate at 108°F for 12–20 hours or until a crust has formed. Flip over the patties and return to the dehydrator without the nonstick sheets to dry the underside for an hour or two. (Climate, temperature, and humidity all affect dehydrating time.) Alternatively, the patties can be dried on a cookie sheet or in a casserole dish in the oven set at the lowest temperature for 4–6 hours until a crust forms. Flip the patties over for an hour to dry the underside. Leave the door slightly ajar if necessary to regulate the temperature.

The patties are best with a crust on the outside and moist inside. The patties can also be dried thoroughly for longer storage and spritzed with fresh water to moisten before serving.

Store in a resealable bag or a covered container in the refrigerator.

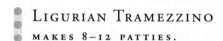

Ligurian Tramezzino
MAKES 8–12 PATTIES.

*Delicious flavors from the Ligurian region of Italy
marry in these delectable patties.*

4 cups chopped crimini mushrooms	1 cup basil
3 tablespoons organic extra-virgin olive oil	2 tablespoons dried oregano
	1 tablespoon dried savory or thyme
3 tablespoons nama shoyu	3 soft dates, pitted
1 tablespoon apple cider vinegar	½ cup pine nuts
1½ cups walnuts	2 tomatoes
1 cup sun-dried tomatoes	1–2 teaspoons sun-dried sea salt, or to taste
2 cloves garlic	
1 zucchini, shredded	

Toss mushrooms with olive oil, nama shoyu, and apple cider vinegar. Allow to marinate for 30 minutes to an hour or until savory and soft.

Soak walnuts in 2 cups fresh water for 1–2 hours. Drain and rinse. Soak sun-dried tomatoes in 1½ cups fresh water until soft (5–15 minutes).

In a food processor, finely chop garlic, zucchini, basil, oregano, and savory or thyme. Add walnuts, sun-dried tomatoes, and pitted dates, and finely chop. Chop pine nuts coarsely with a knife. Cut the tomatoes in half, scoop out the seeds, and dice. Mix in chopped pine nuts, diced tomatoes, and marinated mushrooms and season with sea salt.

Form patties out of ½ cup to 1 cup of mixture. Place patties on nonstick sheets. Dehydrate at 108°F for 12–20 hours or until a crust has formed. Flip over the patties and return to the dehydrator without the nonstick sheets to dry the underside for an hour or two. (Climate, temperature, and humidity all affect dehydrating time.) Alternatively, the patties can be dried on a cookie sheet or in a casserole dish in the oven set at the lowest temperature for 4–6 hours until a crust forms. Flip the patties over for an hour to dry the underside. Leave the door slightly ajar if necessary to regulate the temperature.

The patties are best with a crust on the outside and moist inside. The patties can also be dried thoroughly for longer storage and spritzed with fresh water to moisten before serving.

Store in a zip-lock bag or a covered container in the refrigerator.

Sweet-and-Hot Sauce
makes ¾ cup.

A sweet, spicy sauce for hot sauce lovers. Great to serve on the side of everything for a good kick.

4 dates, pitted
2 tablespoons apple cider vinegar
1 tablespoon nama shoyu
1 tablespoon organic extra-virgin
  olive oil (optional)

1 chili pepper, or 2 teaspoons dried
  chili pepper
Pinch cayenne pepper
Pinch sun-dried sea salt

Soak dates in ½ cup fresh water until very soft (5–10 minutes). Drain the soak water and set aside. Cut off the stem of the chili pepper.

In a blender, blend dates and soak water, apple cider vinegar, nama shoyu, olive oil (if desired), chili pepper, cayenne pepper, and sea salt until smooth. Store in a glass jar with a lid in the refrigerator.

Sun-Dried Tomato Ketchup
MAKES 1 PINT.

For the ketchup lover. An authentic, thick ketchup for your
condiment needs. Add a pinch of cayenne for a wee bit of heat!

½ cup sun-dried tomatoes

1 tomato

2 tablespoons apple cider vinegar

1 tablespoon raw honey or agave
    nectar

1 tablespoon organic extra-virgin
    olive oil

2 teaspoons white miso

1 small clove garlic

1 teaspoon sun-dried sea salt

Pinch cayenne pepper (optional for
    a touch of heat!)

Soak sun-dried tomatoes in just enough fresh water to cover until soft (5–15 minutes). Cut the top out of the tomato. Cut tomato in half and scoop out the seeds with a spoon.

In a blender, blend softened sun-dried tomatoes and soak water, seeded tomato, apple cider vinegar, honey or agave nectar, olive oil, miso, garlic, sea salt, and cayenne pepper (if desired) until smooth. Store in a glass jar with a lid in the refrigerator.

Maple Honey Mustard
MAKES ¾ CUP.

A sweet and savory spicy mustard. Great for sandwiches with
flat breads or to serve with sushi for a sweet, spicy kick.

3 tablespoons brown mustard seeds

2 tablespoons raw honey

2 tablespoons maple syrup

2 tablespoons apple cider vinegar

2 tablespoons nama shoyu

In a blender, blend all ingredients until smooth. Store in a glass jar with a lid in the refrigerator.

AIOLI SAUCE (MAYONNAISE)
MAKES ¾ CUP.

A creamy sauce with whipped oil and a touch of savory tang.
Serve on a sandwich, with crackers, or with steamed artichokes.

½ cup organic extra-virgin olive oil
1 small clove garlic
3 tablespoons apple cider vinegar

2 teaspoons raw honey or brown
  rice syrup
1 teaspoon sun-dried sea salt

In a blender, whip all ingredients for 2–3 minutes on high until sauce thickens. Store in a glass jar with a lid in the refrigerator.

VARIATION: *Garlic Herb Aioli*
Blend in ¼ cup chopped parsley, ¼ cup chopped cilantro, and 2 tablespoons chopped basil.

MISO BBQ SAUCE
MAKES ABOUT I CUP.

A spicy barbecue sauce, savory and rich with miso. Great for
marinating portobello mushrooms to serve as an open-faced
sandwich with flat bread, fresh tomato, and avocado slices.

3 tablespoons red miso
3 tablespoons fresh water
2 tablespoons organic extra-virgin
  olive oil
1 tablespoon raw honey or maple
  syrup
1 clove garlic

2 teaspoons shredded or finely
  minced ginger
1 tablespoon paprika
2 teaspoons chili powder
1 teaspoon black pepper
1 teaspoon celery seed, or
  2 tablespoons minced celery

In a blender, blend all ingredients until smooth. Store in a glass jar with a lid in the refrigerator.

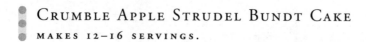

29

Cakes and Frostings

CRUMBLE APPLE STRUDEL BUNDT CAKE
MAKES 12–16 SERVINGS.

This authentic apple strudel is pressed into a doughnut-shaped pan for a gorgeous presentation.

Cake Layer
- 1 cup almonds
- 1 cup walnuts
- 1 cup pecans
- 1 cup dried coconut
- 1 cup pitted soft dates
- ½ cup water
- 1 tablespoon non-alcohol vanilla extract
- 1 tablespoon cinnamon
- 1 tablespoon ideally ground fresh nutmeg
- Pinch sun-dried sea salt

Apple Strudel Layer
- 5 apples
- 1½ cups dried apple rings
- 1 cup currants
- 1 tablespoon cinnamon
- 1 teaspoon ground fresh nutmeg
- 1 tablespoon lemon zest
- 2 tablespoons shredded or finely minced ginger

Crumble
- 1 cup walnuts
- 2 tablespoons maple syrup or raw honey

1 tablespoon cold-pressed coconut
    butter or organic extra-virgin
    olive oil
1 teaspoon cinnamon
1 teaspoon ideally ground fresh
    nutmeg
4 tablespoons date sugar, maple sugar,
    or organic evaporated cane juice
Pinch sun-dried sea salt

Vanilla Glaze

1 cup almonds or raw cashews
¼ cup pitted soft dates
2 tablespoons cold-pressed coconut
    butter
¼ cup lemon juice
1 teaspoon lemon zest
1 tablespoon non-alcohol vanilla
    extract
½ teaspoon cinnamon

To prepare the cake layer: Soak almonds in 2 cups fresh water overnight (about 6–12 hours). Drain and rinse.

In a food processor, grind walnuts, pecans, and soaked almonds into a fine meal. Set aside. Grind the dried coconut into a powder and set aside. Blend dates, water, and vanilla into a smooth paste. In a bowl, mix together ground nuts, coconut, and date paste. Spoon in cinnamon, nutmeg, and sea salt. Mix well. Press into the shape of a doughnut on a platter.

To prepare the apple strudel layer: Peel, core, and shred the apples. Put the shredded apple in a strainer and press to squeeze away excess juice.

In a food processor, grind dried apples. In a bowl, mix shredded apple and ground dried apples with currants, cinnamon, nutmeg, lemon zest, and ginger. Press strudel layer neatly on the cake layer.

To make the crumble: In a food processor, combine walnuts, maple syrup or honey, coconut butter or olive oil, cinnamon, nutmeg, sugar or cane juice, and sea salt. Grind all ingredients into a crumble. Distribute the crumble evenly over the strudel layer.

To make the vanilla glaze: Soak almonds in 2 cups fresh water overnight (about 6–12 hours). Drain and rinse. Alternatively, soak cashews in fresh water for 30 minutes and rinse. Soak dates in ¼ cup fresh water for 5–10 minutes. Drain the soak water and set aside.

In a food processor or blender, blend drained nuts, softened dates, coconut butter, lemon juice, lemon zest, vanilla, and cinnamon into a smooth cream. Add 2 tablespoons of date soak water at a time if necessary to aid in blending smooth. The glaze should be smooth but pourable. Spoon the glaze into a pastry bag or a zip-lock bag with the corner snipped. Drizzle glaze back and forth over the crumble for an authentic glazed presentation.

Traditional Layered Carrot Cake with Lemon Cream Frosting
MAKES 10–12 SERVINGS.

This sweet, moist carrot cake is layered with creamy lemon frosting.
This recipe deliciously transforms carrot pulp left over from
fresh juicing into a moist middle.

2 cups almonds
1½ cups pitted soft dates
2 cups raisins
4 cups carrot pulp (See "Acquiring
    Carrot Pulp" on page 403.)
1 tablespoon non-alcohol vanilla
    extract
1 tablespoon cinnamon
1½ teaspoons fresh ground nutmeg
1 teaspoon cardamom
1 tablespoon lemon zest
1 tablespoon orange zest
Pinch sun-dried sea salt
½ cup chopped walnuts (optional)

Lemon Frosting
1½ cups whole raw cashews (Raw
    cashew pieces can be used.)
1 cup pitted soft dates
1 cup dried shredded coconut
1 cup orange juice
½ cup lemon juice
1 tablespoon lemon zest
1 tablespoon non-alcohol vanilla
    extract
1 cup large dried coconut flakes
    (optional for garnish)

To make the cake batter: Soak almonds in 4 cups fresh water overnight (about 6–12 hours). Drain and rinse. Soak dates in 1½ cups fresh water for 5–10 minutes to soften. Drain the soak water and set aside. Soak raisins in 3 cups fresh water for 10–15 minutes to soften. Drain the soak water and set aside.

In a masticating or triturating juicer (see "Juicing at Home," page 205), with homogenizing "blank" plate," grind almonds, dates, and 1 cup of the raisins into a smooth paste. Alternatively, they can be ground to a paste in a food processor. Mix with carrot pulp, vanilla, cinnamon, nutmeg, cardamom, lemon zest, orange zest, sea salt, walnuts (if desired), and remaining 1 cup of raisins.

To make the lemon frosting: Soak cashews in 2 cups fresh water for 30 minutes. Drain and rinse. Soak dates in 1 cup fresh water for 5–10 minutes to soften. Drain the soak water and set aside.

Acquiring Carrot Pulp

- Rescue the carrot pulp left over from juicing carrots.
- Put shredded or chopped carrot in a food processor. Grind carrot to a pulp. Press the pulp through a fine colander, strainer, or cheese cloth to extract juice. (Retain this juice for drinking.) The pulp should not be too soggy.

In a food processor or blender, grind the dried coconut into a powder and set aside. Blend the cashews, dates, ½ cup of the date soak water, orange juice, lemon juice, lemon zest, and vanilla until smooth. Add a touch more of the date soak water if necessary to aid in blending. Add powdered coconut and blend well. It may be necessary to help the blending along by scraping the sides of the blender with a rubber spatula and continue to blend. Allow to stand in the refrigerator if necessary to thicken.

To layer the cake: Split cake batter in half. Line a serving platter with plastic wrap or waxed paper. Press half of the dough into an even circle. Slip pressed dough on plastic wrap or waxed paper off of the platter. Press remaining dough directly on the platter into an even circle for the bottom layer. Spread just less than half of the frosting on the bottom layer leaving a 1-inch border. Delicately flip over the layer on the plastic wrap or waxed paper onto the frosted layer. Reshape any mishaps and smooth the sides. Spoon the remaining frosting on top of the cake and spread evenly over the top and sides. Garnish with dried coconut flakes, if desired. For best results, allow to chill and set in the refrigerator for an hour or more.

BUDDHA BACK MOCHA CAKE
MAKES 10–12 SERVINGS.

Delicately spiced and sweetened, this cake is so good that it brought the Buddha back! Try garnishing with sifted carob powder for a stunning effect.

½ cup almonds	½ cup whole raw cashews (Cashew
½ cup hazelnuts	pieces can be used.)

½ cup macadamia nuts

1 cup pitted soft dates

½ cup filtered water

1 cup unsulfured apple rings

1 tablespoon non-alcohol vanilla extract

2 tablespoons cold-pressed coconut butter

2 cups carrot pulp (See "Acquiring Carrot Pulp" on page 403.)

½ cup raw carob powder

¼ cup cocoa powder

3 tablespoons grain coffee substitute, or 2 tablespoons organic ground coffee or decaffeinated coffee

1 tablespoon cinnamon

1 tablespoon ideally ground fresh nutmeg

Pinch sun-dried sea salt

Vanilla-Mocha Frosting

½ cup almonds

½ cup hazelnuts

1 cup whole raw cashews

1 cup pitted soft dates

½ cup dried coconut

½ cup orange juice

¼ cup maple syrup or water

1 tablespoon cold-pressed coconut butter (optional)

2 tablespoons non-alcohol vanilla extract

2 teaspoons cinnamon

1 teaspoon ideally ground fresh nutmeg

2 tablespoons raw carob powder

1 tablespoon cocoa powder

1 teaspoon organic grain coffee or coffee substitute

To make the cake batter: Soak almonds and hazelnuts together in 2 cups fresh water overnight (about 6–12 hours). Drain and rinse.

In a food processor, grind almonds, hazelnuts, cashews, and macadamia nuts into a meal. Set aside. Chop apple rings into a fine meal. Set aside. Blend dates, water, coconut butter, and vanilla extract into a paste. By hand, mix ground nuts, ground dried apple, and date paste with carrot pulp, carob, cocoa, grain coffee, cinnamon, nutmeg, and sea salt.

To make the Vanilla-Mocha Frosting: Soak almonds and hazelnuts together in 2 cups fresh water overnight (about 6–12 hours). Drain and rinse. Soak cashews in 1½ cups fresh water for 30 minutes. Drain and rinse. Soak dates in 1 cup fresh water for 5–10 minutes to soften. Drain soak water and set aside.

In a food processor or blender, grind dried coconut into a powder and set aside. Blend hazelnuts, almonds, cashews, dates, orange juice, maple syrup or water, coconut butter (if desired), and vanilla until smooth. Add date soak water as necessary to blend. Spoon in cinnamon, nutmeg, carob, cocoa, and grain coffee, and blend until smooth. Spoon in powdered coconut as it is blending to thicken. It may be necessary to help the blending along by scraping the sides of the processor with a rubber spatula and continue to blend.

To layer the cake: Split cake batter in half. Line a serving platter with plastic wrap or waxed paper. Press half of the dough into an even circle. Slip pressed dough on plastic wrap or waxed paper off of the platter. Press remaining dough directly on the platter into an even circle for the bottom layer. Spread just less than half of the frosting on the bottom layer leaving a 1-inch border. Delicately flip over the layer on the plastic wrap or waxed paper onto the frosted layer. Reshape any mishaps and smooth the sides. Spoon the remaining frosting on top of the cake and spread evenly over the top and sides.

If you wish, this cake can be pressed into one layer. Press the cake dough into an even circle on a serving platter, and frost evenly.

For best results, allow to chill and set in the refrigerator for an hour or more. Stencils can be used to create designs. Cut stars, hearts, and spirals out of cardboard and lay on the cake before sifting. Or sprinkle with ground almonds and cinnamon.

LEMON POPPY SEED CAKE WITH WHIPPED LEMON CREAM FROSTING

MAKES 10–12 SERVINGS.

The classic flavors of lemon and poppy seeds marry in this simple cake, which can be dehydrated or served moist.

1 cup almonds
1 cup whole raw buckwheat
1½ cups pitted dates
½ cup macadamia nuts
2–4 tablespoons raw honey or maple syrup
1½ tablespoons cold-pressed coconut butter or organic extra-virgin olive oil
¼ cup fresh lemon juice
¼ cup lemon zest
2 tablespoons non-alcohol vanilla extract
⅓ cup poppy seeds
Pinch sun-dried sea salt

Whipped Lemon Cream Frosting

2 cups whole cashews
1 cup pitted soft dates
1 vanilla bean (optional) (Whole vanilla beans are expensive but worth the flavor.)
¼ cup raw honey or maple syrup
⅓ cup lemon juice
1 tablespoon lemon zest
2 tablespoons non-alcohol vanilla extract

Garnish

1½ tablespoons poppy seeds
1½ tablespoons lemon zest

To make the cake batter: Soak almonds in 2 cups fresh water overnight (about 6–12 hours). Drain and rinse. Soak whole raw buckwheat in 3 cups fresh water overnight (about 6–12 hours). Drain and rinse in a colander or strainer until the water runs clear. Spread on dehydrator sheets and dehydrate at 108°F for 12–20 hours until dry. Soak dates in 1½ cups fresh water for 5–10 minutes to soften. Drain the soak water and set aside.

In a food processor or blender, grind dried buckwheat into flour. Set aside. Grind macadamia nuts into a fine meal. Set aside.

In a masticating or triturating juicer (see "Juicing at Home," page 205), with the homogenizing "blank" plate, grind drained almonds and softened dates into a smooth paste. Alternatively, the almonds and dates can be ground in a food processor.

In a bowl, mix almond-date mixture with honey or maple syrup, coconut butter or olive oil, lemon juice, lemon zest, vanilla, poppy seeds, and sea salt. Mix in ground buckwheat and macadamia nuts.

Press the dough into a 1½-inch cake. The cake can be dehydrated for 4–8 hours or simply frosted and chilled for an hour before serving.

To make the whipped lemon cream frosting: Soak cashews in 3 cups fresh water for 30 minutes. Drain and rinse. Soak dates in 1 cup fresh water for 5–10 minutes to soften. Drain the soak water and set aside.

Split the vanilla bean and scrape out the seeds with a spoon or a knife. In a blender or food processor, blend cashews, dates, honey or maple syrup, lemon juice, lemon zest, vanilla, and vanilla bean seeds (if desired) into a smooth cream. Add date soak water 1–2 tablespoons at a time only as necessary to aid in blending smooth. Slather frosting evenly over the top and sides of the cake. Garnish with poppy seeds and lemon zest.

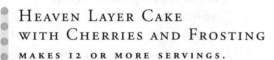

HEAVEN LAYER CAKE
WITH CHERRIES AND FROSTING
MAKES 12 OR MORE SERVINGS.

This sweet and moist layer cake is enhanced by the addition
of sweet cherries and the perfect touch of spices.

1 cup hazelnuts	½ cup apple juice (from pressed
1 cup pecans	apples)
1 cup dried coconut	1 cup pitted soft dates
3–4 apples	½ cup fresh water
⅔ cup dried cherries	½ cup raw carob powder

2 tablespoons cinnamon

2 tablespoons non-alcohol vanilla
extract

Pinch sun-dried sea salt

1 cup dried shredded coconut

½ cup maple syrup or raw honey

2 tablespoons non-alcohol vanilla
extract

Frosting and Cherries

2 cups whole raw cashews (Cashew
pieces can be used), or 1 cup
macadamia nuts and 1 cup
almonds

½ cup pitted soft dates

¾ cup apple juice

2 cups pitted cherries (Thawed frozen
cherries can be used.)

Garnish

⅓ cup chopped hazelnuts

To make the cake batter: Soak hazelnuts in 2 cups fresh water overnight (6–12 hours). Drain and rinse.

In a food processor, grind hazelnuts and pecans into a fine meal. Set aside. Grind dried coconut into a powder. Set aside. Peel apples and remove the cores. Shred the apples and press firmly in a strainer to remove excess juice. (Retain ½ cup of apple juice.) Soak dried cherries in the apple juice to soften. Set aside. Soak dates in ½ cup fresh water for 5–10 minutes to soften. Retain the date soak water.

In a food processor, blend the cherries, apple juice, dates, and date soak water into a smooth paste. In a bowl, mix ground hazelnuts, pecans, and coconut with date-cherry paste. Mix in pressed shredded apple, carob powder, cinnamon, vanilla, and sea salt.

To make the frosting and cherries: Soak cashews in 3 cups fresh water for 30 minutes. Drain and rinse. Alternatively, soak macadamia nuts in 2 cups fresh water for 30 minutes. Drain and rinse. And soak almonds overnight (about 6–12 hours). Drain and rinse. Soak dates in ½ cup apple juice for 5–10 minutes to soften.

In a blender or food processor, grind dried shredded coconut into a powder. Set aside. Blend nuts, dates, apple juice, maple syrup or honey, and vanilla until smooth. Add a few tablespoons of apple juice or fresh water to aid in blending if necessary. Add ground coconut and blend until smooth. It may be necessary to help the blending along by scraping the sides of the blender with a rubber spatula and continue to blend.

To layer the cake: Split cake batter in half. Line a serving platter with plastic wrap or waxed paper. Press half of the dough into an even circle. Slip pressed dough on plastic wrap or waxed paper off of the platter. Press remaining dough directly on the platter into an even circle for the bottom layer. Spread just less than half of the frosting on the bottom layer leaving a 1-inch border. Generously cover with pitted cherries. Delicately flip over the layer on the plastic wrap or waxed paper onto the frosted layer. Reshape any mishaps and smooth the sides. Spoon the remaining frosting on top of the cake and spread evenly over the top and sides.

For best results, allow to chill and set in the refrigerator for an hour or more. Garnish with chopped hazelnuts.

Frostings and Creams

Vanilla Cream Frosting
MAKES 1¼ CUPS.

This velvety vanilla cream fills every frosting need—or you can simply eat it out of the bowl!

1 cup whole cashews (Raw cashew pieces can be used.)
4–6 pitted soft dates
1 tablespoon maple syrup or raw honey
1 tablespoon cold-pressed coconut butter or organic extra-virgin olive oil (optional)

1 tablespoon non-alcohol vanilla extract
½ fresh vanilla bean (optional)

Soak cashews in 1½ cups fresh water for 30 minutes to 1 hour. Drain and rinse. Soak the dates in ½ cup fresh water until very soft (about 5–10 minutes). Drain soak water and set aside. In a blender or food processor, blend cashews, dates, maple syrup or honey, coconut butter or olive oil (if desired), and vanilla (if desired). Add date soak water 2 tablespoons at a time as needed to blend smooth.

Red Raspberry Frosting
MAKES 1½ CUPS.

This creamy red frosting is perfect for any raspberry lover.

1 cup raw whole cashews (Raw cashew pieces can be used.), or 1 cup macadamia nuts

4–6 pitted soft dates

1 tablespoon maple syrup (optional)

½ cup raspberries (Thawed frozen raspberries can be used.)

1 tablespoon shredded beet

1 tablespoon non-alcohol vanilla extract

Soak cashews or macadamia nuts in 2 cups fresh water for 30 minutes. Drain and rinse. Soak dates in ⅓ cup fresh water for 5–10 minutes until very soft. Drain the soak water and set aside.

In a blender or food processor, blend nuts, dates, maple syrup, raspberries, beet, vanilla, and ¼ cup of the date soak water until smooth. Add a few more tablespoons of date soak water if necessary to blend smooth. The less water, the thicker the cream will be.

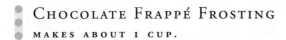

Chocolate Frappé Frosting

MAKES ABOUT 1 CUP.

This smooth chocolate cream frosting is an excellent topping for a berry parfait or strawberry pie.

1 cup whole raw cashews (Raw cashew pieces can be used.)

6 pitted soft dates

1 tablespoon maple syrup

1 tablespoon cold-pressed coconut butter or organic extra-virgin olive oil

1 tablespoon non-alcohol vanilla extract

2 tablespoons raw carob powder

2 tablespoons cocoa powder

Soak cashews in 2 cups fresh water for 30 minutes. Drain and rinse. Soak dates in ⅓ cup fresh water for 5–10 minutes or until very soft. Drain the soak water and set aside.

In a blender or food processor, blend cashews, dates, maple syrup, coconut butter or olive oil, and vanilla. Add ¼ cup of the date soak water to blend smooth. Spoon in carob and cocoa powder and blend into a smooth cream. Add a little extra date soak water if needed to blend smooth.

STRAWBERRIES AND CREAM FROSTING
MAKES ABOUT 1½ CUPS.

This pretty pink frosting is great on any fruit pie or fresh fruit sorbet.

1 cup whole raw cashews (Raw
   cashew pieces can be used.) or 1
   cup macadamia nuts
4–6 pitted soft dates
1 tablespoon maple syrup
   or raw honey
½ cup strawberries (Thawed frozen
   strawberries can be used.)

1 tablespoon cold-pressed coconut
   butter or organic extra-virgin
   olive oil
1 tablespoon shredded beet
1 tablespoon non-alcohol vanilla
   extract

Soak cashews in 2 cups fresh water for 30 minutes. Drain and rinse. Soak dates in ⅓ cup fresh water for 5–10 minutes until very soft. Drain the soak water and set aside.

In a blender or food processor, blend cashews, dates, maple syrup or honey, strawberries, coconut butter or olive oil, beet, and vanilla until smooth. Add date soak water 2 tablespoons at a time as necessary to blend smooth.

VIOLET BLACK RASPBERRY FROSTING
MAKES ABOUT 1 CUP.

*This luscious violet cream is great with fresh berries,
on fresh fruit sorbet, or on any fruit pie.*

1 cup whole raw cashews (Raw
   cashew pieces can be used.) or 1
   cup macadamia nuts
5 pitted, soft dates pitted
1 tablespoon maple syrup or raw
   honey

½ cup black raspberries (Thawed
   frozen black raspberries can
   be used.)
1 tablespoon non-alcohol vanilla
   extract

Soak cashews in 2 cups fresh water for 30 minutes. Drain and rinse. Soak dates in ⅓ cup fresh water for 5–10 minutes to soften. Drain the soak water and set aside.

In a blender or food processor, blend cashews, dates, maple syrup or honey, raspberries, vanilla, and 4 tablespoons of the date soak water until smooth. Add a touch more date soak water as necessary to blend. The less water added, the thicker the frosting. To thin into a sauce, add more water.

GOLDEN LEMON CRÈME
MAKES ABOUT 1½ CUPS.

This lovely lemon cream frosting is perfect for a pie or parfait or simply for dipping sliced apples.

1 cup whole raw cashews	1 lemon
4–5 pitted soft dates	1 tablespoon non-alcohol vanilla
1 tablespoon raw honey	extract
1½ teaspoons lemon zest	1 teaspoon shredded ginger (optional)

Soak cashews in 2 cups fresh water for 30 minutes. Drain and rinse. Soak dates in ⅓ cup fresh water for 5–10 minutes until very soft. Drain the soak water and set aside.

Cut the peel away from the lemon with a small paring knife. Cut the lemon in quarters and remove any seeds.

In a blender or food processor, blend cashews, dates, honey, lemon zest, lemon quarters, vanilla, and ginger (if desired) until smooth. Add date soak water 2 tablespoons at a time as necessary to blend smooth.

NUTTY FROSTED CRÈME
MAKES ABOUT 1½ CUPS.

This classic chocolate hazelnut crème is excellent with raspberries and bananas or as a topping on a fresh fruit sorbet.

1 cup hazelnuts (filberts)	1 tablespoon cold-pressed coconut
5 pitted soft dates	butter or organic extra-virgin
2 tablespoons maple syrup or raw	olive oil
honey	1 tablespoon non-alcohol vanilla
2 tablespoons raw almond butter	extract

1 teaspoon cinnamon

½ teaspoon ground fresh nutmeg

2 tablespoons raw carob powder

1 tablespoon cocoa powder (or 1 additional tablespoon of carob powder)

Soak hazelnuts in 2 cups fresh water overnight (about 6–12 hours). Drain and rinse. Soak dates in ⅓ cup fresh water for 5–10 minutes until very soft. Drain off the soak water and set aside.

In a blender or food processor, blend hazelnuts, dates, date soak water, maple syrup or honey, almond butter, coconut butter or olive oil, vanilla, cinnamon, and nutmeg until smooth. Spoon in carob and cocoa and continue to blend until smooth.

Black Velvet Crème
MAKES ABOUT 1 CUP.

This rich velvet chocolate sauce is divine on anything made with berries.

½ cup pitted soft dates

2 tablespoons maple syrup or raw honey (optional)

½ avocado

1 tablespoon cold-pressed coconut butter or organic extra-virgin olive oil

1 tablespoon non-alcohol vanilla extract

2 tablespoons raw carob powder

2 tablespoons cocoa powder

Soak the dates in ½ cup fresh water for 5–10 minutes until very soft. Drain the soak water and set aside.

In a blender or food processor, blend dates, maple syrup or honey (if desired), avocado, coconut butter or olive oil, vanilla, carob, and cocoa until smooth. Add date soak water 2 tablespoons at a time as necessary to blend smooth. The more liquid added, the thinner the sauce.

Whipped Chai Frosting
MAKES ABOUT 1 CUP.

This whipped cream frosting with traditional chai spices is great on apple slices or sorbet.

1 cup whole raw cashews (Raw cashew pieces can be used.), almonds, or macadamia nuts

4 pitted soft dates

2 tablespoons raw honey

1 tablespoon non-alcohol vanilla extract

2 teaspoons shredded or finely minced ginger

1½ teaspoons cinnamon

½ teaspoon ideally ground fresh nutmeg

¼ teaspoon cardamom

Pinch clove or allspice

Very small pinch black pepper

Pinch sun-dried sea salt

Soak cashews or macadamia nuts in 2 cups fresh water for 30 minutes. If almonds are used, soak almonds in 2 cups fresh water for 4–6 hours. Drain and rinse. Soak the dates in ⅓ cup fresh water for 5–10 minutes until very soft.

In a blender or food processor, blend nuts, dates, date soak water, honey, vanilla, ginger, cinnamon, nutmeg, cardamom, clove or allspice, black pepper, and sea salt until smooth. Add a touch of fresh water if necessary to aid in blending smooth. The less liquid added, the thicker the cream. To thin into a sauce, add more water.

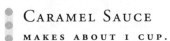

CARAMEL SAUCE
MAKES ABOUT 1 CUP.

Serve this luscious caramel confection on absolutely anything for a sweet treat.

5 tablespoons raw almond butter or raw cashew butter

¼ cup maple syrup

2 tablespoons cold-pressed coconut butter

1 tablespoon vanilla extract

2 pitted soft dates

¼ teaspoon cinnamon

Pinch sun-dried sea salt

In a blender or food processor, blend all ingredients until creamy. Add a touch of fresh water to aid in blending if necessary. The more liquid added, the thinner the sauce will be.

30

Pies, Tortes, and Crusts

Pies

CHOCONOT MOUSSE PIE WITH VANILLA CREAM FROSTING
MAKES 8–10 SLICES.

*This pie came to me in a dream. For a creamy mousse base, the
secret is avocado. It is a truly decadent mousse that will satisfy any
chocolate lover's sweet tooth. Using raw carob powder and a hint
of cocoa powder gives this pie a divine chocolate flavor. The pie also
can be prepared exclusively with carob for sensational results.*

1 pie crust (such as Almond Vanilla
    Crumble Crust on page 425,
    Heavenly Hazelnut Shell on page
    426, or Pecan Graham Cracker
    Crust on page 426)
3 ripe bananas

Choconot Mousse Filling
1¼ cups pitted dates
1½ tablespoons non-alcohol vanilla
    extract
2–4 tablespoons maple syrup
1 tablespoon cold-pressed coconut
    butter or organic extra-virgin olive
    oil (optional)
3 avocados

⅔–¾ cup raw carob powder
¼ cup organic cocoa powder (or
  4 additional tablespoons raw carob
  powder)

Vanilla Cream Frosting
1 cup whole cashews (Raw cashew
  pieces can be used.)
4–6 soft dates, pitted
1 tablespoon maple syrup or raw
  honey

1 tablespoon cold-pressed coconut
  butter or organic extra-virgin olive
  oil (optional)
1 tablespoon non-alcohol vanilla
  extract

Garnish
1 pint strawberries, sliced
2 sprigs fresh mint

To prepare the pie crust: Slice the bananas and layer on the bottom of the crust. With moistened fingers, press the banana slices into a firm, solid layer.

To prepare the Choconot Mousse: Soak the dates in 1½ cups fresh water for 5–10 minutes to soften. Drain the soak water and set aside.

In a food processor, blend the dates, vanilla, and coconut butter or olive oil (if desired) into a smooth paste. It may be necessary to add a few tablespoons of date soak water to blend smooth. Cut the avocados in half. Chop the blade of a chef's knife into the pit. Twist the knife to extract the pits. Scoop the avocados into the food processor with the dates and blend until smooth. Spoon in ⅔ cup of the carob powder and cocoa powder and blend until smooth. For darker Choconot Mousse, add 2 more tablespoons of carob powder or cocoa powder. Spread the mousse evenly over the banana slices.

To make the vanilla cream frosting: Soak cashews in 1½ cups fresh water for 30 minutes to 1 hour. Drain and rinse. Soak dates in ½ cup fresh water until very soft (about 5–10 minutes). Drain soaking water and set aside.

In a blender, blend cashews, softened dates, maple syrup or honey, coconut butter or olive oil (if desired), and vanilla. Add date soak water 2 tablespoons at a time as needed to blend smooth. With a rubber spatula, spread the frosting evenly over the mousse.

For garnish, layer sliced strawberries decoratively on the frosting and place a mint leaf or two on each piece.

The pie serves best after it is chilled in the refrigerator for an hour or two. It keeps fresh for several days.

Mango Papaya Coconut Cream Pie with Raspberry Frosting
makes 8–10 slices.

This beautiful pie presents itself like a sunrise. Papayas are high in pectin, a naturally occurring gelling agent (also found in berries and other fruits), which helps this pie set and serve perfectly.

1 pie crust (such as Pecan Graham Cracker Crust on page 426 or Almond Vanilla Crumble Crust on page 425)
1 medium mango
1–2 medium papayas

Coconut Cream

2 soft dates, pitted or 2 tablespoons maple syrup
1 cup fresh young coconut meat
1 tablespoon non-alcohol vanilla extract
2 teaspoons cold-pressed coconut butter (optional)

Raspberry Frosting

1 cup raw whole cashews (Raw cashew pieces can be used.) or macadamia nuts
4–6 pitted soft dates
1 tablespoon maple syrup (optional)
½ cup raspberries (Thawed frozen raspberries can be used.)
1 tablespoon shredded beet
1 tablespoon non-alcohol vanilla extract

Garnish

1 kiwi, sliced
Several raspberries
2 teaspoons poppy seeds

To prepare the pie crust: Peel the mango, cut the flesh from the pit, and thinly slice. Layer the slices on the bottom of the crust.

To make the coconut cream: Soak the dates in ¼ cup fresh water for 5–10 minutes to soften. Drain the soak water and set aside.

In a blender, blend dates or maple syrup, fresh coconut meat, vanilla, and coconut butter (if desired). Add date soak water 1 tablespoon at a time as needed to blend into a thick cream. Spread the coconut cream evenly on top of mango.

Peel papaya(s) and cut in half. Remove seeds and slice thinly. Layer slices on top of coconut cream.

To make the raspberry frosting: Soak cashews or macadamia nuts in 2 cups fresh water for 30 minutes. Drain and rinse. Soak dates in ⅓ cup fresh water for 5–10 minutes until very soft. Drain the soak water and set aside.

In a blender or food processor, blend nuts, dates, maple syrup (if desired), raspberries, beet, vanilla, and ¼ cup date soak water until smooth. Add a few more tablespoons of date soak water if necessary to aid in blending. The less water, the thicker the cream will be. Spread the raspberry frosting evenly over the papaya. Garnish with kiwi slices, raspberries, and poppy seeds. Allow to stand for an hour or more in the refrigerator to set.

CHERIMOYA RASPBERRY PIE
MAKES 8–10 SLICES.

Mark Twain referred to cherimoyas as "deliciousness itself." This sweet vanilla fruit is married with raspberries in this luscious pie. Try topping this pie with Red Raspberry Frosting (page 408) or Golden Lemon Crème (page 411).

1 pie crust (such as Almond Vanilla Crumble Crust on page 425, Walnut Crumb Crust on page 427, or Heavenly Hazelnut Shell on page 426)

1 tablespoon non-alcohol vanilla extract

Frosting
Red Raspberry Frosting (page 408) or Golden Lemon Crème (page 411)

Filling
2 medium cherimoyas
1 cup dried shredded coconut
1½ cups raspberries

Garnish
½ cup raspberries

To make the filling: Peel and seed the cherimoyas. In a blender or food processor, grind the dried shredded coconut into a powder. Gently mix the ground coconut with the seeded cherimoyas by hand. Gently fold in the raspberries. Spread evenly in the pie crust.

Prepare frosting and spread evenly over the filling. Garnish with raspberries and chill in the refrigerator to set for at least an hour.

EGGFRUIT PIE (PUMPKIN CHEESECAKE)
MAKES 8–10 PIECES.

Eggfruit, or canestelle, can be found in Hawaii and Florida. See "Fruits" (page 83). Latin, Asian, and Phillipino specialty and ethnic food markets may be the best places to forage for this delicacy. It has been intimately named as such for its uncanny resemblance to the creamy consistency and brilliant color of a cooked egg yolk, only sweet like sugar. A velvety bright yellow-orange of incredible sweetness. If the eggfruit is unavailable, I extend my condolences, as there simply is no substitution. Divine in its own right, the closest description of this pie is like the most decadent, creamy pumpkin cheesecake.

1 pie crust (such as Heavenly Hazelnut Shell on page 426 or Pecan Graham Cracker Crust on page 426)
2 cups peeled and pitted eggfruit (canestelle)
½ cup avocado
1½ tablespoons cold-pressed coconut butter or organic extra-virgin olive oil
1 tablespoon cinnamon
1 teaspoon nutmeg
1 tablespoon non-alcohol vanilla extract
Frosting (such as Violet Black Raspberry Frosting on page 410 or Vanilla Cream Frosting on page 408)

Prepare the pie crust. *To make the filling:* Blend cleaned eggfruit, avocado, coconut butter or olive oil, spices, and vanilla into a smooth cream. Spread evenly into pie crust. Prepare frosting and spread evenly over the filling. Chill for at least 1 hour in the refrigerator to set before serving.

PEACHES AND CREAM PIE

MAKES 8–10 SERVINGS.

Peaches are the essence of sweet summer with a light cream for a marriage made in heaven.

1 pie crust (such as Almond-Vanilla Crumble Crust on page 425, Pecan Graham Cracker Crust on page 426, or Buckwheat Crumble Crust on page 428)

6 peaches

1 cup whole raw cashews (Raw cashew pieces can be used.)

¼ cup raw honey

¼ cup lemon juice

1 tablespoon non-alcohol vanilla extract

2 teaspoons cinnamon

2 teaspoons nutmeg

Pinch sun-dried sea salt

Prepare the pie crust. *To make the filling:* Cut the peaches in half and remove the pits. Peel the peaches and slice into thin slices. Soak cashews in 2 cups fresh water for 30 minutes. Drain and rinse.

In a blender or food processor, blend cashews, honey, lemon juice, vanilla, cinnamon, nutmeg, and sea salt until smooth. Fold the cashew sauce into the sliced peaches. Spread the peach and cashew mixture into the pie crust. Allow to chill for an hour or two in the refrigerator before serving.

Tortes

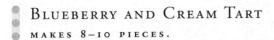

BLUEBERRY AND CREAM TART

MAKES 8–10 PIECES.

This lovely berry tart has a sweet creamy filling. Use a torte pan with a bottom that pops out for a fabulous freestanding masterpiece.

1 pie crust (such as Walnut Crumb Crust on page 427, Pecan Graham Cracker Crust on page 426, or Buckwheat Crumble Crust on page 428)

3 cups fresh blueberries (Raspberries, or blueberries and raspberries, can be used.)

2 teaspoons decorative lemon zest

Cream

2 cups whole raw cashews (raw
  cashew pieces can be used)
6 dates, pitted
5 tablespoons raw honey
2 tablespoons lemon juice
1 teaspoon lemon zest

1½ tablespoons non-alcohol vanilla
  extract
1 tablespoon cold-pressed coconut
  butter or organic extra-virgin olive
  oil (optional)
Pinch sun-dried sea salt

To prepare the pie crust: Press crust into a torte pan with a removable bottom.

To prepare the cream: Soak cashews in 3 cups fresh water for 30 minutes. Drain and rinse. Soak dates in ½ cup fresh water for 5–10 minutes to soften. Drain the soak water and set aside.

In a food processor or blender, blend cashews, dates, honey, lemon juice, lemon zest, vanilla, coconut butter or olive oil (if desired), and sea salt until smooth. It may be necessary to scrape the sides of the food processor with a rubber spatula and continue to blend until smooth. Add a few tablespoons of the dates' soak water to aid in blending if needed. The cream should be thick and very smooth. Spread the cream evenly in the pie crust. Lay the blueberries (and/or raspberries) evenly over the cream. Press the berries gently into the cream. Sprinkle with lemon zest. Chill the pie for a few hours to set before serving.

Mango Vanilla Bean Coconut Flan Torte

MAKES 8–10 PIECES.

*Dried mango gives this creamy coconut flan a succulent
thickness. Use a torte pan with a removable bottom
for a gorgeous presentation.*

1 pie crust (such as Almond-Vanilla
  Crumble Crust on page 425 or
  Pecan Graham Cracker Crust on
  page 426)
1½ cups sliced fresh mango

Mango Vanilla Bean Coconut Flan
1½ cups dried mango (Be sure that
  no sugar or sulfur has been added
  to the fruit.)
1 vanilla bean
2½ cups dried shredded coconut

1 tablespoon non-alcohol vanilla
extract
1 tablespoon cold-pressed coconut
butter (optional)

Garnish
1–2 kiwis, peeled and sliced
Edible flower petals

To prepare the pie crust: Press crust into a torte pan with a removable bottom. Layer the mango slices in the bottom of the crust.

To make the mango vanilla bean coconut flan: With a pair of kitchen scissors, cut the dried mango into pieces. (Be sure to use good sun-dried mango without sugar or sulfur.) In a bowl, cover the dried mango pieces with fresh water and allow to soak until soft (about 5–15 minutes). Split the vanilla bean in half lengthwise. With a knife or the edge of a spoon, scrape out the seeds. Set the seeds aside.

In a food processor, grind the dried coconut into a powder. Set aside. Blend the softened dried mango and soak water until smooth. Add the dried coconut, vanilla extract, vanilla bean seeds, and coconut butter (if desired), and blend until smooth. Spread evenly over the sliced mango. Garnish with kiwi slices and edible flowers.

Allow to set in the refrigerator for at least an hour before serving.

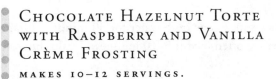

Chocolate Hazelnut Torte with Raspberry and Vanilla Crème Frosting

MAKES 10–12 SERVINGS.

This is a truly decadent moist chocolate torte with smooth hazelnuts and seductive vanilla.

Chocolate Torte
2 cups hazelnuts (filberts)
1½ cups pitted soft dates
2 tablespoons cold-pressed coconut
butter or organic extra-virgin
olive oil
2 tablespoons non-alcohol vanilla
extract

½ cup cocoa powder
1½ cups raw carob powder
2 teaspoons cinnamon

Vanilla Cream Frosting
1½ cups whole raw cashews (Raw
cashew pieces can be used.)
6–8 soft dates, pitted

1 tablespoon coconut butter or
organic extra-virgin olive oil
(optional)
2 tablespoons non-alcohol vanilla
extract

Garnish
1 tablespoon poppy seeds
Edible flower petals (pot marigold
flowers, calendula flowers, or
pansies)

1 pint raspberries

To make the chocolate torte: Soak hazelnuts in 4 cups fresh water overnight (about 6–12 hours). Drain and rinse. Soak dates in 1½ cups fresh water to soften (about 5–10 minutes). Drain the soak water and set aside.

In a masticating or triturating juicer (see "Juicing at Home," page 205) with the homogenizing "blank" plate, grind hazelnuts and dates into a smooth paste. Add some of the date soak water as needed to aid the process. Mix in coconut butter or olive oil and vanilla. Alternatively, the hazelnuts and dates can be ground into a smooth paste in a food processor, adding coconut butter or olive oil, vanilla, and date soak water as necessary to blend smooth.

Add cinnamon, cocoa, and carob powder ¼ cup at a time to avoid clumping. This torte is served without a crust. For best, nonstick serving: Line a platter with plastic wrap or waxed paper. Press in a circle on the lined platter and generously dust with cocoa or carob powder. Slide the plastic or wax paper off the platter. Flip the platter upside down on dusted torte. Flip right-side-up.

To make the vanilla cream frosting: Soak cashews in 2 cups fresh water for 30 minutes. Drain and rinse. Soak the dates in ½ cup fresh water to soften (about 5–10 minutes). Drain the soak water and set aside.

In a blender or food processor, blend cashews, dates, coconut butter or olive oil (if desired), and vanilla. Add date soak water 1 tablespoon at a time as needed to blend smooth. Spread evenly on the torte.

Generously top with raspberries and garnish with a sprinkling of poppy seeds or edible flowers.

WALNUT-PEAR TORTE
MAKES 8–12 SLICES.

*This is a lovely torte with a walnut-spiced crust, layered pears, and
a creamy middle. Any ripe, juicy pears will do; slice with care.
Caramel Sauce (page 413) complements this delicious torte.*

Walnut Crust
- 2 cups walnuts
- 4 soft dates, pitted
- 2 tablespoons raw honey or maple syrup
- 1 tablespoon cinnamon
- 1 teaspoon nutmeg
- Pinch sun-dried sea salt

- ¼ cup lemon juice
- 1 tablespoon non-alcohol vanilla extract
- 1 tablespoon cold-pressed coconut butter or organic extra-virgin olive oil

- 4 firm ripe pears

Cream
- 1½ cups whole raw cashews (Raw cashew pieces can be used.)
- 1 cup pitted soft dates

Garnish
- 2 teaspoons cinnamon
- 1 tablespoon lemon zest

To make the walnut crust: In a food processor, chop walnuts into a fine meal. Add dates, honey or maple syrup, cinnamon, nutmeg, and sea salt and chop until well mixed. Press into the bottom only of a pie plate or torte pan.

To make the cream: Soak cashews in 2 cups fresh water for 30 minutes. Drain and rinse. Soak dates in 1 cup fresh water for 5–10 minutes to soften. Drain the soak water and set aside.

In a blender or food processor, blend cashews, dates, lemon juice, vanilla, and coconut butter or olive oil until smooth. Add date soak water 2 tablespoons at a time only as necessary to blend. The cream should be smooth and thick. Spread the cream evenly over the crust.

To prepare the pears: Peel the pears and cut in half. Cut out the seeds. Cut the pears into slices and fan out decoratively over the cream. Garnish with a sprinkling of cinnamon and lemon zest. Allow to set for at least an hour or two in the refrigerator before serving.

MAPLE-ALMOND MARZIPAN TORTE

MAKES 8–12 PIECES.

This moist maple-sweetened marzipan torte has a touch of vanilla and cinnamon. Try topping this torte with sliced peaches and Caramel Sauce (page 413) for a succulent delight.

Almond Torte
3 cups almonds
1 cup pitted soft dates
¼ cup maple syrup or raw honey
¼ cup organic evaporated cane juice
1 tablespoon cold-pressed coconut
    butter or organic extra-virgin olive
    oil (optional)

1 tablespoon non-alcohol vanilla
    extract
2 teaspoons almond extract
1 tablespoon cinnamon
Pinch sun-dried sea salt

4 peaches
Caramel Sauce (page 413)

To make the almond torte: Soak 2 cups of the almonds in 4 cups fresh water overnight (about 6–12 hours). Drain and rinse. Soak the dates in 1 cup fresh water for 5–10 minutes to soften. Drain the soak water and set aside.

In a food processor, chop the remaining 1 cup of dry almonds (unsoaked) into a powdery-fine meal. Set aside. In a masticating or triturating juicer (see "Juicing at Home," page 205), with the homogenizing "blank" plate, grind the soaked almonds and softened dates into a smooth paste. Mix in maple syrup or honey, cane juice, coconut butter or olive oil (if desired), vanilla extract, almond extract, cinnamon, and sea salt. Fold in ground dry almonds. Alternatively, use a food processor to grind the almonds, dates, maple syrup or honey, coconut butter or olive oil, vanilla extract, almond extract, cinnamon, and sea salt into a smooth paste. Fold in evaporated cane juice and ground dry almonds.

Press the torte into a 1½-inch-thick circle on a platter.

To prepare the peaches: Cut the peaches in half and remove the pits. Peel the peaches and cut into thin slices. Layer the peaches in a circular pattern from the center of the torte out to the edges for a decorative presentation. Allow to set and chill in the refrigerator for an hour or two before serving. Drizzle Caramel Sauce over each piece. This torte is served without a crust.

Crusts

ALMOND-VANILLA CRUMBLE CRUST
MAKES ONE 10-INCH PIE CRUST.

*This is a lovely almond crust that serves as a scrumptious stage
for any filling. Fill with fresh fruit and top with frosting.*

2 cups almonds
1½ cups soaked almonds
½ cup dry almonds
4–6 soft dates, pitted
1 tablespoon maple syrup or raw
   honey

1 tablespoon non-alcohol vanilla
   extract
1 teaspoon almond extract (optional)
2 teaspoons cinnamon
Pinch sun-dried sea salt

Soak 1½ cups of the almonds in 3 cups fresh water overnight (about 6–12 hours). Drain and rinse. Spread almonds on a dry towel and blot dry.

In a food processor, chop the remaining ½ cup dry almonds into a fine meal. Set aside. Chop the soaked almonds into a fine meal. Cut or break the dates into pieces. If the dates are very dry or firm, soak them in ½ cup fresh water for 5 minutes to soften. Add date pieces, maple syrup or raw honey, vanilla, almond extract (if desired), cinnamon, and sea salt to the chopped soaked almonds and chop until well mixed. It may be necessary to scrape the sides of the food processor with a rubber spatula and continue to chop. Add the dry almond meal and chop until well mixed. This will help to dry the dough into a nice, crumbly consistency.

The dough should be crumbly but sticky enough to hold a shape when pressed. If the dough is too dry, add 2 tablespoons fresh water and chop until well mixed. Press the dough evenly into a pie plate or a torte pan. It is best to press the dough to the sides of the plate or pan first and then press into the bottom for even depth.

To scallop the edge of the crust: Use the thumb and forefinger of your dominant hand to pinch the edge of the dough successively around the rim of the plate or pan. Use the forefinger of your other hand to press against the pinches to keep them neat and orderly.

Fill, frost, and serve with love.

HEAVENLY HAZELNUT SHELL
MAKES ONE HEAVENLY 10-INCH PIE CRUST.

*This crust was the house favorite at my restaurant, The Raw
Experience, in Maui, Hawaii.*

1 cup hazelnuts (filberts)
1 cup dry walnuts
4–6 soft dates, pitted
1 tablespoon maple syrup or raw
   honey

2 teaspoons cinnamon
1 teaspoon ideally ground fresh
   nutmeg
2 tablespoons raw carob powder
Pinch sun-dried sea salt

Soak hazelnuts in 2 cups fresh water overnight (about 6–12 hours). Drain and rinse.

In a food processor, chop walnuts into a fine meal. Set aside. Chop hazelnuts into a fine
meal. Cut or break the dates into pieces. If the dates are very dry or firm, soak them in ½ cup
fresh water for 5 minutes to soften. Add date pieces, maple syrup or raw honey, cinnamon,
nutmeg, carob powder, and sea salt to the ground hazelnuts and chop until well mixed. It may
be necessary to scrape the sides of the food processor and continue to chop for a thorough consistency. Add the ground walnuts and chop until well mixed. The dough should be crumbly
but sticky enough to hold a shape when pressed. Press the dough evenly into a pie plate or a
torte pan. It is best to press the dough to the sides of the plate or pan first and then press into
the bottom for even depth.

To scallop the edge of the crust: Use the thumb and forefinger of your dominant hand to pinch
the edge of the dough successively around the rim of the plate or pan. Use the forefinger of
your other hand to press against the pinches to keep them neat and orderly.

PECAN GRAHAM CRACKER CRUST
MAKES ONE CRUMBLY 10-INCH PIE CRUST.

*This graham cracker crust makes a lovely and delicious base for
any fruit pie or mousse.*

2 cups pecans
4–6 soft dates, pitted

1 tablespoon maple syrup or raw
   honey

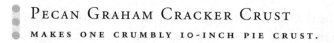

2 tablespoons raw carob powder

1 tablespoon cinnamon

2 teaspoons ideally ground
fresh nutmeg

1 tablespoon non-alcohol vanilla
extract (optional)

Pinch sun-dried sea salt

Soak 1 cup of the pecans in 2 cups fresh water for 2–4 hours. Drain and rinse.

In a food processor, chop 1 cup of dry pecans into a fine meal. Set aside. Chop soaked pecans into a fine meal. Cut or break the dates into pieces. If the dates are very dry or firm, soak them in ½ cup of fresh water for 5 minutes to soften. Add date pieces, maple syrup or honey, carob, cinnamon, nutmeg, vanilla (if desired), and sea salt to the ground soaked pecans and chop until well mixed. It may be necessary to scrape the sides of the food processor with a rubber spatula and continue to chop for a thorough consistency. Add the ground dry pecans and chop until well mixed. The dough should be crumbly but sticky enough to hold a shape when pressed. Press the dough evenly into a pie plate or a torte pan. It is best to press the dough to the sides of the plate or pan first and then press into the bottom for even depth.

To scallop the edge of the crust: Use the thumb and forefinger of your dominant hand to pinch the edge of the dough successively around the rim of the plate or pan. Use the forefinger of your other hand to press against the pinches to keep them neat and orderly.

Fill, frost, and serve with love.

WALNUT CRUMB CRUST
MAKES ONE CRUMBLY 10-INCH PIE CRUST.

*This delicate, crumbly walnut crust is well suited for
any fruit filling, especially pears and figs.*

2 cups walnuts

4–6 soft dates, pitted

1 tablespoon maple syrup or raw
honey

2 teaspoons cinnamon

1 teaspoon nutmeg

Pinch sun-dried sea salt

Soak 1 cup of the walnuts in 2 cups fresh water for 2–4 hours. Drain and rinse.

In a food processor, chop the remaining 1 cup of dry walnuts into a fine meal. Set aside.

Chop soaked walnuts into a fine meal. Cut or break the dates into pieces. If the dates are very dry or firm, soak them in ½ cup fresh water for 5 minutes to soften. Add date pieces, maple syrup or honey, cinnamon, nutmeg, and sea salt to the ground soaked walnuts and chop until well mixed. It may be necessary to scrape the sides of the food processor with a rubber spatula and continue to chop for a thorough consistency. Add the dry ground walnuts and chop until well mixed. The dough should be crumbly but sticky enough to hold a shape when pressed. Press the dough evenly into a pie plate or a torte pan. It is best to press the dough to the sides of the plate or pan first and then press into the bottom for even depth.

To scallop the edge of the crust: Use the thumb and forefinger of your dominant hand to pinch the edge of the dough successively around the rim of the plate or pan. Use the forefinger of your other hand to press against the pinches to keep them neat and orderly.

Fill, frost, and serve with love.

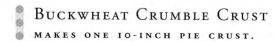

Buckwheat Crumble Crust

MAKES ONE 10-INCH PIE CRUST.

This light crust has a great texture for any fruit filling and frosting.

1½ cups raw buckwheat groats
6 soft dates, pitted
1½ tablespoons raw honey or brown
 rice syrup
1 tablespoon organic cold-pressed
 coconut butter or organic extra-
 virgin olive oil

1 tablespoon non-alcohol vanilla
 extract (optional)
1 tablespoon cinnamon
1½ teaspoons nutmeg
Pinch sun-dried sea salt

Soak raw buckwheat groats in 4 cups fresh water for 2–8 hours. Drain and rinse in a colander or strainer until rinse water runs clear. Give the colander or strainer a good shake to drain well. Spread buckwheat in a thin layer on dehydrator trays. Dehydrate at 108°F for 12 hours or until dry.

In a food processor, grind dried buckwheat into a flour. Cut or break the dates into pieces. If the dates are very dry or firm, soak them in ½ cup fresh water for 5 minutes to soften. Add date pieces, raw honey or brown rice syrup, coconut butter or olive oil, vanilla (if desired), cinnamon, nutmeg, and sea salt and chop until well mixed. It may be necessary to scrape the sides of the food processor with a rubber spatula and continue to chop for a thorough consistency. The dough should be crumbly but sticky enough to hold a shape when pressed. If the dough is too dry, add 2–4 tablespoons fresh water and mix well. Press the dough evenly into a pie plate or a torte pan. It is best to press the dough to the sides of the plate or pan first and then press into the bottom for even depth.

To scallop the edge of the crust: Use the thumb and forefinger of your dominant hand to pinch the edge of the dough successively around the rim of the plate or pan. Use the forefinger of your other hand to press against the pinches to keep them neat and orderly.

Fill, frost, and serve with love.

Good Oat Crust

MAKES ONE 10-INCH PIE CRUST.

This dough dehydrates into a crunchy crust for a classic shell for any fruit filling, especially apples or berries.

1½ cups whole oat groats
4–6 soft dates, pitted
1 tablespoon raw honey or maple
   syrup
2 teaspoons lemon zest

2 teaspoons cinnamon
1 teaspoon nutmeg
½ teaspoon allspice
Pinch sun-dried sea salt

Soak whole oat groats in 3 cups fresh water overnight (about 6–12 hours). Drain and rinse.

In a food processor, chop drained oats, dates, honey or maple syrup, lemon zest, cinnamon, nutmeg, allspice, and sea salt until well mixed. The dough will be quite sticky. Press evenly into a pie plate or torte pan.

To scallop the edge of the crust: Use the thumb and forefinger of your dominant hand to pinch the edge of the dough successively around the rim of the plate or pan. Use the forefinger of your other hand to press against the pinches to keep them neat and orderly.

Dehydrate the crust at 108°F for 12–20 hours or until crunchy.

Fill, frost, and serve with love.

Cookies and Biscotti

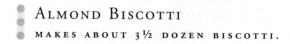

ALMOND BISCOTTI

MAKES ABOUT 3½ DOZEN BISCOTTI.

Sweet almond biscotti are delicious with tea and sliced fruit any time of the day.

2 cups almonds
1 cup pitted dates
2 tablespoons raw almond butter
1 teaspoon non-alcohol vanilla extract
1 teaspoon cinnamon

1 teaspoon almond extract (optional and excellent)
Pinch sun-dried sea salt
30 soaked almonds, cut in half for garnish (optional)

Soak almonds in 4 cups fresh water overnight (about 6–12 hours). Drain and rinse. Soak the dates in 1 cup fresh water for 10–15 minutes until very soft. Drain and set aside soak water.

In a food processor, chop almonds into a fine meal. Add dates, almond butter, vanilla, cinnamon, almond extract (if desired), and sea salt. Blend into a smooth paste. It may be necessary to scrape the sides of the food processor with a rubber spatula and continue to blend for a thorough consistency. Add a few tablespoons of the date soak water as needed to assist in blending smooth.

To form the biscotti: Make approximately 42 balls (about 2 tablespoons of dough each). Place balls on nonstick sheets on dehydrator trays. Use the bottom of a drinking glass to gently press the balls into flat, uniform biscotti. Wipe and wet the bottom of the glass between pressing biscotti to prevent sticking. Gently press almond halves into the biscotti.

Dehydrate at 108°F for 12–20 hours or until quite dry. (Climate, temperature, and humidity all affect dehydrating time.) Flip the biscotti over to dry the underside and return to the dehydrator without the nonstick sheets for 1–2 hours.

Store in a resealable bag in a cool dry place, in the refrigerator, or in the freezer.

PECAN SANDIES
MAKES ABOUT 4 DOZEN COOKIES.

These lovely sweet pecan cookies should be made with a touch of love.

2 cups pecans
½ cup pitted dates
4 tablespoons raw honey
1 teaspoon non-alcohol vanilla extract
Pinch sun-dried sea salt
24 pecan halves for garnish

Soak pecans in 3 cups fresh water for 2–4 hours. Drain and rinse. Soak dates in ½ cup fresh water for 15 minutes or until very soft. Drain off the soak water and set aside.

In a food processor, chop pecans into a fine meal. Add dates, honey, vanilla, and sea salt, and blend into a smooth paste. It may be necessary to scrape the sides of the food processor with a rubber spatula and continue to blend for a smooth consistency. Add a few tablespoons of the date soaking water as needed to assist in blending smooth.

To press the cookies: Make approximately 48 balls (about 1½ tablespoons of dough each). Place balls on nonstick sheets on a dehydrator tray. Use the bottom of a drinking glass to gently press the balls into flat, uniform cookies. Wipe and wet the bottom of the glass between cookies to prevent sticking. Press a pecan half into each cookie.

Dehydrate at 108°F for 12–20 hours or until quite dry. (Climate, temperature, and humidity all affect dehydrating time.) Flip the cookies over to dry the underside and return to the dehydrator without the nonstick sheets for 1–2 hours.

Store in a resealable bag in a cool dry place, in the refrigerator, or in the freezer.

VANILLA BEAN COOKIES
MAKES ABOUT 3 DOZEN COOKIES.

Vanilla bean speckles these sweet creamy cookies for a delicate presentation.

2 cups whole raw cashews (Raw
  cashew pieces can be used.)
⅔ cup pitted dates
1 vanilla bean
¼ cup evaporated cane juice or raw
  honey

2 tablespoons non-alcohol vanilla
  extract
Pinch sun-dried sea salt

Soak cashews in 3 cups fresh water for 1 hour. Drain and rinse. Soak dates in 1 cup fresh water for 15 minutes or until very soft. Drain soak water and set aside. Cut the vanilla bean in half lengthwise. With blade of a small paring knife or the edge of a spoon, scrape out the vanilla bean seeds. Set aside.

In a food processor, chop cashews into a fine meal. Add dates, cane juice or honey, vanilla extract, vanilla bean seeds, and sea salt and blend into a smooth paste. It may be necessary to scrape the sides of the food processor with a rubber spatula and continue to blend for a smooth consistency. Add a few tablespoons of the date soak water as needed to assist in blending smooth. Mix in by hand carob powder, cocoa powder and a tiny pinch of sea salt until well mixed.

To press the cookies: Make approximately 36 balls (about 1½ tablespoons of dough each). Place balls on nonstick sheets on dehydrator trays. Use the bottom of a drinking glass to gently press the balls into flat, uniform cookies. Wipe and wet the bottom of the glass between cookies to prevent sticking.

Dehydrate for 12–24 hours or until quite dry. (Climate, temperature, and humidity all affect dehydrating.) Flip the cookies over to dry the underside and return to the dehydrator without the nonstick sheets for 1–2 hours. The cookies can be dried through and through, or left a little moist inside.

Store in a resealable bag in a cool dry place, in the refrigerator, or in the freezer.

OATMEAL RAISIN COOKIES
MAKES ABOUT 4 DOZEN COOKIES.

*These old-fashioned oatmeal cookies are chock-full of sweet
raisins. Serve fresh from the dehydrator for delicious results.*

2 cups whole oat groats

2 cups raisins

⅔ cup pitted soft dates

2 tablespoons maple syrup or raw
  honey

2 tablespoons cold-pressed coconut
  butter or organic extra-virgin
  olive oil

1 tablespoon lemon zest

1 tablespoon cinnamon

2 teaspoons nutmeg

1 teaspoon allspice

Pinch sun-dried sea salt

½ cup chopped walnuts (optional)

Soak whole oat groats in 4 cups fresh water overnight (about 6–12 hours). Drain and rinse. Soak raisins in 2½ cups fresh water for 15 minutes to soften. Drain the soak water and set aside.

In a food processor, chop oat groats, ½ cup of the raisins, dates, maple syrup or honey, coconut butter or olive oil, lemon zest, cinnamon, nutmeg, allspice, and sea salt thoroughly into a paste. It may be necessary to scrape the sides of the food processor with a rubber spatula and continue to blend for a smooth consistency. Add a few tablespoons of the raisin soak water as needed to assist in blending smooth. By hand, mix in the remaining 1½ cups raisins (and walnuts, if desired).

To press the cookies: Make approximately 48 balls (about 2½ tablespoons of dough each). Place balls on a nonstick sheet on a dehydrator tray. Use the bottom of a drinking glass to gently press the balls into flat, uniform cookies. Wipe and wet the bottom of the glass between cookies to prevent sticking.

Dehydrate at 108°F for 12–24 hours or until fairly dry. (Climate, temperature, and humidity all affect dehydrating time.) Flip the cookies over to dry the underside and return to the dehydrator without the nonstick sheets for 1–2 hours. The cookies should still be moist inside. Serve fresh from the dehydrator.

Store in a resealable bag in a cool dry place, in the refrigerator, or in the freezer.

Coconut Caramel Cookies
MAKES ABOUT 2½ DOZEN COOKIES.

Coconut and caramel marry in these cookies to produce a decadent confection.

3 cups dried shredded coconut
1 cup pitted soft dates
3 tablespoons raw almond butter
2 tablespoons raw honey or maple syrup
2 tablespoons cold-pressed coconut butter or organic extra-virgin olive oil

1 tablespoon non-alcohol vanilla extract
1 tablespoon cinnamon
2 teaspoons nutmeg
Pinch sun-dried sea salt

In a food processor, chop dried coconut, dates, almond butter, raw honey or maple syrup, coconut butter or olive oil, vanilla, cinnamon, nutmeg, and sea salt. The dough should be moist but able to hold a shape. Add a touch more dried coconut if the dough is too moist.

To press the cookies: Make approximately 30 balls (about 1½ tablespoons of dough each). Place balls on nonstick sheets on dehydrator trays. Use the bottom of a drinking glass to gently press the balls into flat, uniform cookies. Wipe and wet the bottom of the glass between cookies to prevent sticking.

Dehydrate at 108°F for 12–24 hours or until fairly dry. (Climate, temperature, and humidity all affect dehydrating time.) Flip the cookies over to dry the underside and return to the dehydrator without the nonstick sheets for 1–2 hours. The cookies should still be moist inside. Serve fresh from the dehydrator.

Store in a resealable bag in a cool dry place, in the refrigerator, or in the freezer.

Ginger Snaps

MAKES ABOUT 3 DOZEN SNAPS.

These spicy, sweet ginger snaps are made with plenty of fresh ginger and just the right spices.

2 cups almonds
1½ cups pitted dates
¼ cup shredded or finely minced ginger
2 tablespoons molasses (optional)

1 tablespoon cinnamon
2 teaspoons nutmeg
½ teaspoon cloves
Pinch sun-dried sea salt

Soak almonds in 4 cups fresh water overnight (about 6–12 hours). Drain and rinse. Soak dates in 1 cup fresh water for 15 minutes. Drain soak water and set aside.

In a food processor, finely chop ginger. Add almonds, dates, molasses (if desired), cinnamon, nutmeg, cloves, and sea salt. Blend into a smooth paste. Add a few tablespoons of date soak water as needed to assist in the blending. It may be necessary to scrape the sides of the food processor with a rubber spatula and continue to blend for a smooth consistency.

To press the cookies: Make approximately 36 balls (about 1½ tablespoons of dough each). Place on nonstick sheets on dehydrator trays. Use the bottom of a drinking glass to gently press the balls into flat, uniform cookies. Wipe and wet the bottom of the glass between cookies to prevent sticking.

Dehydrate at 108°F for 12–24 hours or until quite dry. (Climate, temperature, and humidity all affect dehydrating time.) Flip the cookies over to dry the underside and return to the dehydrator without the nonstick sheets for 1–2 hours. The cookies can be dried to a crisp or left a little moist inside.

Store in a resealable bag in a cool dry place, in the refrigerator, or in the freezer.

Hazelnut Pfeffernüesse
MAKES ABOUT 4 DOZEN COOKIES.

Pfeffernüesse are traditional German spiced holiday cookies.
Serve with warm chai for a warming toast.

2 cups hazelnuts

1 cup whole raw cashews

½ cup raisins

⅓ cup pitted soft dates

¼ cup raw honey or maple syrup

2 tablespoons molasses

1 tablespoon cold-pressed coconut
    butter or organic extra-virgin
    olive oil

2 teaspoons orange zest

2 teaspoons lemon zest

1 tablespoon cinnamon

2 teaspoons nutmeg

Pinch ground cloves

Pinch sun-dried sea salt

Soak 1 cup of the hazelnuts in 2 cups fresh water overnight (about 6–12 hours). Drain and rinse. Soak cashews in 1½ cups fresh water for 1 hour. Drain and rinse. Soak raisins in ½ cup fresh water for 15 minutes to soften. Drain off soak water and set aside.

In a food processor, chop the remaining 1 cup of dry hazelnuts roughly. Set aside. Chop soaked hazelnuts and cashews into a fine meal. Add raisins, dates, honey or maple syrup, molasses, coconut butter or olive oil, orange zest, lemon zest, cinnamon, nutmeg, cloves, and sea salt and blend into a smooth paste. It may be necessary to scrape the sides of the food processor with a rubber spatula and continue to blend for a smooth consistency. Add a little raisin soak water to aid blending if necessary. Mix in dry chopped hazelnuts by hand.

To press the cookies: Make approximately 48 balls (about 2 tablespoons of dough each). Place balls on nonstick sheets on dehydrator trays. Use the bottom of a drinking glass to gently press the balls into flat, uniform cookies. Wipe and wet the bottom of the glass between cookies to prevent sticking.

Dehydrate at 108°F for 12–24 hours or until quite dry. (Climate, temperature, and humidity all affect dehydrating time.) Flip the cookies over to dry the underside and return to the dehydrator without the nonstick sheets for 1–2 hours. The cookies can be dried through and through, or left a little moist inside.

Store in a resealable bag in a cool dry place, in the refrigerator, or in the freezer.

FUDGE COOKIES

MAKES ABOUT 4 DOZEN COOKIES.

*These rich fudge cookies are just right for the chocolate lover
at heart. Try using all carob for a lighter cookie or a blend
of carob and cocoa powder for the real thing.*

1 cup almonds
1½ cups whole raw cashews (Cashew
   pieces can be used.)
1 cup dates, pitted
2 tablespoons maple syrup or raw
   honey
1 tablespoon cold-pressed coconut
   butter or organic extra-virgin
   olive oil

1 tablespoon non-alcohol vanilla
   extract
½ cup raw carob powder
¼ cup organic cocoa powder (or
   4 tablespoons additional raw carob
   powder)
Pinch sun-dried sea salt

Soak almonds in 2 cups fresh water overnight (about 6–12 hours). Drain and rinse. Soak cashews in 2 cups fresh water for 1 hour. Drain and rinse. Soak dates in 1 cup fresh water for 15 minutes or until very soft. Drain soak water and set aside.

In a food processor, chop almonds and cashews into a fine meal. Add dates, maple syrup or honey, coconut butter or olive oil, and vanilla. Blend into a smooth paste. It may be necessary to scrape the sides of the food processor with a rubber spatula and continue to blend for a smooth consistency. Add several tablespoons of the date soak water as needed to blend smooth. Mix in by hand carob powder, cocoa powder, and sea salt until well mixed.

To press the cookies: Make approximately 48 balls (about 1½ tablespoons of dough each). Place balls on nonstick sheets on dehydrator trays. Use the bottom of a drinking glass to gently press the balls into flat, uniform cookies. Wipe and wet the bottom of the glass between cookies to prevent sticking.

Dehydrate at 108°F for 12–24 hours or until quite dry. (Climate, temperature, and humidity all affect dehydrating time.) Flip the cookies over to dry the underside and return to the dehydrator without the nonstick sheets for a few hours. The cookies can be dried through and through, or left a little moist inside.

Store in a resealable bag in a cool dry place, in the refrigerator, or in the freezer.

Valentine Hearts

MAKES ABOUT 5 DOZEN HEART-SHAPED COOKIES.

Be sure to give these sweet raspberry cookies to your sweetheart.
Serve with Vanilla Whole Milk (page 267) or Macadamia
Nut Chocolate Mocha (page 262) for love, sweet love.

1½ cups almonds
1 cup cashews
1 cup pitted dates
1 pint raspberries (Thawed frozen
  raspberries can be used.)
2 tablespoons maple syrup or raw
  honey

2 tablespoons beet powder, or
  2 tablespoons shredded beet
1 tablespoon non-alcohol vanilla
  extract
2 teaspoons cinnamon
Pinch sun-dried sea salt

Soak almonds in 3 cups fresh water overnight (about 6–12 hours). Drain and rinse. Soak raw cashews in 2 cups fresh water for 1 hour. Drain and rinse. Soak dates in 1 cup fresh water for 15 minutes or until very soft. Drain soak water and set aside.

In a food processor, chop almonds and cashews into a fine meal. Add dates, raspberries, maple syrup or honey, beet powder or shredded beet, vanilla, cinnamon, and sea salt, and blend into a smooth paste. It may be necessary to scrape the sides of the food processor with a rubber spatula and continue to blend for a smooth consistency. Add several tablespoons of the date soak water as needed to blend smooth.

To press the cookies: Make approximately 60 balls (about 1½ tablespoons of dough each). Place balls on nonstick sheets on dehydrator trays. Use the bottom of a drinking glass to gently press the balls into flat, uniform cookies. Wipe and wet the bottom of the glass between cookies to prevent sticking. Form the cookies into hearts by hand with clean, moistened fingers: Roll 1½ tablespooons dough into a ball. Place a heart-shaped cookie cutter over the ball of dough and use moist fingers to press the dough into the cookie cutter to make a heart.

Dehydrate at 108°F for 12–24 hours or until quite dry. (Climate, temperature, and humidity all affect dehydrating time.) Flip the cookies over to dry the underside and return to the dehydrator without the nonstick sheets for 1–2 hours. The cookies can be dried through and through, or left a little moist inside.

Store in a resealable bag in a cool dry place, in the refrigerator, or in the freezer.

ALMOND-RASPBERRY THUMBPRINTS
MAKES ABOUT 4 DOZEN COOKIES.

These delicious almond cookies are a wonderful variation of the original.

Almond Dough
2 cups almonds
1 cup pitted dates
2 tablespoons raw almond butter
2 tablespoons raw honey or maple syrup
2 teaspoons cinnamon
1 teaspoon nutmeg

1½ teaspoons almond extract (optional)
Pinch sun-dried sea salt

Jam
1 pint raspberries (Thawed frozen raspberries can be used.)
1 tablespoon non-alcohol vanilla extract

Soak almonds in 4 cups fresh water overnight (about 6–12 hours). Drain and rinse. Soak dates in 1 cup fresh water for 15 minutes or until very soft. Drain soak water and set aside.

In a food processor, chop almonds into a fine meal. Add dates, almond butter, honey or maple syrup, cinnamon, nutmeg, almond extract (if desired), and sea salt, and blend into a smooth paste. It may be necessary to scrape the sides of the food processor with a rubber spatula and continue to blend for a smooth consistency. Add several tablespoons of date soak water as needed to blend smooth. The dough should be firm.

In a food processor, chop raspberries and vanilla until fairly smooth.

To press the cookies: Make approximately 48 balls (about 1½ tablespoons of dough each). Place on nonstick sheets on dehydrator trays. Make a thumbprint in the center of each cookie. Spoon in the raspberry jam to fill the thumbprint.

Dehydrate at 108°F for 12–24 hours or until quite dry. (Climate, temperature, and humidity all affect dehydrating time.) Remove the cookies from the nonstick sheets and return to the dehydrator to dry the underside for 1–2 hours.

Store in a resealable bag in a cool dry place, in the refrigerator, or in the freezer.

Parfaits, Custards,
and Frozen Treats

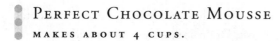

PERFECT CHOCOLATE MOUSSE
MAKES ABOUT 4 CUPS.

This chocolate mousse is simply decadent. Serve in parfait or wine glasses for a lovely presentation, or eat right out of the bowl.

½ cup pitted soft dates
3–4 tablespoons maple syrup
1 tablespoon cold-pressed coconut
    butter (optional)
1½ tablespoons non-alcohol vanilla
    extract

2½ cups mashed avocado (about 3
    medium avocados)
¾ cup raw carob powder
4–6 tablespoons cocoa powder (or
    additional carob powder)

Soak the dates in ½ cup fresh water for 5–10 minutes to soften. Drain the soak water and set aside. In a food processor, blend dates, maple syrup, coconut butter (if desired), and vanilla until smooth. Spoon in avocado and blend until smooth. Add a few tablespoons of date soak water if necessary to aid in blending. Spoon in carob and cocoa powder and blend until smooth.

Spoon mousse into parfait or wineglasses. Keeps fresh for several days.

VARIATION:
Try freezing for a decadent ice cream.

Chocolate Mousse Parfait with Fresh Berries and Vanilla Whip

MAKES 2–4 LAYERED PARFAITS.

This layered parfait with smooth chocolate, creamy vanilla, and fresh berries is divine. The secret in this recipe is the creamy avocados! Carob and cocoa are a sumptuous combination for a rich chocolate flavor. Carob can be used exclusively for lower-impact indulgence.

2 pints raspberries or strawberries, sliced

¾ cup raw carob powder

4–6 tablespoons cocoa powder (or additional carob powder)

Chocolate Mousse

½ cup pitted soft dates

3–4 tablespoons maple syrup

1 tablespoon cold-pressed coconut butter (optional)

1½ tablespoons non-alcohol vanilla extract

2½ cups mashed avocado (about 3 medium avocados)

Vanilla Whip

1 cup whole raw cashews (Raw cashew pieces can be used.)

5 soft dates, pitted

1½ tablespoons non-alcohol vanilla extract

Fresh mint leaves for garnish

To make the chocolate mousse: Soak the dates in ½ cup fresh water for 5–10 minutes to soften. Drain the soak water and set aside. In a food processor, blend dates, maple syrup, coconut butter (if desired), and vanilla until smooth. Spoon in avocado and blend until smooth. Add a few tablespoons of date soak water if necessary to aid in blending. Spoon in carob and cocoa powder and blend until smooth.

To make the vanilla whip: Soak cashews in 2 cups fresh water for 30 minutes. Drain and rinse. Soak dates in ¼ cup fresh water for 5–10 minutes to soften. In a blender, blend drained cashews, dates, date soak water, and vanilla until smooth.

To create a layered effect: Divide mousse in half and spoon into 4–6 parfait or wineglasses. Divide 1 pint of raspberries or sliced strawberries on top of mousse. Spoon remaining mousse on top of the berries. Spoon Vanilla Whip on the second layer of mousse. Top with remaining berries. Garnish with fresh mint.

LIME MERINGUE PARFAIT
WITH MACADAMIA VANILLA BEAN CREAM
MAKES 4–6 LAYERED PARFAITS.

*This is a divine creamy lime meringue with a simple crumble and
luscious vanilla cream. Serve layered in elegant wineglasses.*

1 papaya or mango, diced
1 pint blueberries (optional if
    unavailable)

Crumble
1 cup pecans
1 cup walnuts
¼ cup pitted soft dates
2 teaspoons cinnamon
1 teaspoon nutmeg
Pinch sea salt

Lime Meringue
½ cup pitted soft dates
2 tablespoons raw honey
1½ tablespoons non-alcohol vanilla
    extract
1 tablespoon cold-pressed coconut
    butter (optional)

3 tablespoons lime zest
3 tablespoons lime juice
2½ cups mashed avocado (about 3
    medium avocados)
1 teaspoon spirulina (optional for
    color)
6–12 drops clear stevia (optional)

Vanilla Bean Cream
1 cup macadamia nuts
2 soft dates, pitted
6 tablespoons maple syrup or raw
    honey
1 tablespoon non-alcohol vanilla
    extract
½ vanilla bean

To make the crumble: Soak pecans in 2 cups fresh water for 1–2 hours. Drain and rinse. Spread
the pecans on a dry towel and blot dry or allow to air-dry for 20 minutes.

In a food processor, grind walnuts into a fine meal. Set aside. Grind pecans into a fine meal.
Add dates and pulse-chop until well mixed. Add spices and ground walnuts and pulse-chop until mixed. Divide into 4–6 parfait or wineglasses.

To make the lime meringue: Soak dates in ½ cup fresh water for 5–10 minutes to soften. Drain
the soak water and set aside.

In a food processor or blender, blend dates, honey, vanilla, coconut butter (if desired), lime
zest, and lime juice until smooth. Add 1–2 tablespoons of date soak water if necessary to aid in

blending. Spoon in avocado and spirulina and blend until smooth. Add a few drops of liquid stevia to taste for additional sweetness (if desired). Spoon the meringue on to the crumble.

To make the vanilla bean cream: Soak macadamia nut in 2 cups fresh water for 30 minutes. Drain and rinse. Soak dates in ¼ cup fresh water for 5–10 minutes to soften. Drain the soak water and set aside. Split the vanilla bean lengthwise with a small paring knife. With the edge of a knife or spoon, scrape out all of the tiny seeds. Set aside.

In a blender, blend macadamia nuts, maple syrup or honey, dates, vanilla extract, and vanilla bean until smooth. Add 2 tablespoons or more of date soak water to aid in blending.

Divide the cream and spoon onto meringue. Be sure to cover all of the exposed meringue so it does not brown. Top each parfait with diced papaya or mango and blueberries.

Chill for 1 hour in the refrigerator before serving for best results.

COCONUT CUSTARD FLAN
MAKES 2–4 SERVINGS.

This is simply divine coconut flan with fresh, young coconut meat and a touch of vanilla. Serve in parfait or wineglasses and sprinkle with nutmeg for a lovely presentation.

⅓ cup pitted soft dates or 4–6 tablespoons maple syrup

2 cups fresh young coconut meat

1 tablespoon non-alcohol vanilla extract

2–4 tablespoons coconut water or filtered water as needed

Garnish

2 teaspoons ground fresh nutmeg

Soak dates in ⅓ cup fresh water for 5–10 minutes to soften.

In a blender, blend coconut meat, dates or maple syrup, and vanilla into a smooth cream. Add water 1 tablespoon at a time only as needed to blend. Keep as thick as possible. Spoon into parfait or wineglasses. Garnish with fresh grated nutmeg.

Mango Coconut Flan
MAKES 2–4 SERVINGS.

Fresh coconut meat makes this flan more creamy, though dried coconut can be used if fresh coconut is unavailable. Sweetened simply with dried mango. Serve solo or with sliced fresh mango or kiwi.

1 cup dried mango (Be sure that no sugar or sulfur has been added to the dried fruit.)
1 vanilla bean
1½ cups dried shredded coconut
1 cup fresh young coconut meat (If fresh coconut is unavailable, use

½ cup additional dried mango, cut and soaked, and ½ cup additional dried coconut.)
1 tablespoon non-alcohol vanilla extract

With a pair of kitchen scissors, cut the dried mango into pieces. Soak in 1 cup fresh water until soft (about 5–15 minutes). Retain the soak water. Split the vanilla bean lengthwise with a small paring knife. With the edge of a knife or spoon, scrape out all of the tiny seeds. Set aside.

In a food processor or blender, grind dried coconut into a powder. Set aside. Blend fresh coconut meat as smooth as possible and set aside. Blend softened mango and soak water until smooth. Add ground fresh and dried coconut, vanilla extract, and vanilla bean and blend until smooth. Divide into 2–4 parfait or wineglasses.

Blueberry Nectarine Parfait
MAKES 2–4 PARFAITS.

These parfaits are gorgeously layered with sweet fresh nectarines and succulent blueberries and a creamy violet blueberry custard.

2 ripe nectarines, pitted, peeled, and thinly sliced
1–2 pints fresh blueberries

Violet Custard
1 cup whole raw cashews (Raw cashew pieces can be used.) or macadamia nuts

1 cup dried blueberries (If dried blueberries are unavailable, use ½ cup pitted soft dates and ½ cup fresh blueberries.)
2 tablespoons raw honey or maple syrup
1 tablespoon non-alcohol vanilla extract

To make the violet custard: Soak cashews or macadamia nuts in 2 cups fresh water for 30 minutes. Drain and rinse. Soak the dried blueberries in 1 cup fresh water until soft (about 5–15 minutes). Drain the soak water and set aside. (If dates are being used, pit the dates and soak in ½ cup fresh water for 5–10 minutes to soften. Drain the soak water and set aside.)

In a blender, blend the nuts, blueberries (or dates and fresh blueberries), ¼ cup blueberry soak water, honey or maple syrup, and vanilla until smooth. Add soak water 2 tablespoons at a time to aid in blending.

To assemble the parfait: In 2–4 parfait or wine glasses, place several slices of nectarine. Spoon on some violet custard. Add another a layer of nectarine slices and fresh blueberries. Spoon remaining violet custard and top with remaining blueberries.

SUMMER PEACH PARFAIT
MAKES 2–4 PARFAITS.

This parfait is the essence of sweet summer with its succulent
peaches and creamy almond custard. Add fresh blueberries
for texture and color.

1 cup almonds	1 teaspoon cinnamon
3 peaches	2 teaspoons nutmeg
2 tablespoons almond butter	Pinch sun-dried sea salt
¼ cup raw honey or maple syrup	1 pint blueberries (optional)
¼ cup orange juice	
1 tablespoon non-alcohol vanilla extract	

Soak almonds in 3 cups fresh water overnight (about 6–12 hours). Drain and rinse. Cut the peaches in half and remove the pit. Peel the peaches and thinly slice.

To make the almond custard: In a blender, blend 1 peeled and sliced peach, drained almonds, almond butter, honey or maple syrup, orange juice, vanilla, cinnamon, nutmeg, and sea salt until smooth. Add a few additional tablespoons of orange juice if necessary to aid in blending.

In 2–4 parfait or wine glasses, add a layer of sliced peaches, then a layer of almond custard. Top with another layer of sliced peaches and another layer of custard. Top with fresh blueberries if desired.

Frozen Strawberry-Peach Torte with Blueberries and Orange Crème Whip

MAKES 8–10 SLICES.

This blushing cream pie with whole blueberries and smooth vanilla whip is a perfect treat for a summer birthday.

Strawberry-Peach Torte

6 peaches

1 pint strawberries

4 tablespoons agave syrup or raw honey

1 tablespoon non-alcohol vanilla extract

1 pint blueberries

Orange Crème Whip

1½ cups whole raw cashews (Raw cashew pieces can be used.)

½ cup pitted dates

½ cup orange juice

2 teaspoons orange zest

1½ tablespoons non-alcohol vanilla extract

To make the strawberry peach torte: Cut the peaches in half and remove the pits. Peel the peaches and cut into slices. Cut the tops out of the strawberries. Cut the strawberries in half. Freeze the peaches and strawberries until solid in a zip-lock bag or plastic container.

In a masticating or triturating juicer (see "Juicing at Home," page 205), with the homogenizing "blank" plate, alternate pressing the frozen peaches and strawberries through for a pretty swirl. Mix in agave syrup or honey and vanilla. Gently fold in blueberries. Press the mixture into a 10-inch pie plate and place in the freezer.

To make the orange crème whip: Soak cashews in 2 cups fresh water for 30 minutes. Drain and rinse. Soak the dates in ½ cup orange juice for 5–10 minutes to soften.

In a blender, blend cashews, dates, orange juice, orange zest, and vanilla until smooth. It may be necessary to add a few more tablespoons of orange juice to aid in blending.

Spread the whip on the frozen torte and return to the freezer for an hour or two to chill until firm. The torte can be frozen for several days.

Allow to thaw for 10–15 minutes before serving. Serve each piece with a slice of fresh strawberry.

Crackers, Crisps, and Flat Breads

Crackers and Crisps

SESAME FLAX CRACKERS
MAKES 6–8 CUPS OF CHIPS.

Made with ground and whole sesame seeds, these flax crackers are rich in calcium, protein, and healthy oils for beautiful hair and skin. Serve with soup, salad, or dip.

2 cups flaxseeds
2 cups sesame seeds
1–2 cloves garlic (optional)
1–2 teaspoons sun-dried sea salt

Soak flaxseeds in 4 cups fresh water. The flaxseeds will absorb most or all of the water. In a food processor or blender, grind 1 cup of the sesame seeds into a fine meal. Set aside. Grind the soaked flaxseeds and garlic (if desired) in several batches. It may be necessary to add additional fresh water to aid the grinding. The flaxseeds should be broken, but it is not necessary to blend smooth.

Mix the ground sesame seeds, flaxseeds, whole sesame seeds, and sea salt thoroughly in a bowl with clean, wet hands. Spread the mixture in a thin layer on nonstick sheets to the edges on a dehydrator tray. Use clean, wet hands or a rubber spatula for easy spreading.

Dehydrate at 108°F for 12–20 hours or until mostly dry. Peel away the nonstick sheets and cut the flax sheets into triangles, rectangles, or squares. Return to the dehydrator without the nonstick sheets and dry for 1–2 hours until crispy. (Climate, temperature, and humidity all affect dehydrating time.)

Store in a resealable bag in a cool dry place, in the refrigerator, or in the freezer.

SUN-FIRED TOMATO CRACKERS
MAKES 6–8 CUPS OF CHIPS.

Sun-dried tomatoes lend a sweet and savory flavor to these crunchy crackers. Try a little heat for a kick.

2 cups flaxseeds
1½ cups sun-dried tomatoes
2 cloves garlic
3 tablespoons dried Italian herb
    seasoning

1–2 teaspoons chipotle or chili pepper
    (optional for a touch of heat)
1–2 teaspoons sun-dried sea salt, or to
    taste
3–4 tomatoes, thinly sliced (optional)

Soak flaxseeds in 4 cups fresh water for 15–20 minutes or until saturated. The flaxseeds will absorb most or all of the water. Soak sun-dried tomatoes in 2 cups fresh water until soft (about 5–15 minutes). Reserve the soak water.

In a food processor or blender, blend the sun-dried tomatoes, sun-dried tomato soak water, and garlic until smooth. Set aside.

Grind soaked flaxseeds in several batches. It may be necessary to add additional fresh water to aid the grinding. The flaxseeds should be broken but do not have to be blended until smooth.

Mix the blended sun-dried tomato mixture, ground flaxseeds, dried herbs, chipotle or chili pepper (if desired), and sea salt thoroughly in a bowl with clean, wet hands. Spread the mixture in a thin layer on nonstick sheets to the edges on a dehydrator tray. Use clean, wet hands or a rubber spatula for easy spreading. Lay the sliced tomatoes decoratively on top of the spread flaxseeds mixture, if desired.

Dehydrate at 108°F for 12–20 hours or until mostly dry. Peel away the nonstick sheets and cut the flax sheets into triangles, rectangles, or squares. Return to the dehydrator without the nonstick sheets and dry for 1–2 hours until crispy. (Climate, temperature, and humidity all affect dehydrating time.)

Store in a resealable bag in a cool dry place, in the refrigerator, or in the freezer.

GARLIC-CHILI FLAX CHIPS
MAKES 6–8 CUPS OF CHIPS.

These spicy hot chili chips are rich in healthy omega oils and protein. Turn up the heat as much as you like. Great with guacamole and salsa.

2 cups flaxseeds
4 cloves garlic
1 tablespoon chili pepper
Pinch cayenne pepper
2 teaspoons sun-dried sea salt

Soak flaxseeds in 4 cups fresh water for 15–20 minutes or until saturated. The flaxseeds will absorb most or all of the water. In a food processor or blender, grind the flaxseeds, garlic, chili pepper, and cayenne pepper in several batches. It may be necessary to add additional fresh water to aid the grinding. The flaxseeds should be broken, but it is not necessary to blend smooth.

Mix in sea salt thoroughly with clean, wet hands. Spread the mixture in a thin layer on nonstick sheets to the edges on a dehydrator tray. Use clean, wet hands or a rubber spatula for easy spreading.

Dehydrate at 108°F for 12–20 hours or until mostly dry. Peel away the nonstick sheets and cut the flax sheets into triangles, rectangles, or squares. Return to the dehydrator without the nonstick sheets and dry for 1–2 hours until crispy. (Climate, temperature, and humidity all affect dehydrating time.)

Store in a resealable bag in a cool dry place, in the refrigerator, or in the freezer.

FENNEL PUMPKIN CHIPS
MAKES 4–6 CUPS OF CHIPS.

Pumpkin seeds are rich in protein, vitamin A, phosphorus, and healthy oils. Ginger and fennel seeds help balance blood sugar and promote good digestion.

3 cups pumpkin seeds
1 cup flaxseeds

½ cup lemon juice
¼ cup nama shoyu

2 tablespoons raw honey, maple
    syrup, or 4 soft dates, pitted
3 tablespoons fennel seeds
1 tablespoon chopped ginger

2 cups fresh water, or as necessary to
    blend
Pinch sun-dried sea salt, or to taste

Soak pumpkin seeds in 5 cups fresh water overnight (about 6–12 hours). Drain and rinse. Grind flaxseeds into a meal in a food processor, blender, or coffee mill.

Blend soaked pumpkin seeds, lemon juice, nama shoyu, honey (or maple syrup or dates), fennel seeds, and ginger in a blender or food processor with enough water to blend into a smooth paste.

In a bowl, mix ground flaxseeds into the mixture and season with sea salt. Spread the mixture thinly on nonstick sheets to the edges of the dehydrator trays. Use a rubber spatula for easy spreading.

Dehydrate at 108°F for 12–20 hours or until almost dry. Peel the off the nonstick sheets. Cut into triangles, squares, or rectangles. Return to the dehydrator without the nonstick sheets for a few hours or until crispy. (Climate, temperature, and humidity all affect dehydrating time.)

Store in resealable bags in a cool dry place, in the refrigerator, or in the freezer.

Sweet Potato Crisps
MAKES 4–6 CUPS OF CRISPS.

Seasoned sweet potatoes, nutty flaxseeds, and almonds blend together for sweet and savory crispy chips. Serve with soup or salad or a spread.

3 cups peeled and shredded sweet
    potato
¼ cup lemon juice
1 cup almonds
2 cups flaxseeds
2 cloves garlic

1 cup chopped red onion
1 tablespoon dried rosemary
1 tablespoon savory or thyme
1 tablespoon coriander seeds
1–2 teaspoons sun-dried sea salt

Soak sweet potato in ¼ cup lemon juice and 3 cups fresh water overnight (about 6–12 hours) to leech excess starch. Drain and rinse in a strainer. Soak almonds in 2 cups fresh water overnight (about 6–12 hours). Drain and rinse. Soak flaxseeds in 4 cups fresh water for 15–20 minutes or until saturated. The flaxseeds will absorb most or all of the water.

Grind the sweet potato, almonds, flaxseeds, garlic, red onion, rosemary, savory or thyme, and coriander seeds. This can be done in a masticating or triturating juicer (see "Juicing at Home," page 205), with the homogenizing "blank" plate. Alternatively, they can be ground in a food processor or blender in several batches, adding fresh water as necessary to blend smooth.

In a bowl, mix sea salt into mixture with clean, wet hands. Spread the mixture thinly on nonstick sheets to the edges of the dehydrator trays. Use a rubber spatula for easy spreading.

Dehydrate at 108°F for 12–20 hours or until almost dry. Peel the off the nonstick sheets. Cut into triangles, squares, or rectangles. Return to the dehydrator without the nonstick sheets for a few hours or until crispy. (Climate, temperature, and humidity all affect dehydrating time.)

Store in resealable bags in a cool dry place, in the refrigerator, or in the freezer.

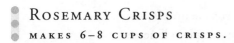

ROSEMARY CRISPS
MAKES 6–8 CUPS OF CRISPS.

Warming, savory rosemary seasons these crunchy crisps.
Serve with soup or salad or any spread or dip.

2 cups sunflower seeds	4–6 tablespoons dried rosemary
2 cups walnuts	4 tablespoons apple cider vinegar
1 cup whole raw cashews (Raw cashew pieces can be used.)	1 cup ground flaxseeds
3 medium tomatoes, diced	1 tablespoon raw honey or maple syrup
1 cup chopped celery	1–2 teaspoons sun-dried sea salt, or to taste
1 clove garlic	
1 cup chopped red onion	

Soak sunflower seeds and walnuts together in 6 cups fresh water overnight (about 6–12 hours). Drain and rinse. Soak cashews in 2 cups fresh water for 1 hour. Drain and rinse. Grind sunflower seeds, walnuts, cashews, diced tomatoes, celery, garlic, red onion, and rosemary. This can be done in a masticating or triturating juicer (see "Juicing at Home," page 205), with the homogenizing "blank" plate. Alternatively, they can be ground in a food processor or blender in several batches, adding the apple cider vinegar and some fresh water as necessary to blend smooth.

In a bowl, mix ground flaxseeds, raw honey or maple syrup, and sea salt thoroughly into mixture. Spread the mixture thinly on nonstick sheets to the edges of the dehydrator trays. Use clean, wet hands or a rubber spatula for easy spreading.

Dehydrate at 108°F for 12–20 hours or until almost dry. Peel the off the nonstick sheets. Cut into triangles, squares, or rectangles. Return to the dehydrator without the nonstick sheets for a few hours or until crispy. (Climate, temperature, and humidity all affect dehydrating time.)

Store in resealable bags in a cool dry place, in the refrigerator, or in the freezer.

CHILI LIME CORN CHIPS
MAKES 4–6 CUPS OF CHIPS.

These fresh corn chips with a kick of chili pepper and lime are great with guacamole or salsa. Add more chili pepper for more heat.

2 cups whole raw cashews	1 cup cilantro leaves
6 ears fresh corn	1 tablespoon lime zest
2 cups ground golden flaxseeds	½ cup lime juice
(Brown flaxseeds can be	1 tablespoon dried chili pepper
substituted.)	1 tablespoon ground coriander seeds
3 cloves garlic	1–2 teaspoons sun-dried sea salt
1 cup parsley leaves	

Soak cashews in 4 cups fresh water for 1–2 hours. Drain and rinse. Cut the corn from the cob. Grind the flaxseeds into a meal in a blender or coffee mill.

Grind the cashews, corn, garlic, parsley, and cilantro. This can be done in a masticating or triturating juicer (see "Juicing at Home," page 205), with the homogenizing "blank" plate. Alternatively, they can be ground in a food processor or blender in several batches, adding some fresh water as necessary to blend smooth.

In a bowl, mix lime zest, lime juice, chili pepper, coriander seeds, and sea salt thoroughly into mixture. Spread the mixture thinly on nonstick sheets to the edges of the dehydrator trays. Use clean, wet hands or a rubber spatula for easy spreading.

Dehydrate at 108°F for 12–20 hours or until almost dry. Peel the off the nonstick sheets. Cut into triangles, squares, or rectangles. Return to the dehydrator without the nonstick sheets for a few hours or until crispy. (Climate, temperature, and humidity all affect dehydrating time.)

Store in resealable bags in a cool dry place, in the refrigerator, or in the freezer.

Flat Breads

RYE FLATS

MAKES 8–10 FLATS.

Rye is unusually rich in fluorine, which is great for healthy teeth and enamel. Chew these rye flats well, and smile bright.

3 cups whole rye for sprouting (yields
    4 cups)
4 tablespoons caraway seeds
2 tablespoons dried dill
2 teaspoons sun-dried sea salt, or
    to taste

To sprout the rye: In a wide-mouth glass jar, covered with screen and secured with a rubber band, soak whole rye in 5 cups fresh water overnight (about 6–12 hours). Drain and rinse. Allow to stand, draining upside down at a 45-degree angle. Rinse and drain two times a day until the sprouting tails are as long as the grain (2–4 days).

Grind the sprouted rye. This can be done in a masticating or triturating juicer (see "Juicing at Home," page 205), with the homogenizing "blank" plate. The sprouted rye can also be ground in two batches in the food processor, adding a little fresh water as necessary to blend into a smooth paste.

Mix the rye with caraway seeds, dill, and sea salt in a bowl with clean, wet hands. Press ½ cup of dough into flat rounds ¼-inch-thick on nonstick sheets on dehydrator trays.

Dehydrate at 108°F for 12–20 hours or until a crust has formed. Flip the flats over to dry the underside for 1–2 hours. (Climate, temperature, and humidity all affect dehydrating time.) The flats can be dried until crisp or left a little moist.

Store in a resealable bag in a cool dry place, in the refrigerator, or in the freezer.

PIZZA CRUSTS
MAKES 6–12 CRUSTS.

Spread with Walnut Pesto (page 302) or Macadamia Nut Ricotta (page 315) and Sun-Fired Tomato Marinara (page 375) and finely chopped vegetables or marinated mushrooms for a dynamic, flavorful pizza.

2 cups spelt, whole kamut, or spring wheat berries for sprouting (yields 3 cups)
2 cloves garlic
1 cup flaxseeds
1 cup minced red onion
1 cup shredded carrot
1 cup diced red bell pepper or shredded beet

½ cup chopped basil
½ cup chopped parsley
1 tablespoon dried rosemary
1 tablespoon dried oregano
2 tablespoons organic extra-virgin olive oil
2 teaspoons sun-dried sea salt, or to taste

To sprout the spelt, kamut, or wheat berries: In a wide-mouth glass jar covered with screen and secured with a rubber band, soak 2 cups whole spelt, kamut, or soft spring wheat berries in 4 cups fresh water overnight (about 6–12 hours). Drain and rinse. Allow to stand, draining upside down at a 45-degree angle. Rinse and drain two times a day until the sprouting tails are as long as the grain (about 2–4 days).

Grind sprouted spelt, kamut, or wheat and garlic. This can be done in a masticating or triturating juicer (see "Juicing at Home," page 205), with the homogenizing "blank" plate. The sprouted spelt, kamut, or wheat and garlic can also be ground in a few batches in the food processor, adding a little fresh water as necessary to blend into a smooth paste.

Soak flaxseeds in 2 cups fresh water for 15 minutes or until saturated. The flaxseeds should absorb most or all of the water. Mix sprouted grain mixture with flaxseeds, red onion, carrot, bell pepper or beet, basil, parsley, rosemary, oregano, olive oil, and sea salt thoroughly in bowl with clean, wet hands. Press into round ¼-inch-thick flats on nonstick sheets on dehydrator trays.

Dehydrate for 12–20 hours at 108°F or until a dry crust forms. Flip over the flats to dry the underside for 1–2 hours. (Climate, temperature, and humidity all affect dehydrating time.) The flats can be dried to a crisp or left a little moist.

Store in a resealable bag in a cool dry place, in the refrigerator, or in the freezer.

COUNSELOR'S STAFF

MAKES 10–12 FLATS.

This recipe comes from the brilliant mind and seasoned palate of our environmental attorney Tom Ballanco. Tom suggests serving it spread with cold-pressed coconut butter or avocado and a pinch of sun-dried sea salt. Our friend Julia Butterfly likes it with a mad amount of garlic, so add a few extra cloves for her.

2½ cups whole kamut for sprouting (yields 4 cups)
2 cups flaxseeds
1 cup hulled hemp seeds or sesame seeds
2–4 cloves garlic
4 green onions, chopped to the top

2–3 tablespoons oregano
¼ cup organic extra-virgin olive oil
Pinch cayenne pepper, or to taste
1 teaspoon sun-dried sea salt
1 cup pitted and chopped kalamata olives

To sprout the kamut: In a wide-mouth glass jar covered with screen and secured with a rubber band, soak 2½ cups whole kamut in 6 cups fresh water overnight (about 6–12 hours). Drain and rinse. Allow to stand, draining upside down on a 45-degree angle. Rinse and drain two times a day until the sprouting tails are as long as the grain (about 2–4 days).

Soak the flaxseeds in 4 cups fresh water for 15 minutes or until saturated. The flaxseeds should absorb most or all of the water. Grind together the sprouted kamut, soaked flaxseeds, hemp or sesame seeds, garlic, green onions, and oregano. This can be done in a masticating or triturating juicer (see "Juicing at Home," page 205), with the homogenizing "blank" plate. Alternatively, they can be ground in the food processor in a few batches, adding a little fresh water as necessary to blend into a smooth paste.

Mix the dough together with olive oil, cayenne pepper, sea salt, and olives using clean, wet hands. Press into round ¼-inch-thick flats on nonstick sheets on dehydrator trays.

Dehydrate for 12–20 hours at 108°F or until a dry crust forms. Flip over the flats to dry the underside for a few hours. (Climate, temperature, and humidity all affect dehydrating time.) The flats can be dried to a crisp or left a little moist. (Tom likes them a little moist.)

Store in a resealable bag in a cool dry place, in the refrigerator, or in the freezer.

Manitok Wild Rice Flat Bread
MAKES 8–10 FLATS.

Nutty wild rice is ground and seasoned to make these hearty flats rich in protein and B vitamins. Serve with a salad or as an open-faced sandwich with hummus or pâté, avocado, tomato, and sprouts.

2 cups long-grain wild rice for
    sprouting (yields 3 cups)
1 cup chia seeds or flaxseeds
1 ear corn
4 soft dates, pitted
¼ cup dulse
2 cloves garlic

4 green onions, chopped to the top
1 cup parsley leaves
1 cup cilantro leaves
1 cup basil leaves
2 tablespoons raw almond butter
1 tablespoon coriander seeds
1 teaspoon sun-dried sea salt

To sprout the long-grain wild rice: In a widemouthed glass jar, covered with screen and secured with a rubber band, soak 2 cups long-grain wild rice in 4 cups fresh water overnight (about 6–12 hours). Drain and rinse. Allow to stand, draining upside down on a 45-degree angle. Rinse and drain two times a day until the sprouting rice is soft and split open (about 2–5 days).

Soak chia seeds or flaxseeds in 2 cups fresh water for 15 minutes or until saturated. The chia seeds or flaxseeds will absorb most or all of the water. Cut the corn from the cob.

Grind the sprouted wild rice with the chia seeds or flaxseeds, dates, corn, dulse, garlic, green onions, parsley, cilantro, and basil. This can be done in a masticating or triturating juicer (see "Juicing at Home," page 205), with the homogenizing "blank" plate. It can also be ground in a few batches in the food processor, adding a little fresh water as necessary to blend into a smooth paste.

Mix with almond butter, coriander seeds, and sea salt with clean, wet hands. Press into round or square ¼-inch flat breads on nonstick sheets on dehydrator trays.

Dehydrate at 108°F for 12–20 hours or until a crust has formed. Flip over and dry the underside for a few hours. (Climate, temperature, and humidity all affect dehydrating time.) These flat breads can be dried to a crisp or preferably left a little moist.

Store in a resealable bag in a cool dry place, in the refrigerator, or in the freezer.

FALAFEL FLATS

MAKES 6–8 FLATS.

This savory garbanzo-bean falafel with all of the authentic herbs and spices can be served with hummus, cucumber, and tomato slices.

2 cups garbanzo beans for sprouting
  (yields 4 cups)
3 cloves garlic
2 cups finely chopped parsley leaves
¼ cup raw tahini

½ cup lemon juice
1 tablespoon lemon zest
1 tablespoon paprika
2 teaspoons sun-dried sea salt

To sprout garbanzo beans: In a widemouthed glass jar covered with screen and secured with a rubber band, soak garbanzo beans in 4 cups fresh water overnight (about 6–12 hours). Drain and rinse. Allow to stand, draining upside down on a 45-degree angle. Rinse and drain two times a day until the sprouting tail is as long as the bean (about 2–3 days).

Grind the sprouted garbanzo beans with garlic and parsley. This can be done in a masticating or triturating juicer (see "Juicing at Home," page 205), with the homogenizing "blank" plate. It can also be ground in a few batches in a food processor, adding lemon juice as necessary to blend into a smooth paste.

Mix ground sprouted garbanzo beans, garlic, and parsley with raw tahini, lemon juice, lemon zest, paprika, and sea salt. Press into round ¼-inch-thick flats on nonstick sheets or dehydrator trays.

Dehydrate at 108°F for 12–20 hours or until a crust forms. Flip over and dry the undersides for 1–2 hours. (Climate, temperature, and humidity all affect dehydrating time.)

Store in a resealable bag in a cool dry place, in the refrigerator, or in the freezer.

CORN BUCKWHEAT TORTILLAS

MAKES 10–12 TORTILLAS.

Sweet corn and buckwheat seasoned with fresh herbs and spices make crunchy tortillas. Great for serving with guacamole and salsa and a fresh salad.

2 cups buckwheat
1 cup almonds

4 ears fresh corn
1 clove garlic

1 cup parsley leaves

1 cup cilantro leaves

1 tablespoon coriander seeds

2 teaspoons cumin seeds

2 teaspoons sun-dried sea salt

Soak buckwheat in 5 cups fresh water overnight (about 6–12 hours). Drain and rinse until the rinse water runs clear. Soak almonds in 3 cups fresh water overnight (about 6–12 hours). Drain and rinse. Cut the corn from the cob.

Grind the buckwheat, almonds, corn, garlic, parsley, and cilantro. This can be done in a masticating or triturating juicer (see "Juicing at Home," page 205), with the homogenizing "blank" plate. It can also be ground in a few batches in the food processor, adding a little fresh water as necessary to blend into a smooth paste.

In a bowl, add coriander seeds, cumin seeds, and sea salt thoroughly into the mixture with clean, wet hands. Press into thin, round flats on nonstick sheets on dehydrator trays.

Dehydrate at 108°F for 12–20 hours or until dry. Flip over and dry the undersides for an hour or two until crunchy. (Climate, temperature, and humidity all affect dehydrating time.)

Store in a resealable bag in a cool dry place, in the refrigerator, or in the freezer.

ZUCCHINI SPELT FLAT BREAD
MAKES 10–12 FLATS.

Fresh zucchini and herbs complement this lovely spelt bread.
Serve with soup, salad, or as an open-faced sandwich.

2 cups whole spelt for sprouting
(yields 3 cups) (Soft spring wheat
berries can be substituted.)

1 cup sunflower seeds

½ cup golden raisins

2 zucchini, chopped

1 cup parsley leaves

1 cup cilantro leaves

½ cup basil leaves

2 teaspoons fennel seeds

2 teaspoons dried dill

2 tablespoons white miso

1 teaspoon sun-dried sea salt

To sprout the spelt: In a widemouthed glass jar covered with screen and secured with a rubber band, soak spelt in 5 cups fresh water overnight (about 6–12 hours). Drain and rinse. Allow to stand, draining upside down on a 45-degree angle. Rinse and drain two times a day until the sprouting tail is as long as the grain (about 2–3 days).

Soak the sunflower seeds in 2 cups fresh water for 2–4 hours. Drain and rinse. Soak the golden raisins in 1 cup fresh water for 15 minutes to soften. Drain the soak water and set aside to aid in grinding.

Grind the sprouted spelt, sunflower seeds, raisins, zucchini, parsley, cilantro, and basil. This can be done in a masticating or triturating juicer (see "Juicing at Home," page 205), with the homogenizing "blank" plate. It can also be ground in a few batches in the food processor, adding a little raisin soak water as necessary to blend into a smooth paste.

In a bowl, mix the fennel seeds, dill, miso, and sea salt into the mixture with clean, wet hands. Press into thin, round or square flats on nonstick sheets on dehydrator trays.

Dehydrate at 108°F for 12–20 hours or until a crust has formed. Flip over and dry the undersides for an hour or two. (Climate, temperature, and humidity all affect dehydrating time.) The flats can be dried to a crisp or left a little moist.

Store in a resealable bag in a cool dry place, in the refrigerator, or in the freezer.

MUESLI FLAT BREAD
MAKES 10–12 FLATS.

This sweet and nutty flat bread with dried fruit and a touch of spices is great with almond butter and sliced fruit or as a snack on the go.

2 cups whole oat groats	1 cup chopped almonds
1 cup buckwheat	½ cup pumpkin seeds
1 cup flaxseeds	½ cup sunflower seeds
1 cup raisins	1 tablespoon cinnamon
1 cup dried apricots	1 teaspoon sun-dried sea salt

Soak whole oat groats in 4 cups fresh water overnight (about 6–12 hours). Soak buckwheat in 3 cups fresh water overnight (about 6–12 hours). Drain and rinse the oats, buckwheat, almonds, pumpkin seeds, and sunflower seeds. The buckwheat may need to be rinsed several times until the rinse water runs clear. Soak almonds in 2 cups of fresh water. Soak pumpkin seeds and sunflower seeds together in 2 cups of fresh water for 2–4 hours. Soak the flaxseeds in 2 cups fresh water for 15 minutes or until saturated. The flaxseeds will absorb most or all of the water. Soak the raisins in 1½ cups fresh water for 15 minutes to soften. With a pair of kitchen scissors, cut the apricots into pieces. Soak in 1½ cups fresh water for 15 minutes or until soft.

Grind the oats, ½ cup of the soaked buckwheat, and the flaxseeds with ½ cup soaked raisins and ½ cup soaked apricots. This can be done in a masticating or triturating juicer (see "Juicing at Home," page 205), with the homogenizing "blank" plate. They can also be ground in a few batches in a food processor, adding a little of the raisin soak water as necessary to blend into a smooth paste.

Mix the remaining buckwheat, raisins, apricots, almonds, pumpkin seeds, sunflower seeds, cinnamon, and sea salt into the mixture with clean, wet hands. Press into round ¼-inch-thick flats on nonstick sheets on dehydrator trays.

Dehydrate for 12–20 hours at 108°F or until a dry crust forms. Flip over the flats to dry the undersides for a few hours. (Climate, temperature, and humidity all affect dehydrating time.) The flats can be dried to a crisp or left a little moist.

Store in a resealable bag in a cool dry place, in the refrigerator, or in the freezer.

SPICED HONEY BREAD
MAKES 6–8 FLAT LOAVES.

These sweet, moist flat loaves with enzyme-rich honey and warming spices can be served with almond butter or a sweet nut cream and fresh fruit.

2 cups whole spelt or spring wheat
    berries for sprouting (yields 3 cups)
½ cup pitted soft dates
1½ tablespoons chopped ginger
1 cup raw honey
2 tablespoons cold-pressed coconut
    butter or organic extra-virgin
    olive oil

1 tablespoon cinnamon
½ teaspoon cloves
Pinch sun-dried sea salt

To sprout the whole spelt or spring wheat berries: In a wide-mouth glass jar covered with screen and secured with a rubber band, soak whole kamut in 4 cups fresh water overnight (about 6–12 hours). Drain and rinse. Allow to stand, draining upside down on a 45-degree angle. Rinse and drain two times a day until the sprouting tails are as long as the grain (about 2–4 days).

Soak the dates in ¾ cup fresh water for 5–15 minutes or until very soft. Drain the soak water.

Grind the sprouted spelt or wheat berries, dates, and ginger. Use some of the date soak water to help the process. This can be done in a masticating or triturating juicer (see "Juicing at Home," page 205), with the homogenizing "blank" plate. They can also be ground in a few batches in a food processor, adding a little date soak water as necessary to blend into a smooth paste.

In a bowl, mix the ground sprouted grain, honey, cold-pressed coconut butter or olive oil, cinnamon, cloves, and sea salt into the mixture with clean, wet hands. Press the dough into 1- to 1½-inch rectangular loaves on nonstick sheets on dehydrator trays.

Dehydrate at 108°F for 20–24 hours or until a crust has formed. Flip the loaves over to dry the undersides for a few hours. (Climate, temperature, and humidity all affect dehydrating time.) The loaves should be well formed and moist.

APPLE WALNUT FLAT LOAVES
MAKES 8–10 FLATS.

*Fresh apple and dried apple are complemented by walnuts and a
touch of spices in this sweet, moist breakfast or dessert bread.
Serve with almond butter and fresh apple or pear slices for
a delicious treat.*

2 cups soaked kamut or spelt
1 cup flaxseeds
1 cup dried apples
4 cups peeled and chopped apples
½ cup chopped celery
1 cup chopped walnuts
2 tablespoons organic extra-virgin
  olive oil

1 tablespoon lemon zest
1 tablespoon cinnamon
½ teaspoon allspice or nutmeg
1 teaspoon sun-dried sea salt
2 apples, peeled and cut into rings or
  thin slices
Sprinkle of cinnamon for garnish

To sprout the kamut or spelt: In a widemouthed glass jar covered with screen and secured with a rubber band, soak the kamut or spelt in 5 cups fresh water overnight (about 6–12 hours). Drain and rinse. Allow to stand, draining upside down on a 45-degree angle. Rinse and drain two times a day until the sprouting tail is as long as the grain (about 2–3 days).

Soak the flaxseeds in 2 cups fresh water for 15 minutes or until saturated. The flaxseeds will absorb most or all of the water. Chop the dried apple and soak in 1½ cups fresh water for 15 minutes to soften. Drain the soak water and use to aid in grinding.

Grind the sprouted grain, flaxseeds, chopped apple, celery, and dried apple. This can be done in a masticating or triturating juicer (see "Juicing at Home," page 205), with the homogenizing "blank" plate. They can also be ground in a few batches in a food processor, adding a little dried apple soak water as necessary to blend into a smooth paste.

Mix walnuts, olive oil, lemon zest, cinnamon, allspice or nutmeg, and sea salt into the mixture with clean, wet hands. Press into round, square, or oval loaves ½ inch to 1 inch thick on nonstick sheets on dehydrator trays. Press apple slices onto the loaves to decorate, and garnish with cinnamon.

Dehydrate at 108°F for 20–24 hours or until a crust forms. Flip over to dry the undersides for 1–2 hours. (Climate, temperature, and humidity all affect dehydrating time.) The bread should be moist. It's best served warm.

34

Dehydrated Extras

Fruit Leather

GOLDEN SPICED APPLE LEATHER
MAKES 2–3 TRAYS.

Fresh apples and spice make everything nice.
Try adding some fresh ginger for a lift.

6 apples, peeled and chopped (Golden
   delicious or fuji apples are excellent
   choices.)
1 tablespoon cinnamon
2 teaspoons nutmeg

Pinch clove
Pinch sun-dried sea salt
1–2 tablespoons chopped ginger
  (optional)
3 cups apple juice or fresh water

Blend apples, cinnamon, nutmeg, clove, salt, ginger (if desired), and juice or water in a food processor or blender until smooth. Pour and spread onto nonstick sheets on dehydrator trays. Dehydrate at 108°F for 12–24 hours or until dry. (Climate, temperature, and humidity all affect dehydrating time.) Peel from sheets and cut to size as desired.

TROPICAL AMBROSIA FRUIT SKIN
MAKES 2–3 TRAYS.

This is a medley of tropical fruits and coconut
for a sweet, chewy snack.

1 mango, peeled and chopped
2 bananas, peeled and chopped
2 kiwis, peeled and chopped
1 cup dried coconut
3 cups apple juice, orange juice,
    coconut water, or fresh water

Blend fruit, coconut, and juice or water in a food processor or blender until smooth. Pour and spread onto nonstick sheets on dehydrator trays. Dehydrate at 108°F for 12–24 hours or until dry. (Climate, temperature, and humidity all affect dehydrating time.) Peel from sheets and cut to size as desired.

PEACH, PEAR, AND APRICOT LEATHER
MAKES 2–3 TRAYS.

Sweet peaches and succulent pears and apricots blend beautifully
in this roll-up for the essence of summer all year long.

6 peaches, peeled and chopped
4 apricots, chopped
2 ripe pears, peeled and chopped
2 cups apple juice, orange juice, or
    fresh water

Blend fruit and juice or water in a food processor or blender until smooth. Pour and spread onto nonstick sheets on dehydrator trays. Dehydrate at 108°F for 12–24 hours or until dry. (Climate, temperature, and humidity all affect dehydrating time.) Peel from sheets and cut to size as desired.

● STRAWBERRY-BANANA LEATHER
● MAKES 2–4 TRAYS.

*Classic flavors of strawberries and bananas blend
into this sweet and chewy treat.*

1 quart strawberries (Thawed frozen
    strawberries can be used out of
    season.)
4 bananas, peeled and chopped
3 cups apple juice or fresh water

Cut the tops off the strawberries. Blend strawberries, bananas, and juice or water in a food processor or blender until smooth. Pour and spread onto nonstick sheets on dehydrator trays. Dehydrate at 108°F for 12–24 hours or until dry. (Climate, temperature, and humidity all affect dehydrating time.) Peel from sheets and cut to size as desired.

● PERSIMMON FRUIT SKIN
● MAKES 2–4 TRAYS.

*Succulent, sweet persimmons and little else blend and
dehydrate into a chewy treat for all ages. (This is a great
use for bruised persimmons.)*

6 persimmons, peeled and seeded
2 cups apple juice, orange juice, or
    fresh water

Blend persimmons and juice or water in a food processor or blender until smooth. Pour and spread onto nonstick sheets on dehydrator trays. Dehydrate at 108°F for 12–24 hours or until dry. (Climate, temperature, and humidity all affect dehydrating time.) Peel from sheets and cut to size as desired.

SWEET ALMOND LEATHER

MAKES 2–4 TRAYS.

Creamy blended almonds, dates, bananas, and a touch
of spice make this fruit leather very satisfying.

1 cup pitted soft dates
2 cups almonds, soaked overnight,
    rinsed and drained
4 bananas
1 tablespoon raw carob powder
    (optional)

2 teaspoons cinnamon
1 teaspoon almond extract (optional)
Pinch sun-dried sea salt
3 cups apple juice or fresh water

Soak dates in 1½ cups fresh water for 15 minutes. (Reserve soak water.) Blend almonds, dates, date soak water, bananas, carob (if desired), cinnamon, almond extract, salt, and juice or water in a food processor or blender until smooth. Pour and spread onto nonstick sheets on dehydrator trays. Dehydrate at 108°F for 12–24 hours or until dry. (Climate, temperature, and humidity all affect dehydrating time.) Peel from sheets and cut to size as desired.

SPIRULINA PROTEIN LEATHER

MAKES 2–3 TRAYS.

Spirulina has the highest percent of protein of any food and graces
this fruit and nutty roll-up with charm and a rich green color.

2 cups almonds
1 cup raisins
2 apples, peeled and chopped
2 bananas
2–3 tablespoons spirulina
1 tablespoon cinnamon
3 cups apple juice, orange juice, or
    fresh water

Soak almonds in 4 cups fresh water overnight (about 6–12 hours). Rinse and drain. Soak raisins in 1½ cups fresh water for 15 minutes to soften. (Reserve soak water). Blend almonds, raisins, raisin soak water, apples, bananas, spirulina, cinnamon, and juice or water in a food processor or blender until smooth. Pour and spread onto nonstick sheets on dehydrator trays. Dehydrate at 108°F for 12–24 hours or until dry. (Climate, temperature, and humidity all affect dehydrating time.) Peel from sheets and cut to size as desired.

Sweet Snacks and Energy Bars

SWEET SESAME BARS

MAKES ABOUT 1 DOZEN BARS.

*These crunchy and chewy sesame bars are packed with
protein and calcium. A great snack for on the go.*

2 cups sesame seeds
6 tablespoons raw honey
2 tablespoons lemon juice
Pinch sun-dried sea salt

Mix sesame seeds, honey, lemon juice, and salt thoroughly in bowl. The texture should be sticky and able to hold a shape when pressed. Using wet hands to prevent sticking, press the mixture into thin bars about 1½ x 3 inches onto nonstick sheets on dehydrator trays. Dehydrate at 108°F for 12–20 hours or until quite dry. Flip over the bars to dry the undersides and return to the dehydrator without the nonstick sheets for 2–4 hours until dry.

3-6-9 BARS

MAKES ABOUT 2 DOZEN BARS.

*This is a sweet snack for beautiful skin, hair, and sustainable
energy. The seeds are rich in healthy omega 3, 6, and
9 oils and protein. Hemp seeds are one of the most
nutritious and balanced of all seeds and nuts.*

1 cup pumpkin seeds
1 cup flaxseeds
6 dates, pitted
4 tablespoons raw honey or maple syrup
1 tablespoon non-alcohol vanilla extract (optional)

1 teaspoon cinnamon (optional)
Pinch sun-dried sea salt
1 cup hulled hemp seeds or sesame seeds
½ cup raisins (optional)

Soak pumpkin seeds in 2 cups fresh water for 2–4 hours. Drain and rinse. Soak ½ cup flaxseeds in 1 cup fresh water for 15–20 minutes or until saturated. (The flaxseeds will absorb all or most of the water.) Soak dates in ½ cup fresh water for 5–10 minutes or until very soft. Drain the soak water. Grind the remaining ½ cup of dry flaxseeds in a food processor or blender until broken. Set aside. Chop pumpkin seeds, flaxseeds, dates, honey or maple syrup, vanilla (if desired), cinnamon (if desired), and sea salt in a food processor or blender. By hand, mix in hemp seeds or sesame seeds, ground flaxseeds, and raisins (if desired). The texture should be sticky, but the mixture should be able to hold a shape when pressed.

Using wet hands to prevent sticking, press the mixture into thin bars about 1½ inch by 3 inches on nonstick sheets on dehydrator trays. Dehydrate at 108°F for 12–20 hours or until quite dry. Flip over the bars to dry the undersides and return to the dehydrator without the nonstick sheets for 2–4 hours until dry.

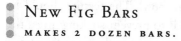 NEW FIG BARS

MAKES 2 DOZEN BARS.

These chewy, sweet fig bars have evolved from the original.

Dough

2 cups raw buckwheat groats
1½ cups whole oat groats
1½ cups pitted soft dates
2 tablespoons organic extra-virgin olive oil
1 tablespoon non-alcohol vanilla extract

1 tablespoon cinnamon
Pinch sun-dried sea salt

Fig Filling

3 cups dried figs, cut into quarters, hard stems removed
1½ cup raisins
1 tablespoon lemon zest

To make the dough: Soak raw buckwheat groats in 5 cups fresh water for 4–6 hours. Drain in a colander or a strainer and rinse until the water runs clear. Give the colander or strainer a good shake to help drain. Spread the drained buckwheat in a thin layer on dehydrator sheets and dehydrate at 108°F overnight (about 6–12 hours) or until dry. Also soak whole oat groats in 4 cups fresh water overnight (about 6–12 hours). Drain and rinse. Soak dates in 1 cup fresh water for 5–10 minutes until very soft.

In a food processor, grind dried buckwheat into flour. Set aside. In a food processor, chop oats, dates, olive oil, vanilla, cinnamon, and sea salt into a paste. Mix in buckwheat flour by hand. The dough should be sticky but dry enough to hold a shape when pressed.

To make the fig filling: Soak the figs and raisins in 3 cups fresh water for 5–15 minutes until very soft. Drain the soak water and set aside. This can be used to sweeten a smoothie or as an ingredient in marinades or sauces. In a food processor, chop the figs, raisins, and lemon zest into a smooth paste. Split the dough into four equal parts. With wet hands, press each quarter of the dough into a thin layer on a nonstick sheet on a dehydrator tray. Spread the fig filling evenly over two quarters of the dough. Gently flip the remaining two quarters of dough on top of the fig filling. Gently press edges together neatly.

Dehydrate at 108°F for 12–20 hours or until a crust has formed. The fig bars should still be moist inside. Cut into bars and return to the dehydrator without the nonstick sheets or plastic wrap for 2–3 hours.

TROPICAL AMBROSIA BARS
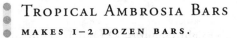
MAKES 1–2 DOZEN BARS.

This is a tropical ambrosia of macadamia nuts, coconut, and fruits dried into a power-packed snack. Try adding fresh ginger for a lift or Brazil nuts or cashews for a delicious variation.

1 cup dried pineapple
½ cup dried mango (Be sure that no sugar or sulfur has been added to the dried fruit.)
2½ cups dried coconut

1 cup macadamia nuts, Brazil nuts, or raw cashews
1 tablespoon non-alcohol vanilla extract (optional)
Pinch sun-dried sea salt

With a pair of kitchen scissors, cut the pineapple and mango into pieces. Soak the pineapple and mango pieces in 1½ cups fresh water until softened (about 5–15 minutes). Drain the soak water and set fruit aside.

In a food processor, chop the nuts roughly. Set aside. Chop the softened pineapple and mango, coconut, vanilla (if desired), and sea salt. Mix in chopped macadamia nuts by hand. Using wet hands to prevent sticking, press 2–4 tablespoons of the mixture into ¼-inch-thick bars on nonstick sheets on dehydrator trays. Dehydrate at 108°F for 12–20 hours or until quite dry. Flip over the bars to dry the undersides and return to the dehydrator without the nonstick sheets for 1 to 2 hours until dry.

Cereals

▪ Basic Buckwheat Crunch Cereal
MAKES ABOUT 4 CUPS.

Alkaline buckwheat is soaked and dehydrated for a simple crunchy
cereal. Serve with Almond Milk (page 266) and fresh fruit, or use
to top fresh-fruit sorbet.

  3 cups whole buckwheat groats
      (untoasted)
  6 cups fresh water

Soak whole buckwheat groats in 6 cups fresh water overnight (about 6–12 hours). Drain and rinse in a colander or strainer until the rinse water runs clear. Shake the colander or strainer to help drain. Allow buckwheat to stand for 10 minutes to drain well.

Spread the buckwheat in a thin layer on dehydrator trays (no need for nonstick sheets) and dehydrate at 108°F for 12–20 hours or until completely dry. (Climate, temperature, and humidity all affect dehydrating time.)

Store in clean glass jars with lids or in resealable bags in a cool, dry place or in the freezer.

HONEY-NUT CEREAL
MAKES ABOUT 4 CUPS.

*Lightly spiced, honey-nut buckwheat is a great crunchy cereal
for all times. Serve with Almond Milk (page 266) and
sliced bananas, or eat plain.*

2½ cups whole buckwheat groats
   (untoasted)

Honey-Nut Sauce
4 tablespoons raw almond butter
6 tablespoons raw honey

1 cup orange juice
1 tablespoon cinnamon
1 teaspoon nutmeg
½ teaspoon sun-dried sea salt

Soak whole buckwheat groats in 6 cups fresh water overnight (about 6–12 hours). Drain and rinse in a colander or strainer until the rinse water runs clear. Shake the colander or strainer to help drain. Allow buckwheat to stand for 10 minutes to drain well.

To make the honey-nut sauce: Mix almond butter, raw honey, orange juice, cinnamon, nutmeg, and sea salt in a bowl. Place the drained buckwheat in a generously sized bowl. Pour honey-nut sauce over the buckwheat and fold with clean, wet hands or a large spoon until well coated.

Spread the buckwheat mixture into a thin layer on nonstick sheets on dehydrator trays. Dehydrate at 108°F for 12–20 hours or until dry. After 12 hours, remove the buckwheat from the nonstick sheets and return to the dehydrator for 2 hours until very dry. (Climate, temperature, and humidity all affect dehydrating time.)

Store in clean glass jars with lids or in resealable bags in a cool, dry place or in the freezer.

HEMP NUT AND SPICE CEREAL
MAKES 4 CUPS.

Hemp seeds are one of the most nutritious and balanced of all seeds and nuts. They are rich in healthy omega oils and protein, and have a great nutty flavor.

2 cups whole buckwheat groats (untoasted)
1½ cups hulled hemp seeds
½ cup flaxseeds
4 tablespoons maple syrup, agave syrup, or raw honey

1 tablespoon non-alcohol vanilla extract
1 tablespoon cinnamon
1 teaspoon nutmeg
1 teaspoon sun-dried sea salt

Soak whole buckwheat groats in 5 cups of fresh water overnight (about 6–12 hours). Drain and rinse in a colander or strainer until the rinse water runs clear. Shake the colander or strainer to help drain. Allow buckwheat to stand for 10 minutes to drain well.

Mix buckwheat, hemp seeds, flaxseeds, maple or agave syrup or honey, vanilla, cinnamon, nutmeg, and sea salt in a bowl.

Spread the mixture into a thin layer on dehydrator trays (it should not be necessary to use nonstick sheets). Dehydrate at 108°F for 12–24 hours or until dry. (Climate, temperature, and humidity all affect dehydrating time.)

Store in clean glass jars with lids or in resealable bags in a cool, dry place or in the freezer.

And More!

CRUNCHY ONION RINGS
MAKES 2 CUPS.

Marinated dehydrated onion rings are delicious as a salad topping or as the base of French onion soup, or simply enjoy as a savory snack.

2 yellow onions, thinly sliced
3 tablespoons nama shoyu
2 tablespoons apple cider vinegar

2 teaspoons maple syrup or raw honey (optional)
Pinch sun-dried sea salt

Toss sliced onions with nama shoyu, vinegar, syrup or honey (if desired), and sea salt. Allow to marinate at least 30 minutes until savory and soft. Drain off marinade (the marinade can be used again for other recipes such as a vinaigrette salad dressing).

Spread onion rings on dehydrator trays and dehydrate at 108°F for 12–20 hours or until crispy and dry. (Climate, temperature, and humidity all affect dehydrating time.)

Store in a resealable bag in a cool, dry place.

CRUNCHY SHOYU PUMPKIN SEEDS
MAKES 3 CUPS.

Enzyme-rich pumpkin seeds are seasoned with shoyu and dried into a crunchy snack or topping for a salad or soup. They are rich in protein and healthy oils, and are easy to digest. They make a great alternative to roasted seeds. Try adding 4 tablespoons shredded or finely minced fresh ginger for a spicy variation.

3 cups pumpkin seeds
¼ cup nama shoyu

Soak pumpkin seeds in 4 cups fresh water for 2–4 hours. Drain and rinse. Toss pumpkin seeds with nama shoyu and allow to marinate for 30 minutes to an hour, mixing occasionally. Spread on dehydrator trays and dehydrate at 108°F for 12–20 hours or until dry. (Climate, temperature, and humidity all affect dehydrating time.)

Store in a resealable bag in a cool, dry place.

SWEET AND SPICY CRUNCHY CASHEWS
MAKES 3 CUPS.

Crunchy, creamy cashews are seasoned and dried with a touch of sweet and a kick of spice. This is a dynamic snack that can be served as a small side dish with salsa.

3 cups raw cashews (whole or in pieces)
2 tablespoons raw honey or maple syrup

2 teaspoons chipotle pepper or dried chili pepper
1 teaspoon chili powder
2 teaspoons sun-dried sea salt

Soak cashews in 4 cups fresh water for 1 hour. Drain and rinse. Toss cashews with honey or syrup, pepper, chili powder, and sea salt and allow to marinate for 30 minutes to an hour, mixing occasionally.

Spread on dehydrator trays and dehydrate at 108°F for 12–20 hours or until dry. (Climate, temperature, and humidity all affect dehydrating time.)

Store in a resealable bag in a cool, dry place.

Sweet Wood Almonds
MAKES 3 CUPS.

*Sweet, savory, spicy almonds dried to a satisfying crunch
make a great snack salad or topping.*

2 cups almonds
2 tablespoons nama shoyu
1 tablespoon raw honey or maple
   syrup
1 clove garlic, minced

1 tablespoon shredded or finely
   minced ginger
1 teaspoon chipotle pepper or chili
   powder
Pinch sun-dried sea salt

Soak almonds in 4 cups fresh water overnight (about 6–12 hours). Drain and rinse. Spread almonds onto a dry towel and blot dry. Toss almonds with nama shoyu, honey or syrup, garlic, ginger, pepper or powder, and sea salt. Allow to marinate 30 minutes to an hour to develop flavor. (They can be marinated as long as a day and stored in the refrigerator.)

Spread almonds on dehydrator trays and dehydrate at 108°F for 12–20 hours or until dry. (Climate, temperature, and humidity all affect dehydrating time.)

Store in a resealable bag in a cool, dry place.

Sweet Spiced Walnuts
MAKES 2 CUPS.

Sweetness and spice are infused into these crunchy walnuts. Excellent for topping a parfait or served with juicy pear slices.

2 cups walnuts
3 tablespoons raw honey or maple
   syrup

2 teaspoons cinnamon
1 teaspoon nutmeg
Pinch sun-dried sea salt

Soak walnuts in 4 cups fresh water overnight (about 6–12 hours). Drain and rinse. Spread walnuts onto a dry towel and blot dry. Toss with honey or syrup, cinnamon, nutmeg, and sea salt. Allow to marinate 30 minutes to an hour. (The walnuts can be marinated for up to a day in the refrigerator to really absorb the flavor.)

Spread on dehydrator trays and dehydrate at 108°F for 12–20 hours or until dry. (Climate, temperature, and humidity all affect dehydrating time.)

Store in a resealable bag in a cool, dry place.

CARAMELIZED PECANS
MAKES 2 CUPS.

*Sweet crunchy pecans are caramelized with vanilla and
a touch of magic for a divine topping or treat.*

- 2 cups pecans
- 2 tablespoons raw honey or maple syrup
- 1 tablespoon non-alcohol vanilla extract
- 1 teaspoon cinnamon
- Pinch nutmeg
- 3–6 drops liquid stevia (optional)
- Pinch sun-dried sea salt

Soak pecans in 4 cups fresh water overnight (about 6–12 hours). Drain and rinse. Spread pecans onto a dry towel and blot dry. Toss with honey or syrup, vanilla, cinnamon, nutmeg, stevia (if desired), and sea salt. Allow to marinate 30 minutes to 1 hour to absorb flavor.

Spread on dehydrator trays and dehydrate at 108°F for 12–20 hours or until dry. (Climate, temperature, and humidity all affect dehydrating time.)

Store in a resealable bag in a cool, dry place.

PARMESAN CRUMBLE
MAKES 2 CUPS.

*Crumbled seasoned pine nuts and cashews make a
fantastic Parmesan-like topping for salad or soup.*

- 3 cups cashews
- ½ cup pine nuts
- 2 cloves garlic
- 3 tablespoons nutritional yeast
- 2 teaspoons sun-dried sea salt

Soak cashews in 4 cups fresh water for 1 hour. Drain and rinse. In a food processor, chop garlic, cashews, and pine nuts into a fine meal. Add nutritional yeast and sea salt, and mix well.

Spread on dehydrator trays and dehydrate at 108°F for 12 hours or until dry and crumbly. (Climate, temperature, and humidity all affect dehydrating time.)

Store in a resealable bag or glass jar with a lid in a cool, dry place or in the refrigerator.

CORN AND SCALLION HERB CROUTONS
MAKES 4 CUPS.

A dried medley of sweet fresh corn and scallions seasoned with fresh herbs makes an excellent salad or soup topping or a simple snack.

    4 ears fresh corn
    4 green onions, finely chopped
    ¼ cup chopped cilantro
    ¼ cup chopped parsley
    2 teaspoons sun-dried sea salt

Cut the corn from the cobs and discard the cobs. Toss corn, green onions, cilantro, parsley, and sea salt to mix.

Spread on dehydrator trays and dehydrate at 108°F for 12–20 hours or until dry. (Climate, temperature, and humidity all affect dehydrating time.)

Store in a resealable bag or glass jar with a lid in a cool, dry place or in the refrigerator.

REFERENCES

Alliance for Food and Fiber. *Food Safety Information Kit.* Sacramento, CA, 1989.

Anderson, E., et al. *North America's Only Native Grain.* Cass Lake, MN: Northern Lakes Wild Rice Co., 1988.

Beleme, John. "The Miso Master's Apprentice." *East West Journal,* April 1981.

Center for Science in the Public Interest. *Guess What's Coming to Dinner: Contaminants in Our Food.* Washington, D.C., March 1987.

Clark, H. *The Cure for All Diseases.* Chula Vista, CA: New Century Publishing, 1995.

Colbin, A. *Food and Healing.* New York: Ballantine Books, 1986.

DeLangre, S., and Marie, S. *A Grain of Salt* newsletter. The Grain & Salt Society, Asheville, NC.

DK Publishing. *101 Essential Tips: Cooking with Spices.* New York: DK Publishing, 1998.

Earthworks, et al. *The Next Step: 50 More Things You Can Do to Save the Earth.* Kansas City, MO: Andrews McMeel Publishing, 1991.

Eden Foods. *Traditional Japanese Foods.* Clinto, MI, 1984.

Eden Foods. *Ume Plum Concentrate.* Clinto, MI, 1984.

Erasmus, U. *Fats That Heal, Fats That Kill.* Vancouver, B.C.: Canada Alive Books, 1986.

Food and Drug Administration Pesticide Program. *Residues in Foods: 1987.* Washington, D.C., 1987.

Food and Marketing Institute. *Pesticides in Our Food Supply.* Washington, D.C., 1987.

Fresh Produce Council and Alliance for Food and Fiber. *Issues in Food Safety.* Los Angeles, CA, Winter 1989.

Gundersen, E.P. *The Handy Physics Answer Book.* Canton, MI: Visible Ink Press, 1999.

Herbst, S.T. *The New Food Lover's Companion.* Hauppage, NY: Barrons, 2001.

Hill, C. (ed.) *Medical Discoveries of Japanese Doctors.* Boulder Creek, CA: University of the Tress Press, 1980.

Ingram, C. *Vegetable Identifier.* Anness Publishing, 1997.

Jacobson, M.F. *Eater's Digest: The Consumer's Factbook of Food Additives.* Garden City, NY: Doubleday, 1972.

Kilham, C. *The Whole Food Bible.* Rochester, VT: Healing Arts Press, 1997.

MacNeil, Karen. *The Book of Whole Foods: Nutrition & Cuisine.* New York: Vintage Books, 1981.

Morris, R.D. "Chlorination & Cancer: A Medical Analysis," *American Journal of Public Health* 82(7) (1992): 955–963.

Mrieb, A.N. *Essentials of Human Anatomy and Physiology.* n.p.: Benjamin/Cummings, 1997.

Murray, M. *The Complete Book of Juicing.* Roseville, CA: Prima Publishing, 1998.

National Coalition Against the Misuse of Pesticides. *Pesticide and You* newsletter. Washington, D.C., 1987.

Null, G. *The Joy of Juicing.* New York: 1992.

Olson, E.D. *Think Before You Drink.* New York: Natural Resources Defense Council, September 1993.

Pitchford, P. *Healing with Whole Foods.* Berkeley, CA: North Atlantic Books, 1993.

Santillo, H. *Food Enzymes.* Scottsdale, AZ: Hohm Press, 1987.

Schnider, E. *The Vegetables from Amaranth to Zucchini: Essential Reference.* New York: HarperCollins, 2001.

Shurtleff, W., and Akiko, A. *The Book of Miso.* New York: Ballantine Books, 1975.

Steinman, D., and Wisner, R. *Living Healthy in a Toxic World.* New York: Berkley, 1996.

Tickell, J. *From the Fryer to the Fuel Tank.* Jacksonville, FL: Veggie Van Publications, 2000.

Tobin, R.S., et al. "Effects of Activated Carbon and Bacteriostatic Filters on Microbial Quality of Drinking Water," *Applied and Environmental Microbiology* (March 1981).

Troxler, R., and Saffer, B. Harvard School of Dental Research. Paper delivered to the International Association for Dental Research General Session, 1987.

Waker, N.W. *Fresh Vegetable and Fruit Juices.* Norwalk Press, 1978.

Waker, N.W. *Raw Vegetable Juices.* Jove, 1970.

Wildfeuer, ed. *Stella Natura 2001: Kimberton Hills Agricultural Calendar.* San Francisco: Biodynamic Farming and Gardening Association, 2001.

Wood, R. *The Whole Foods Encyclopedia.* New York: Prentice Hall Press, 1988.

Worthington-Roberts, B. *Putting Carbohydrates in Perspective.* Washington, D.C.: The Wheat Industry Council, 1985.

RESOURCE GUIDE

Natural Foods

DEER GARDEN REJUVENATIVE FOODS
P.O. Box 8464
Santa Cruz, CA 95061
1-800-805-7957
www.rejuvenative.com
Organic, cold-pressed, live nut butters; sauerkraut; kimchi; and organic chocolate spreads.

EDEN FOODS
701 Tecumseh Road
Clinton, MI 49236
1-888-441-3336
1-888-424-3336
www.edenfoods.com
Organic bulk, seaweed, vinegars, oils, and condiments.

FRONTIER NATURAL BRANDS
P.O. Box 299
3021 78th Street
Norway, IA 52318
1-800-669-3275
www.frontiernaturalbrands.com
Bulk herb and spices, vanilla extracts, and organic coffees and teas.
Storage containers and body-care products are also available.

GOLD MINE NATURAL FOOD CO.
7805 Arjons Drive
San Diego, CA 92126
858-537-9830
1-800-475-FOOD
www.goldminenaturalfood.com
Organic foods, macrobiotics, and natural foods. American-made products and Japanese imports. Nonfood items are also available.

GOVINDA'S
2651 Ariane Drive
San Diego, CA 92117
1-858-270-0691
www.govinda-foods.com
Raw crackers, cookies, and snack bars.

GREAT EASTERN SUN
92 McIntosh Road
Asheville, NC 28806
1-800-334-5809
www.great-eastern-sun.com
Organic and natural foods, macro foods, and kitchen tools.

GUAYAKÍ
684 Clarion Court
San Luis Obispo, CA 93401
1-888-482-9254
www.guayaki.com
Yerba maté tea, bulk and bags; gourds for yerba maté.

JAFFE BROTHERS
28560 Lilac Road
Valley Center, CA 92082
www.organicfruitsandnuts.com
Organic nuts, seeds, grains, beans, and dried fruits.

LIVING TREE COMMUNITY FOODS
1-800-260-5534
www.livingtreecommunity.com
Raw organic nut butters, olives, and dried fruits.

LYDIA'S ORGANICS
81 Upland Avenue
Mill Valley, CA 94941
1-707-576-1330
lydiasfoods@care2.com
www.lydiasorganics.com
Dehydrated organic live crackers, cookies, and cereals.

MOUNTAIN ARK TRADING COMPANY
P.O. Box 3170
Fayetteville, AR 72702
1-800-643-8909
Organic and natural foods. Nonfood items are also available.

NATURAL LIFESTYLE MARKET
16 Lookout Drive
Asheville, NC 28804
1-800-752-2775
www.natural-lifestyle.com
Essentials for natural living, kitchen, home care, food, and tools.

SMOKEY MOUNTAIN NATURAL FOODS
15 Aspen Court
Ashville, NC 28806
1-800-926-0974
Organic and natural foods. Nonfood items are also available.

WALNUT ACRES (ORGANIC FOOD COMPANY)
www.walnutacres.com
Certified organic foods.

Oils

OMEGA NUTRITION
6515 Aldrich Road
Bellingham, WA 98226
1-800-661-3529
www.omeganutrition.com
Organic, cold-pressed oils, spreads, probiotics, and enzymes.
Nonfood items are also available.

Seeds

SEEDS OF CHANGE
P.O. Box 15700
Santa Fe, NM 87506
1-888-762-7333
www.seedsofchange.com
Heirloom and organic gardening seeds (non-GMO).

Sea Salts

THE GRAIN & SALT SOCIETY
273 Fairway Drive
Asheville, NC 28805
1-800-TOP-SALT (867-7258)
www.celtic-seasalt.com
Sun-dried sea salts, natural foods, and condiments.

Sea Vegetables

MAINE SEAWEED COMPANY
P.O. Box 57
Steuben, ME 04680
1-707-546-2875
High-quality, hand-harvested kelp, alaria, dulse, digitata kelp, and wild nori.

MENDOCINO SEA VEGETABLE COMPANY
P.O. Box 372
255 Welding Street
Navarro, CA 95463
1-707-895-3741

OCEAN HARVEST SEA VEGETABLES
P.O. Box 1719
Mendocino, CA 95460
1-707-936-1923
*Wild nori, sea lettuce, wakame, sea whip, fucus tip, ocean ribbons,
sea palm fronds, and grapestone.*

RISING TIDE SEA VEGETABLES
P.O. Box 1914
Mendocino, CA 95460
1-707-964-5663

Organic American Miso and Soy Manufacturers

California

MIYAKO ORIENTAL FOODS
Terno Shimizu
4287 Puente
Baldwin Park, CA 91706
1-626-926-9633

YAMAZAKI MISO
Kazuko Yamazaki
4192 Countu Road South
Orlando, CA 95963
1-530-865-5979

Hawaii

AMERICAN HAWAIIAN SOY
John Morita
274 Kalihi Street
Honolulu, HI 96819
1-808-841-8435

HAWAIIAN MISO & SOY
William Higa
1714 May Street
Honolulu, HI 96819
1-808-841-7354

Massachusetts

SOUTH RIVER MISO COMPANY
Christian Elwell
South River Farm
Conway, MA 01341
1-413-369-4057
Three-year barley, black soy bean, adzuki, dandelion-leek, golden millet, and chick pea.

New York

MSB FOOD ENTERPRISES
Michael Lee
710 Longfellow Avenue
Bronx, NY 10474
1-718-617-4105

North Carolina

AMERICAN MISO CO.
Greg Gonzales
4225 Maple Creek Road
Rutherfordton, NC 28139
1-704-287-2940

Wisconsin

EARTH FIRE PRODUCTS
Bob Ribbens
P.O. Box 92
Gays Mills, WI 54631
1-800-267-6918

General Products

HARMONY (GIAM)
360 Interlocken Boulevard, Suite 300
Broomfield, CO 80021
1-800-869-3446
www.giam.com
Green products, organic clothing, and household products.

LEHMAN'S HARDWARE & APPLIANCES
One Lehman Circle
P.O. Box 41
Kidron, OH 44636
1-216-857-5757
Non-electric appliances.

REAL GOODS
966 Mazzoni Street
Ukiah, CA 95482
1-800-762-7325
Gardening books, efficient appliances, and nontoxic cleaning products.

Organic and Biodynamic Farming

ANTHROPOSOPHICAL SOCIETY IN AMERICA (BIODYNAMICS)
1923 Geddes Avenue
Ann Arbor, MI 48104
1-734-662-1727
information@anthroposophy.org
www.anthroposophy.org

ATTRA (APPROPRIATE TECHNOLOGY TRANSFER FOR RURAL AREAS) (BIODYNAMICS)
P.O. Box 3657
Fayetteville, AR 72702
1-800-346-9140
www.attra.org

CALIFORNIA CERTIFIED ORGANIC FARMERS
P.O. Box 8136
Santa Cruz, CA 95061

THE DEMETER ASSOCIATION, INC. (BIODYNAMICS)
Britt Road
Aurora, NY 13026
1-315-364-5224
www.demeter-usa.org

FARM VERIFIED ORGANIC PROGRAM (FVO)
Mercantile Development Inc.
P.O. Box 2747
274 Riverside Avenue
Westport, CT 06880

JOSEPHINE PORTER
Institute for Applied Biodynamics
P.O. Box 133
Woolwine, VA 24185-1033
1-540-930-2463

LAND STEWARDSHIP PROJECT
1717 University Avenue
St. Paul, MN 55104

MICHAEL FIELDS AGRICULTURE INSTITUTE (BIODYNAMICS)
W2493 County Road ES
East Troy, WI 53120
1-262-642-3303

NATURAL ORGANIC FARMERS ASSOCIATION (NOFA)
4 Park Street
Concord, NH 03301

ORGANIC BUYERS AND GROWERS ASSOCIATION
P.O. Box 9747
Minneapolis, MN 55440

ORGANIC FOOD ALLIANCE (OFA)
211 Wilson Boulevard, Suite 531
Arlington, VA 22201

ORGANIC FOODS PRODUCTION ASSOCIATION OF NORTH AMERICA (OFPANA)
P.O. Box 1078
23 Ames Street
Greenfield, MA 01301

THE PFEIFFER CENTER (BIODYNAMICS)
260 Hungry Hollow Road
Chestnut Ridge, NY 10977
1-914-352-5020, ext. 20
info@pfeiffercenter.org

Healing, Education, and Rejuvenation Centers

ANN WIGMORE INSTITUTE
P.O. Box 429
Rincon, PR 00677
1-787-868-6307

ANN WIGMORE FOUNDATION
P.O. Box 399
San Fidel, NM 87049
1-505-552-0595

HIPPOCRATES HEALTH CENTER
1443 Palmdale Court
West Palm Beach, FL 33411
1-800-842-2125

OPTIMUM HEALTH INSTITUTE
6970 Central Avenue
Lemon Grove, CA 91945
1-619-464-3346

TREE OF LIFE REJUVENATION CENTER
P.O. Box 778
Patagonia, AZ 85624
1-520-394-2520
www.treeofliferejuvenation.com

OPTIMUM HEALTH INSTITUTE
Route 1 Box 339-J Cedar Road
Cedar Creek, TX 78612
1-512-303-4817

Education and Information

Information about hazardous agricultural chemicals:

CENTER FOR SCIENCE IN THE PUBLIC INTEREST
1501 16th Street NW
Washington, D.C. 20036

NATIONAL COALITION AGAINST THE MISUSE OF PESTICIDES
530 7th Street SE
Washington, D.C. 20003

PESTICIDE ACTION NETWORK NEWSLETTER
965 Mission Street, #541
San Fransisco, CA 94103

UNITED STATES GENERAL ACCOUNTING OFFICE
Washington, D.C. 20548

Make Your Views Known!

Write your congressional representatives and senators!

YOUR CONGRESSIONAL REPRESENTATIVE
U.S. House of Representatives
Washington, D.C. 20515

YOUR SENATOR
U.S. Senate
Washington, D.C. 20510

Food Information

AMERICAN ASSOCIATION OF MEAT PROCESSORS
P.O. Box 269
224 E. High Street
Elizabethtown, PA 17022

FOOD AND DRUG ADMINISTRATION
Consumer Communications
5600 Fishers Lane
Rockville, MD 20857

NATIONAL DAIRY COUNCIL
10255 W. Higgins Rd., Suite 900
Rosemont, IL 60018

Food Safety

AMERICANS FOR SAFE FOOD
1501 16th Street NW
Washington, D.C. 20036

CENTER FOR SCIENCE IN THE PUBLIC INTEREST (CSPI)
1501 16th Street NW
Washington, D.C. 20036

CLEAN WATER ACTION PROJECT
317 Pennsylvania Avenue SE
Washington, D.C. 20003

COMMUNITY NUTRITION INSTITUTE
2001 S. Street NW, Suite 530
Washington, D.C. 20009

FOOD RESEARCH AND ACTION CENTER
1319 F Street, Suite 500
Washington, D.C. 20004

INSTITUTE FOR FOOD AND DEVELOPMENT POLICY
145 9th Street
San Francisco, CA 94103

NATIONAL COALITION AGAINST THE MISUSE OF PESTICIDES (NCAMP)
530 7th Street SE
Washington, D.C. 20003

PESTICIDE ACTION NETWORK
965 Mission Street, #514
San Fransisco, CA 94103

PUBLIC CITIZEN HEALTH RESEARCH GROUP
2000 P Street NW, Suite 700
Washington, D.C. 20036

PUBLIC VOICE FOR FOOD AND HEALTH POLICY
1001 Connecticut Avenue NW, Suite 522
Washington, D.C. 20036

INDEX